LIFE UNIVERSITY
1269 BARCLAY CIRCLE
MARIETTA, GA 30060
(770) 426-2688

LIFE UNIVERSITY
1269 BARCLAY CIRCLE
MARIETTA, GA 30060
(770) 426-2688

1999
YEAR BOOK OF
PSYCHIATRY AND
APPLIED MENTAL HEALTH®

Statement of Purpose

The YEAR BOOK Service

The YEAR BOOK series was devised in 1901 by practicing health professionals who observed that the literature of medicine and related disciplines had become so voluminous that no one individual could read and place in perspective every potential advance in a major specialty. In the final decade of the 20th century, this recognition is more acutely true than it was in 1901.

More than merely a series of books, YEAR BOOK volumes are the tangible results of a unique service designed to accomplish the following:

- to *survey* a wide range of journals of proven value
- to *select* from those journals papers representing significant advances and statements of important clinical principles
- to provide *abstracts* of those articles that are readable, convenient summaries of their key points
- to provide *commentary* about those articles to place them in perspective

These publications grow out of a unique process that calls on the talents of outstanding authorities in clinical and fundamental disciplines, trained literature specialists, and professional writers, all supported by the resources of Mosby, the world's preeminent publisher for the health professions.

The Literature Base

Mosby and its Editors survey approximately 500 journals published worldwide, covering the full range of the health professions. On an annual basis, the publisher examines usage patterns and polls its expert authorities to add new journals to the literature base and to delete journals that are no longer useful as potential YEAR BOOK sources.

The Literature Survey

The publisher's team of literature specialists, all of whom are trained and experienced health professionals, examines every original, peer-reviewed article in each journal issue. More than 250,000 articles per year are scanned systematically, including title, text, illustrations, tables, and references. Each scan is compared, article by article, to the search strategies that the publisher has developed in consultation with the 270 outside experts who form the pool of YEAR BOOK editors. A given article may be reviewed by any number of editors, from one to a dozen or more, regardless of the discipline for which the paper was originally published. In turn, each editor who receives the article reviews it to determine whether or not the article should be included in the YEAR BOOK. This decision is based on the article's inherent quality, its probable usefulness to readers of that YEAR BOOK, and the editor's goal to represent a balanced picture of a given field in each volume of the YEAR BOOK. In addition, the editor indicates when to include figures and tables from the article to help the YEAR BOOK reader better understand the information.

Of the quarter million articles scanned each year, only 5% are selected for detailed analysis within the YEAR BOOK series, thereby assuring readers of the high value of every selection.

The Abstract

The publisher's abstracting staff is headed by a seasoned medical professional and includes individuals with training in the life sciences, medicine, and other areas, plus extensive experience in writing for the health professions and related industries. Each selected article is assigned to a specific writer on this abstracting staff. The abstracter, guided in many cases by notations supplied by the expert editor, writes a structured, condensed summary designed so that the reader can rapidly acquire the essential information contained in the article.

The Commentary

The YEAR BOOK editorial boards, sometimes assisted by guest commentators, write comments that place each article in perspective for the reader. This provides the reader with the equivalent of a personal consultation with a leading international authority—an opportunity to better understand the value of the article and to benefit from the authority's thought processes in assessing the article.

Additional Editorial Features

The editorial boards of each YEAR BOOK organize the abstracts and comments to provide a logical and satisfying sequence of information. To enhance the organization, editors also provide introductions to sections or individual chapters, comments linking a number of abstracts, citations to additional literature, and other features.

The published YEAR BOOK contains enhanced bibliographic citations for each selected article, including extended listings of multiple authors and identification of author affiliations. Each YEAR BOOK contains a Table of Contents specific to that year's volume. From year to year, the Table of Contents for a given YEAR BOOK will vary depending on developments within the field.

Every YEAR BOOK contains a list of the journals from which papers have been selected. This list represents a subset of the approximately 500 journals surveyed by the publisher and occasionally reflects a particularly pertinent article from a journal that is not surveyed on a routine basis.

Finally, each volume contains a comprehensive subject index and an index to authors of each selected paper.

The 1999 Year Book Series

Year Book of Allergy, Asthma, and Clinical Immunology: Drs. Rosenwasser, Boguniewicz, Borish, Routes, Spahn, and Weber

Year Book of Anesthesiology and Pain Management®: Drs. Tinker, Abram, Chestnut, Roizen, Rothenberg, and Wood

Year Book of Cardiology®: Drs. Schlant, Collins, Gersh, Graham, Kaplan, and Waldo

Year Book of Chiropractic®: Dr. Lawrence

Year Book of Critical Care Medicine®: Drs. Parrillo, Balk, Calvin, Franklin, and Shapiro

Year Book of Dentistry®: Drs. Meskin, Berry, Jeffcoat, Leinfelder, Roser, Summitt, and Zakariasen

Year Book of Dermatology and Dermatologic Surgery™: Drs. Thiers and Lang

Year Book of Diagnostic Radiology®: Drs. Osborn, Birdwell, Dalinka, Groskin, Maynard, Pentecost, Ros, Smirniotopoulos, and Young

Year Book of Emergency Medicine®: Drs. Wagner, Dronen, Davidson, King, Niemann, and Hamilton

Year Book of Endocrinology®: Drs. Bagdade, Fitzpatrick, Braverman, Horton, Kannan, Landsberg, Molitch, Morley, Odell, Poehlman, and Rogol

Year Book of Family Practice®: Drs. Berg, Bowman, Davidson, Dexter, and Scherger

Year Book of Gastroenterology: Drs. Aliperti and Fleshman

Year Book of Hand Surgery®: Drs. Amadio and Hentz

Year Book of Medicine®: Drs. Klahr, Frishman, Malawista, Mandell, Jett, Young, Barkin, and Bagdade

Year Book of Neonatal and Perinatal Medicine®: Drs. Fanaroff, Maisels, and Stevenson

Year Book of Nephrology, Hypertension, and Mineral Metabolism: Drs. Schwab, Bennett, Emmett, Hostetter, and Moe

Year Book of Neurology and Neurosurgery®: Drs. Bradley and Gibbs

Year Book of Nuclear Medicine®: Drs. Gottschalk, Blaufox, Coleman, Strauss, and Zubal

Year Book of Obstetrics, Gynecology, and Women's Health: Drs. Mishell, Herbst, and Kirschbaum

Year Book of Oncology®: Drs. Ozols, Eisenberg, Glatstein, Loehrer, and Urba

Year Book of Ophthalmology®: Drs. Wilson, Augsburger, Cohen, Eagle, Grossman, Laibson, Maguire, Nelson, Penne, Rapuano, Sergott, Spaeth, Tipperman, Ms. Gosfield, and Ms. Salmon

Year Book of Orthopedics®: Drs. Morrey, Beauchamp, Currier, Tolo, Trigg, and Swiontkowski

Year Book of Otolaryngology–Head and Neck Surgery®: Drs. Paparella, Holt, and Otto

Year Book of Pathology and Laboratory Medicine®: Drs. Raab, Cohen, Dabbs, Olson, and Stanley

Year Book of Pediatrics®: Dr. Stockman

Year Book of Plastic, Reconstructive, and Aesthetic Surgery®: Drs. Miller, Bartlett, Garner, McKinney, Ruberg, Salisbury, and Smith

Year Book of Psychiatry and Applied Mental Health®: Drs. Talbott, Ballenger, Frances, Lydiard, Meltzer, Jensen, and Tasman

Year Book of Pulmonary Disease®: Drs. Jett, Castro, Maurer, Peters, Phillips, and Ryu

Year Book of Rheumatology, Arthritis, and Musculoskeletal Disease™: Drs. Panush, Hadler, Hellman, LeRoy, Pisetsky, and Simon

Year Book of Sports Medicine®: Drs. Shephard, Drinkwater, Eichner, Torg, Alexander, and Mr. George

Year Book of Surgery®: Drs. Copeland, Bland, Deitch, Eberlein, Howard, Luce, Seeger, Souba, and Sugarbaker

Year Book of Urology®: Drs. Andriole and Coplen

Year Book of Vascular Surgery®: Dr. Porter

The Year Book of PSYCHIATRY AND APPLIED MENTAL HEALTH®

Editor in Chief
John A. Talbott, M.D.

Professor and Chair, Department of Psychiatry, University of Maryland School of Medicine; Director, Institute of Psychiatry, University of Maryland Medical System, Baltimore, Maryland

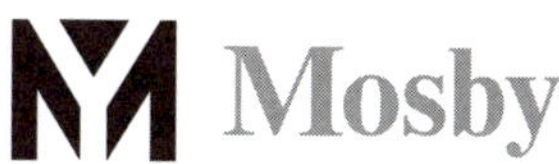

Mosby

St. Louis Baltimore Boston Carlsbad Naples New York Philadelphia Portland London
Madrid Mexico City Singapore Sydney Tokyo Toronto Wiesbaden

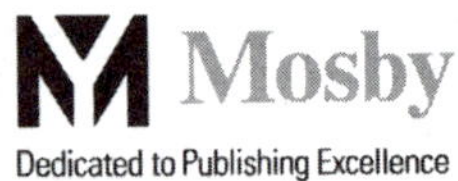

Publisher: Theresa Van Schaik
Developmental Editor: Laura C. Berendson
Manager, Periodical Editing: Kirk Swearingen
Production Editor: Amanda Maguire
Project Supervisor, Production: Joy Moore
Production Assistant: Laura Bayless
Manager, Literature Services: Idelle L. Winer
Illustrations and Permissions Coordinator: Phyllis K. Thompson

1999 EDITION
Copyright © May 1999 by Mosby, Inc.

Printed in the United States of America
Composition by Reed Technology and Information Services, Inc.
Printing/binding by Maple-Vail

Mosby, Inc.
11830 Westline Industrial Drive
St. Louis, MO 63146
Customer Service: customer.support@mosby.com
www.mosby.com/Mosby/CustomerSupport/index.html

International Standard Serial Number: 0084–3970
International Standard Book Number: 0–8151–9734–9

Editors

James C. Ballenger, M.D.

Professor and Chair, Department of Psychiatry and Behavioral Sciences; Director, Institute of Psychiatry; Executive Director, Center for Drug and Alcohol Programs, Medical University of South Carolina, Charleston, South Carolina

Richard J. Frances, M.D., F.A.C.P., F.A.P.A.

Clinical Professor, New York University; Adjunct Professor, University of Medicine and Dentistry of New Jersey; President and Medical Director, Silver Hill Hospital, New Canaan, Connecticut

Peter S. Jensen, M.D.

Associate Clinical Professor of Psychiatry, Uniformed Services, University of the Health Sciences, Bethesda, Maryland

R. Bruce Lydiard, Ph.D., M.D.

Professor of Psychiatry and Behavioral Sciences, Medical University of South Carolina; Director, Clinical Psychopharmacology Research Division, Institute of Psychiatry, Medical University of South Carolina, Charleston, South Carolina.

Herbert Y. Meltzer, M.D.

Bixler Professor of Psychiatry and Pharmacology; Director, Division of Psychopharmacology, Vanderbilt University Medical Center, Nashville, Tennessee

John E. Schowalter, M.D.

Albert J. Solnit Professor of Child Psychiatry and Pediatrics, Yale Child Study Center, New Haven, Connecticut

Allan Tasman, M.D.

Professor and Chair, Department of Psychiatry and Behavioral Sciences, University of Louisville School of Medicine, Louisville, Kentucky

Table of Contents

Journals Represented

Mosby and its Editors survey approximately 500 journals for its abstract and commentary publications. From these journals, the Editors select the articles to be abstracted. Journals represented in this YEAR BOOK are listed below.

Acta Psychiatrica Scandinavica
Administration and Policy in Mental Health
Alzheimer Disease and Associated Disorders
American Journal of Epidemiology
American Journal of Medicine
American Journal of Physiology
American Journal of Preventive Medicine
American Journal of Psychiatry
American Journal of Psychotherapy
American Journal of Public Health
Annals of Internal Medicine
Annals of Neurology
Archives of Disease in Childhood
Archives of Family Medicine
Archives of General Psychiatry
Archives of Pediatrics and Adolescent Medicine
Archives of Psychiatric Nursing
Biological Psychiatry
Brain
British Journal of Cancer
British Journal of General Practice
British Journal of Psychiatry
British Medical Journal
Canadian Journal of Psychiatry
Canadian Medical Association Journal
Child Development
Clinical Journal of Pain
Community Mental Health Journal
Comprehensive Psychiatry
Developmental Medicine and Child Neurology
Diabetes Care
Digestive Diseases and Sciences
Endocrinology
General Hospital Psychiatry
Gerontologist
Harvard Review Psychiatry
International Journal of Epidemiology
International Journal of Geriatric Psychiatry
International Journal of Group Psychotherapy
Journal of Affective Disorders
Journal of Behavior Therapy and Experimental Psychiatry
Journal of Child Psychology and Psychiatry and Allied Disciplines
Journal of Clinical Psychiatry
Journal of Clinical Psychopharmacology
Journal of Consulting and Clinical Psychology
Journal of Family Practice
Journal of Nervous and Mental Disease

Journal of Nuclear Medicine
Journal of Pharmacology and Experimental Therapeutics
Journal of Psychiatric Research
Journal of Psychotherapy Practice and Research
Journal of the American Academy of Child and Adolescent Psychiatry
Journal of the American Academy of Psychiatry and the Law
Journal of the American Board of Family Practice
Journal of the American Geriatrics Society
Journal of the American Medical Association
Lancet
Magnetic Resonance Imaging
Medical Care
Medical Journal of Australia
New England Journal of Medicine
Obstetrics and Gynecology
Pediatrics
Proceedings of the National Academy of Sciences
Psychiatric Services
Psychiatry
Psychiatry Research
Psychological Medicine
Psychosomatic Medicine
Psychotherapy and Psychosomatics
Schizophrenia Bulletin
Schizophrenia Research
Science

STANDARD ABBREVIATIONS

The following terms are abbreviated in this edition: acquired immunodeficiency syndrome (AIDS), cardiopulmonary resuscitation (CPR), central nervous system (CNS), cerebrospinal fluid (CSF), computed tomography (CT), deoxyribonucleic acid (DNA), electrocardiography (ECG), health maintenance organization (HMO), human immunodeficiency virus (HIV), intensive care unit (ICU), intramuscular (IM), intravenous (IV), magnetic resonance (MR) imaging (MRI), and ribonucleic acid (RNA).

NOTE

The YEAR BOOK OF PSYCHIATRY AND APPLIED MENTAL HEALTH® is a literature survey service providing abstracts of articles published in the professional literature. Every effort is made to assure the accuracy of the information presented in these pages. Neither the editors nor the publisher of the YEAR BOOK OF PSYCHIATRY AND APPLIED MENTAL HEALTH® can be responsible for errors in the original materials. The editors' comments are their own opinions. Mention of specific products within this publication does not constitute endorsement.

To facilitate the use of the YEAR BOOK OF PSYCHIATRY AND APPLIED MENTAL HEALTH® as a reference tool, all illustrations and tables included in this publication are now identified as they appear in the original article. This change is meant to help the reader recognize that any illustration or table appearing in the YEAR BOOK OF PSYCHIATRY AND APPLIED MENTAL HEALTH® may be only one of many in the original article. For this reason, figure and table numbers will often appear to be out of sequence within the YEAR BOOK OF PSYCHIATRY AND APPLIED MENTAL HEALTH®.

1 Child and Adolescent Psychiatry

Introduction

This section presents a series of articles on investigators' attempts to improve the clinical characteristics and assessment procedures used in determining children's psychiatric conditions. Some of these characteristics might be ascertained during a clinical evaluation, such as behavioral inhibition vs. withdrawal (Kerr et al.,), diagnostic criteria such as age of onset (Barkley and Biederman), physical stigmata (Buckley), or specific cognitions pertaining to suicidal ideation and behavior (Negron et al.). Still other forms of clinical information might only be available through the use of new technologies (Berns et al.; Just et al.; Leung and Connolly; Turner et al.; Valla et al.).

The gamut of these articles reflects the need for a process I call "breaking apart the phenotype." In other words, what kind of information do we need to go beyond our superficial *Diagnostic and Statistical Manual*-based descriptions of our patients in order to get a better handle on the underlying etiologic and developmental processes, pathophysiology, and contextual factors that give rise to a child's disorder? The success of such efforts is absolutely necessary if we are to achieve adequate understanding of our patients' "disorders." More importantly, such insights will lay the foundation for more optimal treatments as well as knowledge-based and effective preventive intervention.

Peter S. Jensen, M.D.

Evaluation and Assessment of Clinical Characteristics

Boys' Behavioral Inhibition and the Risk of Later Delinquency

Kerr M, Tremblay RE, Pagani L, et al (Univ of Montreal)
Arch Gen Psychiatry 54:809–816, 1997   1–1

Background.—Studies of the protective effects of shyness, anxiety, and social withdrawal in boys at risk of delinquency have yielded conflicting results. This may be because behavioral inhibition, which is the protective factor, has been confounded with social withdrawal and other constructs. Behavioral inhibition and the risk of later delinquency in boys were further investigated.

1

Methods.—Boys of low socioeconomic status in Montreal, Quebec, were studied. Predictors at ages 10–12 years were peer-rated inhibition, social withdrawal, and disruptiveness. Outcomes at 13–15 years were self-rated depressive symptoms and delinquency. Eight behavioral profiles obtained between the ages of 10 and 12 years were compared with 4 outcome profiles at 13–15 years of age.

Findings.—Inhibition appeared to protect against delinquency in disruptive and nondisruptive boys. Disruptive, uninhibited boys were likely to become delinquent, whereas disruptive, inhibited boys were not. Among the disruptive boys, inhibition did not increase the risk for depression. Among nondisruptive boys, only those who were inhibited were significantly less likely (than chance) to become delinquent. However, withdrawal did not protect against delinquency. Boys who were disruptive and withdrawn had the greatest risk of becoming delinquent, with or without depressive symptoms.

Conclusions.—Although behaviorally similar, inhibition and social withdrawal are associated with different risks for subsequent outcomes. Thus, they should be differentiated conceptually and empirically.

▶ This study draws an important distinction between anxiety resulting from behavioral inhibition, and apparent shyness and social withdrawal that occur for other, nonanxious reasons. The importance of this distinction becomes more apparent when we consider the authors' findings that behavioral inhibition acts as a protective factor in children who are disruptive, whereas among nonbehaviorally inhibited children, the combination of both disruptive and withdrawn behavior conveys increased risk. Obviously, the constructs of overt social and behavioral withdrawal, behavioral inhibition and anxiety could be easily confused, yet these data as well as other sources of converging evidence suggest that such children differ not only in behavior, but also in underlying biological processes. It is comforting (though infrequent) that our ways of categorizing children lead to distinctions that have predictive meaning. The subtleties of these clinical distinctions may also suggest that even in today's cost-conscious, managed care environment, there is still a need for careful history taking and good clinical interviewing skills.

P.S. Jensen, M.D.

Toward a Broader Definition of the Age-of-Onset Criterion for Attention-Deficit Hyperactivity Disorder
Barkley RA, Biederman J (Univ of Massachusetts, Worcester; Harvard Med School, Boston)
J Am Acad Child Adolesc Psychiatry 36:1204–1210, 1997   1–2

Introduction and Methods.—The characteristics of attention-deficit hyperactivity disorder (ADHD), estimated to be present in 3% to 11% of children, are thought to arise early in childhood, and follow-up studies suggest that the disorder persists into adolescence in 40% to 80% of cases.

In addition, there is emerging recognition of ADHD in adults. Using historical, empirical, conceptual, and pragmatic perspectives, investigators critique the age-of-onset criterion (AOC) for the diagnosis of ADHD.

Results.—A requirement for ADHD is that sufficient symptoms that have caused impairment arise before the age of 7 years. This requirement may be established easily in childhood cases, but recall of the precise age of onset of symptoms is poor as time passes. It is possible, however, to challenge the requirement of any precise AOC for ADHD in diagnostic taxonomies such as *Diagnostic and Statistical Manual (DSM)-IV.* No rationale for selecting an AOC of 7 years was ever published; a precise AOC for ADHD did not appear until *DSM-III;* and the validity of the AOC was not evaluated. Results of field trials do not support the traditional AOC of 7 years, but these data were not available for *DSM-IV.* Few other childhood disorders and no adult disorders require so precise an AOC as that for ADHD. The recommended AOC limits the number of children with diagnosed ADHD, and would probably limit the number of adults as well. Reliance on the current AOC requirement will restrict the opportunity to study ADHD in older adolescents and adults as a valid diagnostic entity.

Discussion.—Several lines of argument support dispensing with a precise AOC for the diagnosis of ADHD. Until there is empirical justification for a requirement of symptom onset or onset of impairment before the age of 7 years, the current AOC should be abandoned or broadened.

▶ Too often we reify our psychiatric diagnoses as if they were "real things"—entities cast in stone rather than works in progress, shaped as much by culture, perception, and learning processes as by genes and brain development. This tendency to reify is a danger, particularly for those trained in the era of the *DSM-III, DSM-IIIR,* and *DSM-IV,* when nosologic systems have raised to an art form the highly structured approach to establishing the presence of diagnostic criteria. ADHD is no exception to the rule. While this is not exactly the authors' point (more mine, in fact), they do call into question the artificial, before-age-7, age-on-onset cut-off criterion in *DSM-IV* ADHD. The arbitrariness of this cut-off has become a particularly pressing issue, given the increased recognition of the high proportion of ADHD children who become ADHD adults, subtleties of determining when a symptom is really a symptom, frequent delays in help seeking and appropriate diagnostic workups in children and adolescents, and problems with the retrospective determination of exact age of onset. In this instance, however, the structured nature of the DSM has been helpful, because it allowed the empirical demonstration of the lack of usefulness of the age cut-off.

P.S. Jensen, M.D.

Test of Two Views of Impulsivity in Hyperactive and Conduct-disordered Children

Leung PWL, Connolly KJ (Chinese Univ of Hong Kong, Shatin; Univ of Sheffield, England)
Dev Med Child Neurol 39:574–582, 1997   1–3

Introduction.—One of the diagnostic features of hyperactivity is impulsivity, in which the child trades accuracy for speed. Studies examining first-response as a measure of impulsivity have been inconclusive. Hyperactive children may have a general tendency to minimize delay, but it is still unknown whether hyperactive children have a general, trait-like tendency to trade accuracy for speed. The 2 alternative views of impulsivity were tested in hyperactive children. In hyperactive and conduct-disordered children, the nature of impulsivity was examined.

Methods.—There were 2 experiments, 1 involving a primary task and the other involving a delayed reaction time task. The primary task was simple and did not involve any demanding perceptual analysis, and the delayed reaction time task was used to examine disinhibition. The children, aged 7–8 years, with normal intelligence quotients, were divided into 4 groups: a pure hyperactive group, a hyperactive-conduct-disordered group, a pure conduct-disordered group, and a normal control group.

Results.—None of the 3 clinical groups showed any sign of impulsivity at the input/perceptual stage when the stimulus configuration and presentation were simple and well organized. There was no tendency to rush responding, such as trading of accuracy for speed, before adequate consideration of the relevant stimuli. At the output/motor stage, the pure hyperactive group were found to be disinhibited, failing to temporarily withhold activated responses. This deficit was found only in the pure hyperactive group.

Conclusion.—Previous studies have suggested that hyperactive children would trade accuracy for speed in situations of considerable ambiguity. In situations with clear-cut and well-organized cues, hyperactive children can attend to the relevant information and avoid premature responses, according to the results of this study. Hyperactive children will have difficulty in delaying or inhibiting responses, however, if a piece of behavior is activated and a response prepared. Minimal waiting or delaying should be employed in tasks assigned to hyperactive children.

▶ Unfortunately (to my mind, at least), many of our current diagnoses comprise curious admixtures of symptoms with varying combinations of behavioral characteristics that have no clear theoretical or neuroscientific underpinnings. Attention deficit-hyperactivity disorder (ADHD), with its classic triad of symptoms (inattention, hyperactivity, impulsivity) is a good case in point, where any of several combinations of these major symptom clusters can yield a diagnosis. This tendency to lump what may be etiologically and neuroscientifically different behaviors into a common syndrome is a proclivity of clinicians, but not of basic scientists. Arguably, the field of learning disabilities research has made rapid strides in the last several years because researchers have carefully attended to the problem that standard classification systems introduced a good deal of "noise" (i.e., error) into the precision and validity of much learning disabilities research. But as investigators began to break apart the learning disabilities phenotype into its component parts, such as phonemic awareness, exciting new genetic and basic neuroscience findings emerged. In essence, Leung and Connolly have begun attempts to break apart the ADHD phenotype by carefully constructing measures of "impulsivity" in children, and comparing them in 4 different groups: ADHD only, ADHD plus conduct disorder, conduct disorder only, and normals. While this study had fairly small sample sizes, the authors found theoretically meaningful differences in the ADHD-only group compared to the normal and other 2 clinical groups in some (but not all) aspects of impulsivity. A good start, and just the type of research we will need to catch up with our learning disabilities colleagues.

P.S. Jensen, M.D.

Case Study: An Infection-triggered, Autoimmune Subtype of Anorexia Nervosa
Sokol MS, Gray NS (Menninger Clinic, Topeka, Kan; Univ of Pittsburgh, Pa)
J Am Acad Child Adolesc Psychiatry 36:1128–1133, 1997   1–4

Background.—A subtype of childhood-onset obsessive-compulsive disorder has been reported recently and hypothesized to be a pediatric infection-triggered autoimmune neuropsychiatric disorder. Certain cases of anorexia nervosa appear to be similar to this subtype. Three such patients were seen.

Patients.—The patients were 2 boys aged 12 and 16 years, respectively, and a girl, 14 years. Anorexia nervosa worsened acutely after a group A β-hemolytic streptococcal infection in the first patient. Antibiotic treatment alleviated this patient's symptoms. The second boy had a history of upper respiratory tract infections, sudden onset of obsessive symptoms, and failure to gain weight as expected as he grew taller. Assessment showed a moderately elevated anti-DNase B. The last patient had had a severe Epstein-Barr virus infection about 1 year previous to her current evaluation. She had no history of an eating disorder or other psychiatric symptoms. Postinfectious autoimmune migratory polyarthritis developed, at which time she became obsessed about eating and being overweight. Her antinuclear antibody titer was 1:320 and showed a diffuse pattern.

Conclusions.—An anorexia nervosa subgroup characterized by a postinfectious acute onset or significant worsening of clinical symptoms may exist. Such cases may be distinguished clinically by pediatric onset; a sudden onset of clinically significant symptoms or a pattern of sudden, recurrent symptom exacerbations and remissions; increased, pervasive symptoms that do not occur only during stress or illness; and evidence of an antecedent or concomitant infection. Additional research is needed.

▶ These 3 case studies offer an intriguing hypothesis that will require further confirmation with more controlled study approaches, but the more general point is inescapable: the brain is the organ of the mind. The cases illustrate the rapid conceptual changes that continue to sweep psychiatry, as well as the importance of carefully obtained clinical details. Not only must we inquire about our patients' life experiences, current living situation, and general health and mental health status, but even "subtleties" such as recent infection status.

P.S. Jensen, M.D.

Adolescent Sexual Behavior, Drug Use, and Violence: Increased Reporting With Computer Survey Technology

Turner CF, Ku L, Rogers SM, et al (Research Triangle Inst, Washington, DC; Urban Inst, Washington, DC; Univ of Illinois, Urbana)
Science 280:867–873, 1998   1–5

Introduction.—Audio computer-assisted self-interviewing (audio-CASI) can be used to administer complex survey questionnaires and to record respondents' answers without the direct participation of a survey interviewer. Surveys of risk behaviors are compromised by their reliance on respondents to report accurately about behaviors that are highly sensitive and possibly illegal. The ability of audio-CASI technology to measure sensitive behaviors in adolescent respondents was assessed.

Methods.—A multistage area probability sample of 15–19-year-old boys was taken from households in the continental United States. There was oversampling of Black and Hispanic boys. A total of 1,690 respondents were questioned about sexual behavior, drug use, and violence. Respondents were randomized to answer questions using either audio-CASI or a self-administered questionnaire. For those randomized to audio-CASI, digitally recorded questions were asked through headphones and respondents answered in complete privacy by pressing numbered keys on a laptop computer keyboard.

Results.—Respondents interviewed with audio-CASI were more likely (by factors of 3 or more, using estimates of prevalence) than those who completed a self-administered questionnaire to report male-male sex, injection drug use, and sexual contact with intravenous drug users. Other high-risk behaviors were also reported with increased frequency in the audio-CASI group.

Conclusion.—Audio-CASI interviews provided estimates, more accurate than previous estimates collected in less private interviews, regarding high-risk behaviors in adolescent boys. These data give a disturbing picture of the biological and social risks currently confronting young men in the United States.

▶ One of the challenges of psychiatric studies is that human beings are active participants in the research process, whether we like it or not. Thus, the degree to which a subject is fully willing to tell his or her story obviously affects the quality of the information that researchers can obtain. This article nicely illustrates that some of our new technologies can facilitate participants' reporting of sensitive or stigmatized information, such as information about drug use and sexual behavior. The method, known as "audio-CASI," allows participants to report highly sensitive information through interview questions stored on computer and the opportunity to respond in complete privacy via computer. Amazingly, positive responses to sensitive questions were higher on the audio-CASI by threefold, while nonsensitive and/or nonstigmatized information showed equivalent prevalences in paper self-report.

P.S. Jensen, M.D.

Reliability of the Dominic-R: A Young Child Mental Health Questionnaire Combining Visual and Auditory Stimuli
Valla J-P, Bergeron L, Bidaut-Russell M, et al (Riviere-des-Prairies Hosp, Montreal; Univ of North Texas, Fort Worth)
J Child Psychol Psychiatry 38:717–724, 1997   1–6

Background.—Collecting data from young children on their own mental health in a standardized manner has been challenging. Questionnaires developed for adults involving verbal questions only are problematic when used with young children. The *Dominic-R* is a structured picture-based questionnaire in which a boy or girl named Dominic is pictured in situations intended to illustrate the abstract emotional and behavioral content of *DSM-III-R* criteria. A revised version of this instrument includes additional questions to provide auditory as well as visual symptom queries. The reliability of the *Dominic-R* was tested.

Methods and Findings.—Three hundred forty community children aged 6–11 years participated in the study. The *DSM-III-R* disorders covered were simple phobias, separation anxiety disorder, overanxious disorder, depression-dysthymia, attention deficit hyperactivity disorder, oppositional defiant disorder, and conduct disorder. The test-retest reliability of symptoms of these disorders and of symptom scores of these disorders was established. Most symptoms were associated with kappa scores of more than 0.40. The intraclass correlations ranged from 0.74 to 0.81.

Conclusions.—The *Dominic-R* questionnaire permits reliable standardized assessment of children as young as 6 years of age. This instrument increases young children's understanding of questions that evaluate mental health symptoms using a combination of visual and auditory signals. It also avoids time-related questions to the child. This questionnaire brings the structured interview of young children in line with standard clinical practice.

▶ Many clinicians are challenged by the daunting assessment issues with younger children. Although a play therapy evaluation often yields interesting clinical inisights, our "clinical insights" are often not replicable when undertaken by other, similarly skilled clinicians. Thus, tools that offer a reliable assessment of young children adapted to their cognitive capacities while drawing upon the communication modalities often used by this age group would appear to offer obvious advantages. Look for further studies with this and similar innovative assessment methods.

P.S. Jensen, M.D.

Toward a Developmental-Contextual Model of the Effects of Parental Spanking on Children's Aggression
Gunnoe ML, Mariner CL (Calvin College, Grand Rapids, Mich; Child Trends Inc, Washington, DC)
Arch Pediatr Adolesc Med 151:768–775, 1997   1–7

Background.—The effects of spanking on children between the ages of 2 and 11 years are unclear. The effects of spanking may depend on the meaning that children ascribe to it. This "developmental-contextual model" was posited as a challenge to the application of an unqualified social learning model.

Methods.—Population-based survey data were obtained from 1,112 children, aged 4–11 years. Data were controlled for several family and child factors, including children's baseline aggression.

Findings.—Spanking predicted fewer fights for children aged 4–7 years and for black children, as well as more fights for 8- to 11-year-olds and for white children. In subgroup regression analyses, spanking appeared to foster no aggression in children younger than 6 years. In addition, increased aggression was evident in only 1 subgroup: 8- to 11-year-old white boys in single-mother families.

Conclusions.—Claims that spanking teaches aggression seem to be unfounded for most children. Other preventive and harmful effects may occur depending on the child and family context. Additional research is needed to identify moderators of the effects of spanking on children's adjustment.

▶ In an interesting study that challenges the political correctness of the saying "never spank a child," these findings suggest that a variety of factors, including the child's age and the meaning of spanking within a given context or culture, are related to the degree to which spanking invariably leads to later behavioral problems or aggression. Context and meaning matter. So how are we going to incorporate them more thoughtfully into our diagnostic and clinical assessments?

P.S. Jensen, M.D.

Microanalysis of Adolescent Suicide Attempters and Ideators During the Acute Suicidal Episode

Negron R, Piacentini J, Graae F, et al (East Ridge Health Systems, Martinsburg, WV; Univ of California, Los Angeles; Cornell Univ, NY; et al)
J Am Acad Child Adolesc Psychiatry 36:1512–1519, 1997   1–8

Background.—A better understanding of the internal psychological states, responses, and coping styles of suicidal adolescents would be of value. The psychological and event-related contingencies characterizing and differentiating adolescent suicidal ideation and attempts were compared.

Methods.—Sixty-seven teenagers, aged 12–17 years, referred consecutively to a suicide disorders clinic were assessed. Thirty-five had expressed suicidal ideation, and 32 had attempted suicide. A semistructured interview was administered to elicit data on current and past emotional, cognitive, and behavioral states.

Findings.—Before the precipitant stressor, suicide attempters reported significantly more feelings of hopelessness than teens with suicidal ideation. Compared with ideators, suicide attempters spent more time thinking about suicide during the suicidal episode, were more likely to isolate themselves, and were less likely to tell anyone what they were thinking. Teens with suicidal ideation reported significantly more residual anger after the episode than suicide attempters. A stressful event preceded all episodes of ideation and attempts. The 2 groups had comparable scores on the Beck Depression Inventory.

Conclusions.—Teens having suidicidal ideation and those attempting suicide can be differentiated by degree of preexisting hopelessness, a tendency toward isolation, not talking about ideation, and longer periods of thinking about suicide during suicidal episodes. Such findings may be useful in preventing and treating suicidal adolescents.

► Despite the frequency of adolescent suicide attempts, little is known about why adolescents progress from thinking about suicide (a very common behavior) to attempting suicide. This study is unique and appears to be the first ever to explore the nature of the specific events, mood changes, cognitions, and coping strategies of ideators vs. attempters. This work is novel and opens the way for an area of future study that may yield new methods for identifying youth at greatest risk for suicide attempts, and possibly, in preventing suicide attempts.

P.S. Jensen, M.D.

The Clinical Stigmata of Aberrant Neurodevelopment in Schizophrenia
Buckley PF (Case Western Reserve Univ, Cleveland, Ohio)
J Nerv Ment Dis 186:79–86, 1998   1–9

Background.—The neurodevelopmental hypothesis is a major etio-pathologic model for schizophrenia. The clinical stigmata of aberrant neurodevelopment in schizophrenic patients are reviewed.

Obstetric Complications.—Obstetric complications (OCs) have been studied extensively and are now recognized risk factors for the development of schizophrenia. However, the association between OCs and clinical aspects or etiologic risk factors for schizophrenia is complex. Many studies report that OCs occur more often in males. Obstetric complications have also been associated with earlier age of onset and with evidence of early developmental problems and symptomatic precursors of schizophrenia. In monozygotic twins discordant for schizophrenia, OCs and minor physical anomalies have been associated with neurologic soft signs. Other studies attempting to relate OCs to genetic predisposition for schizophrenia have demonstrated either an inverse relationship or no relationship between OCs and genetic risk.

Minor Physical Anomalies.—Minor physical anomalies may be an external marker of abnormal CNS development. Several studies have demonstrated an excess of minor physical anomalies in schizophrenic patients. Clinical correlates include poor premorbid adjustment, earlier disease onset, genetic predisposition, and cognitive impairment.

Other Stigmata.—Several researchers have reported that finger and palm print examination in schizophrenic patients may be useful in providing evidence of developmental disturbance. Evidence also suggests that premorbid abnormalities can be identified in patients who subsequently develop schizophrenia, the most prominent abnormalities being attention, motor function, coordination, sensory integration, and social deficits. In addition, the occurrence of structural brain lesions of clear neurodevelopmental origin in schizophrenic patients may support the notion that observed brain abnormalities are caused by a neurodevelopmental process.

Conclusions.—Clinical stigmata of neurodevelopmental arrest include OCs, minor physical anomalies, abnormal dermatoglyphics, and childhood neuromotor precursors of adult-onset schizophrenia. Epidemiologic, postmortem, and brain imaging data support the importance of these stigmata in schizophrenia.

▶ As our appreciation of factors related to brain development increases, along with appreciation that some psychiatric disorders might be appropriately understood as disorders of brain development, this article is a useful overview of what findings have yielded concerning the importance of assessing children for history or presence of obstetric complications (or both), minor physical anomalies, abnormal dermatoglyphics, and other clinical stigmata of aberrant neurodevelopment. Such findings appear to be overrepresented in patients with schizophrenia, but they may be even more common in patients with pervasive developmental disorders or frank cognitive dysfunction. Growing understanding of such factors increasingly juxtaposes the fields of neurology and psychiatry, and enhances our appreciation of the usefulness of the medical model for selected psychiatric disorders.

P.S. Jensen, M.D.

Cognitive Deficits in Parents From Multiple-incidence Autism Families
Piven J, Palmer P (Univ of Iowa, Iowa City)
J Child Psychol Psychiatry 38:1011–1021, 1997   1–10

Introduction.—There is general agreement regarding the significance of genetic factors in autism. Definition of the phenotype is under debate. It is also not known if cognitive deficits in relatives include an expression of the underlying genetic liability for autism. The cognitive abilities in parents of at least 2 siblings with autism and parents with a Down syndrome child were compared.

Methods.—Parents of 50 autistic probands and 30 Down syndrome probands underwent assessment of intelligence, reading and spelling, and executive function.

Results.—Parents of children with autism performed significantly worse in measures of performance IQ (a test of executive function) and in reading measures (passage comprehension and rapid automatized naming).

Conclusion.—Genetically related cognitive deficits may exist in nonautistic relatives of persons with autism. These findings and future investigations of cognitive deficits in relatives may offer insights into the fundamental neuropsychological deficits in autism.

▶ I expect that as we become more sophisticated with our diagnostic systems, we will find that many of our "disorders" are spectrum conditions, present to varying degrees in family members of an affected proband. Such a notion is in concert with the likelihood that multiple genes lead to the expression of most psychiatric disorders, and that single genes, while not leading to disorder per se, may be related to the presence of specific traits that vary within the population. These authors illustrate these points very nicely with their study of families of children with autism, showing that there appears to be a broader phenotype that characterizes family members of persons with autism, such that these family members may exhibit a range of specific cognitive deficits, compared with non-autism-related controls. These areas will likely remain important to discussion and controversy over the next decade, as we continue to grapple with the question of what a "mental disorder" really is.

P.S. Jensen, M.D.

Salivary Cortisol and Cardiovascular Activity During Stress in Oppositional-Defiant Disorder Boys and Normal Controls

van Goozen SHM, Matthys W, Cohen-Kettenis PT, et al (Utrecht Univ, The Netherlands; Rudolph Magnus Inst, Utrecht, The Netherlands)
Biol Psychiatry 43:531–539, 1998   1–11

Introduction.—Arousal-regulating mechanisms are especially important in explaining individual differences in antisocial behavior. The hypothalamic-pituitary-adrenal (HPA) axis is a primary mediator of stress; thus, factors associated with stress cause alterations in adrenal steroid metabolism. The responses of cortisol and cardiovascular activity during stress were assessed in boys with oppositional-defiant disorder (ODD).

Methods.—Alterations in salivary cortisol concentration and cardiac activity were assessed in 21 ODD research subjects and 31 normal controls (NC). Mean ages of the ODD and NC groups were 10.2 and 9.6 years, respectively. Boys underwent a situation of induced stress that involved frustration, provocation, and aggression in a general setting of competition between the research participant and a videotaped opponent. The opponent was of similar age and the same sex and competed with the participant during the session. Salivary cortisol was collected within 30 minutes of induced stress. An armcuff was fixed to the nondominant arm for cardiovascular registration.

Results.—Baseline heart rate was significantly lower in the ODD than in the NC group. Provocation and frustration produced higher heart rate in ODD than in NC participants. Cortisol levels were lower for the ODD than for the NC group overall. Individual differences were great. Because anxiety is important in mediating cortisol response, research participants were placed in 1 of 4 groups, based on the intensity of their externalizing behavior and anxiety levels. Cortisol increase caused by stress exposure was greatest in highly externalizing and highly anxious participants. Cortisol decreases were greatest in boys with high externalizing behavior and low anxiousness.

Conclusion.—This is the first known article describing salivary cortisol and autonomic activity determinations in a series of clearly defined ODD boys and normal controls. Cortisol may be an important marker of anxiety, inhibition, and conduct disorder; it may reflect neurohormonal processes involved in the expression of ODD. These findings support need for further investigation of HPA-axis sympathetic autonomic functioning in the maintenance of aggression in boys.

▶ In recent years, the HPA has been consistently implicated in the onset and severity of child psychiatric disorders such as depression, anxiety disorders, the disruptive disorders (attention-deficit hyperactivity disorder, conduct disorder), and co-morbid states. This article takes us a step further toward understanding the HPA's role, by examining the responsivity of the HPA to stressors in ODD children vs. normal controls, and positing that ODD children with anxiety would have the highest responses, in heart rate and cortisol levels, to a stressor. Indeed, such findings were demonstrated, contrasting remarkably with the findings of lowest physiologic responses in children who were aggressive or conduct disordered but without anxiety. This article nicely illustrates the importance of co-morbidity and its potential role in exacerbating or ameliorating psychopathologic and pathophysiologic characteristics of disorder. This area of research will help to refine our diagnostic and etiopathophysiologic understanding in the next few years.

P.S. Jensen, M.D.

Brain Regions Responsive to Novelty in the Absence of Awareness
Berns GS, Cohen JD, Mintun MA (Univ of Pittsburgh, Pa; Washington Univ, St Louis)
Science 276:1272–1275, 1997   1–12

Background.—Detecting novelty is a cognitive function necessary for survival. It requires an assessment of expectedness and context. Positron emission tomography was used to map brain regions responsive to novelty, without awareness.

Methods and Findings.—Ten volunteers performed a simple reaction-time task in which all stimuli were equally likely but that followed a complex sequence, unknown to the participants. Behavioral performance measures indicated that participants learned the sequences, although they were not aware that any order existed. After the volunteers were trained, a subtle, unperceived change in the nature of the sequence resulted in increased blood flow in a network that comprised the left premotor area, left anterior cingulate, and right ventral striatum. Decreases in blood flow were recorded in the right dorsolateral prefrontal and parietal regions.

Conclusions.—The time course of the changes observed suggests that the ventral striatum is responsive to novel information and that the right prefrontal region is related to the maintenance of contextual information. Both processes apparently occur without the individual's awareness.

▶ Using use-of-art neuroimaging techniques, these investigators documented the ability of the human brain to learn and respond to complex patterns, despite the lack of conscious awareness. In particular, special cortical regions appear to be activated in response to novel stimuli, determining the specific contexts for which the stimuli should be attended to, and used by the human in complex perceptual judgments that increase accuracy of prediction in responses to future environmental stimuli. While this study was not of children per se, it does help us understand children's (adults') abilities to perceive and respond to contextual information. This is an exciting finding, and its ramifications are likely to be far reaching. How do children sense safety? Acceptance? Rejection? Social relations? As we increasingly expand our capacity to map the human cortex, our ability to understand the neural bases of these subtle yet very important factors that make us human will likewise increase. Fascinating, eh?

P.S. Jensen, M.D.

Brain Activation Modulated by Sentence Comprehension

Just MA, Carpenter PA, Keller TA, et al (Carnegie Mellon Univ, Pittsburgh, Pa; Univ of Pittsburgh, Pa)
Science 274:114–116, 1996   1–13

Background.—Comprehending visually presented sentences induces brain activation that increases with the linguistic complexity of the sentence. Comprehension demand was manipulated using 3 sentence types that differed in structural complexity but were similar superficially, containing 2 clauses and the same number of words.

Methods and Findings.—Fifteen college-age participants responded to active conjoined sentences with no embedded clause, sentences with subject relative clauses, and sentences with object relative clauses. Volume of neural tissue activated during sentence comprehension was determined using echoplanar functional MRI. Modulation of the volume of activation by sentence complexity was recorded in a network of 4 regions: the classic left-hemisphere language areas and their homologous right-hemisphere regions. Volumes of activation were much smaller in the right areas than in the left.

Conclusions.—The amount of neural activity engendered by a given cognitive process depends on the computational demand imposed by the task. Any mapping between brain site and cognitive function is a variable function between 2 levels of description of a dynamic system that is modulated by the demand of the task. Thus, it cannot be a static cartography of brain anatomy.

▶ In this study by Just and colleagues, investigators demonstrated that the degree of brain activation set in motion by language and sentence comprehension is related to the linguistic complexity of the sentence. In view of the increasing knowledge concerning the plasticity of the human cortex, these findings further illustrate that human ability to learn and comprehend language is not simply a static ability, but very much a function of the complexity of the task and the degree to which the brain efficiently "recruits" additional neural tissue across an entire network or cortical brain areas.

P.S. Jensen, M.D.

Case Series: Pediatric Seasonal Affective Disorder: A Follow-up Report

Giedd JN, Swedo SE, Lowe CH, et al (Natl Inst of Mental Health, Bethesda, Md)
J Am Acad Child Adolesc Psychiatry 37:218–220, 1998   1–14

Introduction.—Few trials have examined seasonal affective disorder (SAD) in children. Prevalence rates of SAD in the pediatric population range from 3% to 5% for fourth to sixth graders. Reported is a 7-year follow-up of the course of illness and response to treatment in 7 research participants who were diagnosed with SAD during childhood.

Methods.—All patients experienced at least 2 weeks' duration of sadness, anxiety, or irritability during winter and at least 3 symptoms of either fatigue, sleep changes, altered appetite, carbohydrate craving, or headaches. All children had dysfunction in school. Symptoms diminished in spring and summer. Light therapy was used over a 2-year period when symptoms were pronounced enough to cause severe dysfunction. At 7-year follow up, patients were assessed by questionnaires and interviewed by a psychiatrist. Parents participated in a telephone interview.

Results.—All patients continued to experience seasonal symptoms. The symptoms were stable and responded to light therapy. Two patients with hypomania or mania responded to light therapy. Two patients required antidepressants in conjunction with light therapy. All patients reported benefit from learning about their illness and continued to make consistent efforts to increase their light exposure in the fall and winter months.

Conclusion.—These findings indicate that seasonal symptoms persist. Parents, teachers, and clinicians need to understand the importance of early recognition and intervention to prevent unnecessary suffering in children with SAD. Children whose school performance is best in the first and last quarters and worst in the second and third quarters may have SAD.

▶ I have never been fully convinced by the presumed phenomenon of seasonal affective disorder, especially in children. This series of case reports casts the phenomenon in continued doubt, to my mind, because most of this series of 7 patients had fairly benign outcomes. The authors also raise the possibility that 3% of chldren have seasonal affective disorder, with symptoms especially pronounced during the school year and winter months. Although light therapy appears to be beneficial in such patients, most of us do note that we feel better during the summer than during the winter, and we prefer sun over rain, all things being equal. So how are we going to draw boundaries between health and disease?

P.S. Jensen, M.D.

Risk, Pathophysiology, and Outcomes

INTRODUCTION

This section highlights a number of important principles. The most obvious 1 is that a host of early factors—some innate, some contextual and interactional, some biological, and some social—coalesce into a complex, marvelous, and seemingly inseparable mixture that progressively builds the child's brain and fashions his/her psychological substrate. These factors are usually developmental, that is, new structures are built on the foundations of earlier brain-behavior patterns. While continuities across time are commonplace and expectable, discontinuities and qualitative shifts in function and behavior occur as well. Obviously, longitudinal studies shed valuable light on such issues. Correlational studies are far weaker in providing satisfactory information on these topics, so I include them only when they contribute truly unique information. Otherwise, the design of the studies presented in this section are either longitudinal, experimental, or both. Some articles highlight the cumulative nature and adverse public health impact of various risk factors over time, even to the point of substantial repercussions on physical health (Felitti et al.).

Just as I note the importance of "breaking apart the phenotype" in the previous section on evaluation and assessment of clinical characteristics, many of the articles here illustrate the need to better understand and break apart "environtypes." Which *specific* aspects of our environments affect us adversely or beneficially, and how do they do this? How do various extrinsic-environmental and innate factors combine? Why are some but not all persons similarly affected by exposures to "psychotoxic" risk factors? For example, the study by O'Hearn and colleagues identifies which aspects of marital conflict have the greatest effects on children.

Some may question my inclusion of a number of animal studies. However, important links in our knowledge of what constitutes truly "causal" risk factors must come from experimental studies, a feat rarely, if ever, possible using child subjects. The risk factors we are most concerned about cannot ethically be "tweaked" in studies with children. Studies of other mammalian species such as primates (with whom we share about 95% of our genetic material) are critical for accurate understanding. Some of this is tough reading, but as I have struggled with it over time, I have found it increasingly worthwhile.

Lastly, a number of the studies illustrate new technologies that are allowing us to better understand brain-behavior-environment relations (e.g, Pine, Coplan, Wasserman, et al., Rapoport et al., Whitaker et al.).

Peter S. Jensen, M.D.

Maternal Deprivation and Stress Induce Immediate Early Genes in the Infant Rat Brain
Smith MA, Kim S-Y, Van Oers HJJ, et al (Natl Inst of Mental Health, Bethesda, Md; Univ of Delaware, Newark)
Endocrinology 138:4622–4628, 1997   1–15

Introduction.—During postnatal days 4–14, neonatal rats have little or no adrenocortical response to most stimuli that create responses later in life. The attenuated pituitary and adrenal responses to stress observed during this stress-hyporesponsive period are well described. The hypothalmic-pituitary-adrenal (HPA) axis can be disinhibited by maternal deprivation (DEP), allowing the rat to respond to mild stressors. Changes in the expression of stress-responsive genes in the brains of neonatal rats were measured by in situ hybridization to determine how DEP can alter HPA axis sensitivity.

Methods.—Rats were maternally deprived and removed from the home for 24 hours at postnatal day 11 or 19. Food and water were not made available during the deprivation period. Nondeprived controls were left with the mother rat until the time of testing. Neonates were stressed by administration of a single injection of saline and placed on a heating pad for 30 or 120 minutes before being sacrificed. Trunk blood was collected for determination of ACTH and corticosterone. Frozen brain sections from the rat brain, including the level of the hypothalmic paraventricular (PVN), underwent in situ hybridization. The messenger (mRNA) levels of 2 immediate-early genes (IEGs; c-fos and NGFI-B) and CRH were determined in rats killed at 30 minutes after injection. In rats killed at 2 hours after injection, CRH mRNA was analyzed.

Results.—Even in the presence of a minimal HPA axis response, the mild stress of a single saline injection significantly increased mRNA levels of c-fos and NGFI-B in the hypothalmic PVN and cerebral cortex in nondeprived rats during postnatal day 12. In deprived rats, induction of IEGs in response to stress was greatly enhanced in the PVN of postnatal day 12 neonates. In rats matured beyond the stress-hyporesponsive period, DEP attenuated the effects of stress on IEG induction. Deprivation diminished basal levels of CRH mRNA in the PVN in both postnatal day 12 and postnatal day 20 rats.

Conclusion.—There was a marked difference between stress-hyporesponsive period rats at postnatal day 12 and more mature rats at postnatal day 20. Maternal DEP potentiated the ability of stress to produce IEGs in the PVN in the younger rats.

▶ In our quest to understand risk factors for abnormal neurodevelopment, careful attention must be paid to the impact of the maternal HPA on the developing fetus. Experimental studies are not feasible or ethical in humans, but animal models can shed important light on how such factors may be related to brain development and later outcomes. These authors demonstrate that maternal deprivation facilitates the "turning on" of specific early genes in young rats exposed to specific painful stressors, while animals not subjected to separation from the mother appear to be buffered from the effects of the same stressors. Interestingly, these effects were time sensitive and time specific, so that young rats that had matured beyond 20 days postnatal did not respond differentially to the stress exposure. Findings suggest that the presence of the caregiving rat moderates the neonate's response to early exposure to stressors, and that the combination of the 2 risk factors (stressor exposure plus maternal deprivation) may be related to later, long-lasting forms of dysfunction in mammalian species. My grandmother always knew this, of course, so it is nice that we scientists are finally catching up.

P.S. Jensen, M.D.

Maternal Care, Hippocampal Glucocorticoid Receptors, and Hypothalamic-Pituitary-Adrenal Responses to Stress

Liu D, Diorio J, Tannenbaum B, et al (McGill Univ, Montreal)
Science 277:1659–1662, 1997

1–16

Introduction.—Experimental studies indicate that animals handled during infancy show reduced responses to stress compared with animals who do not have this attention during the first weeks of life. These studies conclude that development of hypothalamic-pituitary-adrenal (HPA) responses to stress are modified by early environmental events. In rats, differences between handled and nonhandled animals persist as late as 24 to 26 months. Other authors propose that the effects of postnatal handling are mediated by changes in mother-to-pup interactions. Researchers evaluated the question of how this maternal mediation might occur and whether such factors contribute to naturally occurring individual differences in HPA responses to stress.

Methods.—The behavior of mothers of handled or nonhandled litters was assessed during the first 10 days of life. The relation between naturally occurring individual differences in maternal care and HPA development was evaluated.

Results.—Mothers in the handled pups group showed increased levels of licking and grooming and were more likely to nurse in the arched-back posture than mothers in the nonhandled pups group. Adult rats who had been handled as pups (and consequently licked by their mothers) showed reduced plasma adrenocorticotropic hormone and corticosterone responses to acute stress, increased hippocampal glucocorticoid receptor messenger RNA expression, enhanced glucocorticoid feedback sensitivity, and decreased levels of hypothalamic corticotropin-releasing hormone messenger RNA. A significant correlation was noted between each measure and the frequency of maternal licking and grooming.

Conclusion.—Findings support the hypothesis that the effect of postnatal handling on HPA development is mediated by effects on mother-pup interaction. Handling increases the frequency of licking and grooming, and these maternal activities are associated with reduced HPA responsivity to stress. This tactile stimulation regulates pup physiology and affects development of the CNS.

▶ In animal studies, Liu and colleagues have demonstrated that variations in maternal care in neonatal rat pups affect the further development of stress-responsive neuroendocrine systems. These early maternal–care-related factors serve to program the nature of the young organism's current and longer-lasting responses to threatening stimuli. They, likely, help in shaping the organism's responses in providing a better fit for its particular "ecological niche" and for environments it is likely to face during subsequent development. Better understanding of these processes and their applicability to humans may eventually help researchers to design specific care-giving and environmental modifications that will prevent later problems in behavior and emotion, resulting because of the development of early defensive processes in otherwise healthy organisms.

P.S. Jensen, M.D.

Moderate Alcohol Consumption and Psychological Stress During Pregnancy Induce Attention and Neuromotor Impairments in Primate Infants

Schneider ML, Roughton EC, Lubach GR (Univ of Wisconsin, Madison)
Child Dev 68:747–759, 1997   1–17

Introduction.—The behavioral and physical effects of high levels of maternal alcohol consumption during pregnancy are well known. The effects of lower levels of exposure have not been defined, however. Prenatal stress and its influence on prenatal alcohol exposure also have not been adequately addressed. The effects of moderate alcohol consumption and psychological stress during pregnancy on offspring growth and behavior were assessed in 33 rhesus monkey infants.

Methods.—Healthy female monkeys were assigned to 1 of 3 groups: 1) alcohol consumption, 0.6 g/kg daily, beginning 5 days before breeding and continuing throughout gestation (the equivalent of 1–2 drinks per day) 2) alcohol consumption, as already described, and exposure to mild psychological stress (removal from home cage and exposure to 3 random noise bursts), and 3) sucrose consumption equivolemic and equicaloric to alcohol consumption, and no psychological stress. At 4 days postpartum and weekly thereafter, infants underwent brief weekly separations from their mothers for determination of growth, behavior, and facial dimensions.

Results.—All infants were within normal limits in weight at 5 months, in gestational length, and in facial dimensions. Birth weight of males in the alcohol/stress condition was significantly lower, compared to birth weight of males in other conditions. This significant interaction must be interpreted with the understanding that there were 6 males in the alcohol/stress group and 3 each in the control and alcohol-only groups, respectively. Compared to controls, infants exposed to moderate alcohol consumption and those exposed to alcohol and stress had significantly lower scores in measures of orientation, motor maturity, and infant behavior state. Alcohol-induced neuromotor impairments were aggravated by maternal exposure to psychological stress. There was a 23% fetal loss rate (abortion and stillbirths) in the alcohol/stress group.

Conclusion.—Moderate levels of alcohol consumption during pregnancy can affect the developing nervous system of the primate fetus and cause neurobehavioral deficits. Primates in this series experienced impaired attention and neuromotor functioning. However, gestation length and morphology were not affected by moderate levels of alcohol consumption.

▶ One of the critical questions facing child and adolescent psychiatrists and others is how various risk factors work together in leading to the onset of mental disorders in children and adults. It is unclear exactly what dose of various risk factors is required to precipitate disorder or impairment. In this interesting article, the investigators studied rhesus monkeys to explore the effects of the equivalent of 1–2 drinks daily of alcohol, coupled with environmental stressors (exposure to 3 random noise bursts during removal from the monkeys' accustomed surroundings). While fetal alcohol syndrome characteristics were not produced in the experimental monkeys exposed to alcohol and environmental stressors, results indicated that the 2 risk factors exerted independent and additive effects leading to subtle attentional and neuromotor deficits. Animals exposed to both stressors were significantly impaired, compared to controls and alcohol-only exposed primates. Of note, these dual risk factor primates did *not* show evidence of an overt fetal alcohol syndrome, but low to moderate levels of alcohol consumption, coupled with environmental stressors, were sufficient to produce a range of deficits. These findings have implications for health care providers interested in how low socioeconomic status may interact with low to moderate alcohol consumption to explain variations in adverse pregnancy outcomes in at-risk children.

P.S. Jensen, M.D.

Developmental Outcome of Infants Born With Biological and Psychosocial Risks

Laucht M, Esser G, Schmidt MH (Central Inst of Mental Health, Mannheim, Germany; Univ of Potsdam, Germany)
J Child Psychol Psychiatry 38:843–853, 1997   1–18

Objective.—The application of "child at risk" has been extended from children with prematurity or other complications of pregnancy and delivery to include children facing other threats to their mental development. Some researchers have suggested that these biologic and psychosocial influences are not independent of each other—that adverse family settings are associated with a greater frequency of complications of pregnancy and delivery. A growing number of potential risk factors during child development have been identified in recent years, but the factors' etiologic significance is unknown. This prospective, longitudinal study examined the impact of biologic and psychosocial risk factors on early child development.

Methods.—Three hundred fifty infants with risk factors for developmental disorders were studied from birth to school age in the Mannheim Study of Risk Children. The children were selected for their different combinations of biologic and psychosocial risks. The children's motor, cognitive, and social-emotional functioning were assessed at the ages of 3, 24, and 54 months.

Results.—As a group, children who had prenatal and perinatal complications or who were raised in adverse family environments showed unfavorable early childhood development. Children with multiple risk factors had significant developmental lags, compared to children without risk factors: by preschool age, motor development lagged by more than 1.5 standard deviation, while cognitive and social-emotional development lagged by nearly 1.0 standard deviation. Psychosocial risk factors posed the greatest threat to child development, accounting for one third of attributable variance in motor development, two thirds of variance in cognitive development, and four fifths of variance in social-emotional outcome. Most of the impact of organic risks was on motor impairment; the social-emotional effects had mostly resolved by preschool age. Throughout development, the effects of biologic and psychosocial risks were additive. The severity of stress factors mainly accounted for their detrimental effects. However, most children developed favorably, regardless of risk: no more than 20% of the variance in developmental outcome could be linked to prenatal and perinatal complications or to adverse family settings.

Conclusions.—Psychosocial risk factors outweigh biologic risk factors in their impact on child development through the preschool years, these results suggest. Preventive approaches should seek to reduce psychosocial stresses in families with young children, while promoting health resources and protective resources in families at risk. Early parent-child interaction appears to be a particularly important mediator of family stressors. With a few exceptions, measures to prevent adverse developmental outcomes after prenatal and perinatal complications appear to be effective.

▶ Most studies of risk factors for child and adolescent psychopathology have been plagued by the problem of "nonspecificity," the action of any risk factor producing diverse outcomes (rather than a specific type of disorder). Further, risk factors' effects seem to be best understood and most visible when additive: their effects become more apparent as 3, 4, or more risk factors accumulate. Lastly, examination of the risk factors for a given disorder has found little evidence that the risk factors leading to that disorder are at all unique, compared with those leading to other disorders. This article takes our understanding a bit further, showing that all risk factors are not equal, either in terms of the magnitude of their effects, or in terms of the types of adverse outcomes they produce. Thus, in the longitudinal Mannheim Study of Risk Children from birth to 4 and one-half years later, children exposed to initial biologic risk factors fared better, especially in cognitive and socio-emotional outcomes, than children exposed to early psychosocial family risk factors. Teasing apart the potential effects of intervening variables will be an important next step, but this article highlights the baseline psychosocial and family risk factors in the child's life as an area especially important for future interventions.

P.S. Jensen, M.D.

Family Conflict and Slow Growth

Montgomery SM, Bartley MJ, Wilkinson RG (Royal Free Hosp, London; Univ College London; Univ of Sussex, Brighton, England)
Arch Dis Child 77:326–330, 1997   1–19

Background.—Previous studies have shown that slow growth in childhood is related to later difficulty in the labor market. This finding suggests that slow growth in children could be an indicator of a process that is damaging to future mental and physical health. This study examined the effects of family conflict on growth rate in children.

Methods.—The analysis included British National Child Development Study data on 6,574 children born in 1 week in 1958. This continuing longitudinal study has collected detailed data on the children at birth and ages 7, 11, 16, 23, and 33 years. Their growth at age 7 years was noted, with short stature defined as the lowest one fifth of the height distribution. The effects of family conflict—including domestic tension, divorce, separation, or desertion—on childhood growth were assessed, independent of material disadvantage. Multivariate analysis was performed to adjust for full adult height as a measure of genetically predetermined height.

Results.—The rate of short stature was 31% for children with a history of family conflict vs. 20% for those without family conflict: relative odds 1.79, 95% confidence interval 1.39–2.30. This figure was slightly reduced after adjustment for social class, crowding, sex, and predetermined height: relative odds 1.62, 95% confidence interval 1.18–2.23. Short stature was noted in 44% of children from the most crowded households, compared with 16% of those from the least crowded households. This relationship was reduced but still significant after adjustment for potential confounders: relative odds 3.07, 95% confidence interval 2.08–4.51. Though low social class was initially related to short stature, this relationship was not significant after adjustment.

Conclusions.—Slow growth during childhood is independently related to family conflict. The findings suggest that family conflict may have lasting consequences for children, and that slow growth could be a sensitive indicator of emotional disturbance and chronic stress for children. The link between slow growth in childhood and difficulty in the labor market during adulthood could reflect adverse psychological and cognitive outcomes of psychosocial and material adversity during childhood.

▶ This article springs from analyses from the longitudinal National Child Development Study, a British study of a birth cohort begun in 1958. Even after controlling for socioeconomic status, parental smoking, participants' eventual adult height, and crowding variables, findings indicated that early family conflict resulted in delayed growth at age 7 years. Since domestic conflict has been shown to be related to a range of effects—early developmental, psychological, physical health-related, and even economic—we must turn increasing attention to practical and palatable approaches to reducing these health risks in the general population.

P.S. Jensen, M.D.

Antecedents of Preschool Children's Internalizing Problems: A Longitudinal Study of Low-income Families

Shaw DS, Keenan K, Vondra JI, et al (Univ of Pittsburgh, Pa; Univ of Chicago)
J Am Acad Child Adolesc Psychiatry 36:1760–1767, 1997   1–20

Introduction.—There are few trials available to guide the understanding of the developmental precursors of internalizing problems in young children. However, there is considerable evidence that the causes of such internalizing problems are multifactoral and include child, parental, and family elements. The antecedents of preschool-age internalizing problems were evaluated, using the construct of emotion regulation as a guide.

Methods.—Longitudinal data were gathered in 86 low-income mother-infant dyads. Assessment visits were made when infants were 12, 15, 18, 24, 36, and 60 months old. Risk factors relating to internalizing problems were measured by the Child Behavior Checklist.

Results.—Negative emotionality, disorganized attachment classification, negative life events, exposure to childrearing disagreements, and parenting hassles assessed during infancy were related to the development of preschool-age internalizing problems. The interaction of high negative emotionality and exposure to childrearing disagreements added distinctive variance to the prediction of scores on the Child Behavior Checklist Withdrawal and Depression/Anxiety subscales.

Conclusion.—Several risk factors identified in the first 2 years of life were correlated with development of preschool-age internalizing problems. These findings are an important contribution to the recognition of precursors of early internalizing problems.

▶ One area where more research understanding is urgently needed is the study of infants, toddlers, and preschoolers, and more particularly their internalizing disorders, where very little work has been done to date. Although most child and adolescent psychiatrists acknowledge the importance of early environmental factors on shaping later outcomes, it has been less clear which child-specific characteristics might also be identified as possible markers for later adverse outcomes, and as indicators of need for more immediate intervention. This article addresses this gap, demonstrating the importance and relevance of child, parent, and environmental factors to later internalizing outcomes. Because the authors studied children ages 1–5, better understanding of children's preschool and early school-readiness was demonstrated by early behavioral measures. So how are we going to heighten public awareness that "school readiness" is better viewed as largely behavioral and emotional, rather than simply cognitive in origin?

P.S. Jensen, M.D.

Can Cognitive Distortions Differentiate Between Internalising and Externalising Problems?

Leung PWL, Wong MMT (Chinese Univ of Hong Kong, Shatin)
J Child Psychol Psychiatry 39:263–269, 1998   1–21

Introduction.—Earlier reports of internalizing problems have focused on the relationship between internalizing problems and personalizing, but no studies have the specificity of this relationship versus other forms of psychopathology, such as externalizing problems. Moreover, fewer studies have included other forms of cognitive distortion, such as overgeneralization, catastrophizing, and selective abstraction. All 4 forms of cognitive distortion were examined in a community sample of adolescents to assess the specificity of cognitive distortions with internalizing problems.

Methods.—Four hundred and five students randomly selected from 3 mainstream high schools in Hong Kong completed the Youth Self-Report Form and the Children's Negative Cognitive Errors Questionnaire. Mean age of 189 boys and 216 girls was 15 years.

Results.—Internalizing problems were specifically correlated with selective abstraction, personalizing, overgeneralization, and catastrophizing. As the severity of internalizing rose, the magnitude of cognitive distortions increased positively at a quadratic rate.

Conclusion.—There are specific event/schema-linked cognitive distortions represented in the Children's Negative Cognitive Errors Questionnaire that can distinguish internalizing from externalizing problems. It cannot be assumed that externalizing problems are free from cognitive distortions, however.

▶ In the last few years, increasing research methodologic sophistication has yielded important findings concerning treatments (particularly cognitive behavioral treaments) for internalizing conditions. An important component of such treatments is the targeting and modification of problematic internal representations, attributions, and schemas potentially indicative of cognitive distortions and bad habits of thinking. This article shows that as children exhibit more internalizing problems, the steepness of curve relating these symptoms to cognitive distortions increases, suggesting increasing relevance of such cognitive factors in the severe end of the spectrum of internalizing disorders. The authors noted a degree of specificity of these findings relative to internalizing disorders. Although specificity was not absolute, the findings do demarcate the relevance of therapies targeting cognitive distortions in the internalizing vs. externalizing disorders.

P.S. Jensen, M.D.

Impact of Family Type and Family Quality on Child Behavior Problems: A Longitudinal Study
Najman JM, Behrens BC, Andersen M, et al (Univ of Queensland, St Lucia, Australia; Queensland Health, Brisbane, Australia; Mater Children's Hosp, Brisbane, Australia)
J Am Acad Child Adolesc Psychiatry 36:1357–1365, 1997   1–22

Background.—Substantial changes have occurred recently in types and quality of families. The extent to which family type and quality affects child behavior problems was studied.

Methods.—A total of 8,556 pregnant women were enrolled in a prospective, longitudinal study. Details of changes in family type and quality were assessed on the Spanier Dyadic Adjustment Scale. These data were used to predict 3 second-order syndromes developed from the Child Behavior Checklist and administered to mothers when their children were 5 years of age.

Findings.—Mothers reporting no partner changes (married and single) had the lowest rates of child behavior problems. Mothers who more often described their relationship with their partner as poor reported the highest rate of child behavior problems in all 3 syndromes. Adjustment for possible confounding variables did not affect these results.

Conclusions.—Changes of partner and dyadic conflict appear to result in child behavior problems. The latter appears to have a greater effect than the former. The fewest child behavior problems are reported by mothers with no partner changes and no conflict.

▶ While it is widely known that both marital conflict and marital disruption (e.g., partner changes) are important risk factors for child behavior problems, relatively less is known about the independence of these factors. This longitudinal study began when prospective mothers were seen for their first visit for prenatal care. Not surprisingly, both marital conflict and partner status changes were related to later behavior problems, with marital conflict emerging as the most important risk factor. These findings held, even after controlling for socioeconomic status, income, and maternal age. But 1 finding may surprise some (at least it did me): children of single parents fared better in terms of later behavior problems than reconstituted families. Better understanding of how families function optimally across various cultural settings, and how family factors affect children of different ages and genders will be an important area of continuing study over the next decade.

P.S. Jensen, M.D.

Supportive Parenting, Ecological Context, and Children's Adjustment: A Seven-Year Longitudinal Study

Pettit GS, Bates JE, Dodge KA (Auburn Univ, Ala; Indiana Univ, Bloomington; Vanderbilt Univ, Nashville, Tenn)
Child Dev 68:908–923, 1997   1–23

Background.—In certain models of parenting effectiveness, different aspects of supportive parenting (SP) are expected to be associated with different types of child outcome. Two major questions about the possible effect of early SP on children's school adjustment were addressed: (1) whether SP assessed before kindergarten predicts grade 6 adjustment after adjustment for early harsh parenting (HP); and (2) whether SP buffers the effects of early family adversity on grade 6 adjustment.

Methods and Findings.—Data on parenting and family adversity were obtained from home-visit interviews with 585 mothers before their children entered kindergarten. Four SP measures were assessed: mother-to-child warmth, proactive teaching, inductive discipline, and positive involvement. The use of harsh physical discipline defined HP. Indicators of family adversity were socioeconomic disadvantage, family stress, and single parenthood. Behavior problems, social skills, and academic performance were assessed using teacher ratings and school records in kindergarten and in grade 6. Supportive parenting predicted adjustment in grade 6, even after controlling for kindergarten adjustment and HP. High levels of SP moderated the impact of family adversity on subsequent behavior problems.

Conclusions.—These and previous findings suggest that SP assessed in early childhood predict successful adaptation through the elementary school years. Supportive parenting appears to be linked with child outcomes both directly, as additive main effects, and indirectly, by mitigating the effects of adversity.

▶ Just what is "supportive parenting"? As operationalized by these investigators, it includes 4 constructs: parents' observed warmth, use of inductive disciplinary strategies, interest in their children's peer contacts, and proactive teaching of social skills. Of note, SP benefited children across a range of outcomes, including academic, behavioral, and social adjustment at both kindergarten and grade 6. Moreover, especially among children at risk for adverse outcomes (by virtue of the presence of other risk factors), SP appeared especially important, capable of offsetting other potential disadvantageous life circumstances. Some evidence of age-, gender-, and ethnicity-specific effects were seen, but will require independent confirmation.

P.S. Jensen, M.D.

Role of Parenting in Adolescent Deviant Behavior: Replication Across and Within Two Ethnic Groups

Forehand R, Miller KS, Dutra R, et al (Univ of Georgia, Atlanta; Ctrs for Disease Control and Prevention, Atlanta, Ga)
J Consult Clin Psychol 65:1036–1041, 1997

1–24

Introduction.—There is a growing rate of deviant behavior in adolescents. Parenting is a major influence on such behavior, particularly parental monitoring and positive communication between parents and adolescents. It is important to understand the cultural context in which parenting occurs. This study examined the effects of parental monitoring and communication on adolescent behavior across and within ethnic groups.

Methods.—The study included 907 adolescents and their mothers, identified from the Family Adolescent Risk Behavior and Communication Study. All participants were African-Americans living in Montgomery, Ala. or the Bronx, NY, or Hispanics living in the Bronx or San Juan, Puerto Rico. All of the adolescents were 14–16 years old. The participants responded to study instruments assessing parental monitoring and parent-adolescent communication, which were analyzed for their relationship to adolescent deviance. Deviant behaviors included aggression, sexual intercourse with 2 or more partners, and drug and alcohol abuse.

Results.—The rate of deviant behavior was consistently higher for boys than for girls. In all 4 samples, increased parental monitoring was related to lower levels of deviant behavior on multiple regression analysis. However, parent-adolescent communication was not significantly related to adolescent deviance.

Conclusions.—The results support research in other populations which has suggested that high levels of parental monitoring are associated with reduced levels of adolescent deviant behavior. This relationship is noted across ethnic groups and geographic locations. Parental monitoring may simply reduce opportunities for deviant behavior, though other explanations are possible as well. Parent-adolescent communication was not significant in this analysis, but should still be addressed in programs for prevention of and intervention in adolescent deviance.

▶ One of the problems with many studies concerning psychosocial risk factors is that it is rarely clear if the purported risk or protective factors are situation or culture specific, and whether the reported relations are equally applicable in different settings or ethnic groups. Forehand and colleagues examined the simple, additive, and interactive effects of parental monitoring and parent-adolescent communication variables on deviant behavior in 4 different samples, 2 composed of Hispanic and 2 of African-American ethnic groups. Not surprisingly, gender (being male) was consistently related to behavioral deviance (e.g., drug use, aggression, etc.) across all 4 samples. But most importantly, findings indicated that parental monitoring was consistently related to reduced adolescent behavior problems across samples, whereas parent-adolescent communication was less consistently related to deviant behavior. These findings are cross-sectional (hence, causality cannot be inferred), so follow-up intervention studies designed to enhance parental monitoring should be done to determine the extent to which increased monitoring results in decreased behavioral deviance, and the extent to which such interventions are effective across cultural and geographic contexts.

P.S. Jensen, M.D.

Family Functioning and Parent General Health in Families of Adolescents With Major Depressive Disorder

Tamplin A, Goodyer IM, Herbert J (Univ of Cambridge, England)
J Affect Disord 48:1–13, 1998   1–25

Introduction.—The extent of agreement among family members about family function is not known. How much families with a depressed member vary as a group from other families is also not clear. Family functioning and parents' mental health in families of adolescents with major depression were compared to those in families in a community control sample.

Methods.—The McMaster Family Assessment Device and the General Health Questionnaire were administered to 61 families of adolescents with major depression and to 34 families in a community control sample.

Results.—The mean Family Assessment Device and General Health Questionnaire scores for families of adolescents with major depression were significantly worse than for control families; 56% and 29%, respectively, met criteria for current dysfunction. In families of adolescents with major depressive disorder, family dysfunction was correlated with the additive effects of co-morbid Oppositional Defiant Disorder in the depressed adolescent and with mother's current poor mental health. The father's current mental health had no correlation with family functioning.

Conclusion.—In families of depressed adolescents, there was a high level of agreement among all family members regarding their perceptions of functioning problems. Co-morbid diagnosis of Oppositional Defiant Disorder in the depressed adolescent and poor mental health in the mother were major characteristics in families of adolescents with major depression. Awareness of these 2 potential indicators of family functioning problems could help in the recognition of and intervention in families for whom assistance could be efficacious.

▶ It has become increasingly clear that children and adolescents with depression are exposed to a range of risk factors and potentially depression-exacerbating conditions. Although the relation between maternal depression and infant/toddler functioning is well established, less has been known about family relations in adolescents who meet full criteria for depression. This article fills an important void, demonstrating not only the relationship between depressed adolescents and their families, but also that depressed adolescents with co-morbid Oppositional Defiant Disorder or a depressed mother are at greater risk and might warrant more systematic targeting for additional treatment resources. Although not all families displayed significant functioning difficulties, the 56% prevalence of such difficulties among families of depressed adolescents may provide an important clue as to why many depressed adolescents do not respond to medication. Are we missing part of the picture when we deliver medication but do not address other intercurrent and ongoing relationship difficulties?

P.S. Jensen, M.D.

Depressive Symptoms in Children and Adolescents: Etiological Links Between Normality and Abnormality: A Research Note
Eley TC (Inst of Child Health, London)
J Child Psychol Psychiatry 38:861–865, 1997 1–26

Background.—It has been clearly shown that children and adolescents can develop extreme depression, leading to academic and psychosocial problems and persisting into adulthood. It is uncertain, however, whether pediatric depression is better considered as one end of a continuum or as qualitatively different from the normal range of depressive symptoms. This study compared the etiologic factors causing normal and abnormal depressive symptoms in a sample of child and adolescent twins.

Methods.—The study included 395 same-sex twin pairs, recruited from the Register for Child Twins. Depressive symptoms were evaluated using the Children's Depressive Inventory. The findings in monozygotic and dizygotic twin pairs were analyzed to assess the contributions of genetic and environmental factors to depressive symptoms. Multiple cutoff points were used to define the abnormal group.

Results.—Analysis of individual differences confirmed the importance of genetic factors, with a nonsignificant common-environment component. Genetic factors contributed to a similar extent to abnormal-group membership as defined using multiple cutoff points. Again, common environment was not significant, though it seemed to contribute more to abnormal-group membership than to individual differences.

Conclusions.—Genetic factors appear to play an etiologic role in both individual differences and abnormal-group membership for self-reported depressive symptoms in children and adults. This and previous studies suggest that specific environmental influences may be linked to abnormally high levels of depressive symptoms. The author calls for further studies to replicate these findings, and to identify the environmental influences on pediatric depressive symptoms.

▶ One of the interesting arguments between various factions in child and adult psychopathology has been about whether Diagnostic and Statistical Manual-style disorders (such as very severe depressive disorder identified using traditional psychiatric interviews) differ qualitatively from symptoms identified using psychologists' traditional checklists/or rating scales (such as milder forms of depression). In this study of 395 same-sex child twin pairs,

Eley demonstates that depression heritability estimates are similar when comparing individual differences and "extreme group membership" (scoring above a high cutoff on the Child Depression Inventory) across differing thresholds of severity (13, 15, or 17). Interestingly, data indicated that the heritability estimates of children's scores above the cutoff were less than variations in self-reported depressive symptoms across the entire sample (individual differences between monozygotic and dizygotic twin pairs), suggesting that the highest levels of depression were caused by common environmental factors. As Sir Peter Medawar has said, "genes propose, but environments dispose." So exactly what are these "environtypes"? If nothing else, certainly a focus for future research!

P.S. Jensen, M.D.

The Risk for Early-adulthood Anxiety and Depressive Disorders in Adolescents With Anxiety and Depressive Disorders
Pine DS, Cohen P, Gurley D, et al (Columbia Univ, New York; Univ of Colorado, Denver)
Arch Gen Psychiatry 55:56–64, 1998   1–27

Background.—It is important to understand the relationship between anxiety and depressive disorders in adolescents and those in adults, because anxiety and depressive disorders are common psychiatric conditions in adolescents. Only longitudinal research can directly measure the risk of adult disorders in adolescents, however. This article addresses 2 limitations in previous research on this issue and uses epidemiological and longitudinal data to deal with these limitations.

Methods.—An epidemiological sample of 776 participants between 9 and 18 years old were given psychiatric evaluations in 1983, 1985, and 1992. The degree of longitudinal association between adolescent and adult anxiety and depressive disorders was determined, using odds ratios from logistic regression analyses and a set of latent Markov analyses. The focus was on associations among narrowly defined anxiety and depressive disorders.

Results.—Simple logistic models showed that adolescent anxiety or depressive disorders predicted a twofold to threefold higher risk of adult anxiety or depression. Analysis showed some degree of specificity in the courses of simple and social phobias, but less specificity in the courses of other disorders. Analysis using latent variables showed that most adolescent disorders did not persist into young adulthood, although most adult disorders were preceded by adolescent disorders.

Conclusions.—Adolescents with anxiety and depressive disorders have a strong risk for recurrent disorders as young adults. Most anxiety and depressive disorders in early adulthood are preceded by the same disorders in adolescence.

► Previous studies of adults, such as the Epidemiologic Catchment Area study, have indicated that the child and adolescent years constitute epochs of peak ages of onset of adult anxiety and depressive disorders. Yet few (if any) articles have actually documented this in longitudinal studies of children and adolescents examined into the adult years. This article nicely demonstrates a relative degree of specificity of particular anxiety and depressive syndromes, such as adolescent phobias predicting adult phobias, but not of other anxiety disorders. Most anxiety and depressive disorders warranting intervention in the adult years had their onset in adolescence. However, many adolescent disorders resolved and did not persist into adulthood.

P.S. Jensen, M.D.

The Parenting and Family Functioning of Children With Hyperactivity

Woodward L, Taylor E, Dowdney L (Univ of Auckland, New Zealand)
J Child Psychol Psychiatry 39:161–169, 1998   1–28

Introduction.—Psychosocial factors have typically been viewed as peripheral to an understanding of the nature and etiology of childhood hyperactivity. However, it is increasingly evident that psychosocial factors are important in the development and prognosis of the behavioral and interpersonal problems of children with hyperactivity. Parenting and family-life factors associated with childhood hyperactivity were assessed in a community sample of London school children.

Methods.—Age range of 30 boys with pervasive hyperactivity and 28 comparison controls was 7–10 years. Parenting and family functioning measures were evaluated during a home-visit assessment.

Results.—Poor parent coping and aggressive disciplinary actions were significantly correlated with hyperactivity, after adjusting for effects of conduct disorder and parents' mental health. Disciplinary aggression was the best parenting predictor of hyperactivity in children.

Conclusion.—Children who were hyperactive were more often exposed to parenting behaviors that were aggressive and less proactive, even after allowing for the confounding influence of child conduct disorder and parents' mental health. These findings challenge the notion that psychological factors are unimportant in hyperactivity. We need to assess the role of these factors in the course, prognosis, and treatment outcomes of children with hyperactivity.

► One of my pet peeves is the degree to which many of us (including a fair number of researchers) seem to have reified our diagnostic categories, and oversimplified the role of inborn (supposedly non-malleable) biologic factors in the onset and etiology of these conditions, particularly attention-deficit hyperactivity disorder (ADHD). Thus, I am pleased when someone challenges existing wisdom by demonstrating the importance of environmental factors in the onset and severity of ADHD. These authors do challenge existing theory, showing that parental disciplinary aggression and problematic parental coping were significantly related to hyperactivity. To my mind, more such studies are needed, not just to balance the biologic oversimplication of ADHD, but to address possibly important mechanisms of pathophysiology that we have not adequately studied. For example, why is it that children from neglecting or abusive backgrounds appear to have higher levels of ADHD-like behaviors? Should we regard these as merely phenocopies of "true ADHD," or explore what such findings might mean for our larger understanding of patholophysiologic mechanisms in the development and regulation of attention mechanisms, motor behavior, and impulse control?

P.S. Jensen, M.D.

Attention Deficit Hyperactivity Disorders and Other Psychiatric Outcomes in Very Low Birthweight Children at 12 Years
Botting N, Powls A, Cooke RWI, et al (Liverpool Univ, England; St Michael's Hosp, Bristol, England)
J Child Psychol Psychiatry 38:931–941, 1997   1–29

Introduction.—Increased incidences of hyperactivity and attention deficits have been reported in very low birth weight (VLBW) infants. The frequency of psychiatric symptoms was assessed in 12-year-old VLBW children. Their behavior was analyzed for overactivity and poor attention, antisocial behavior, anxiety, and depression.

Methods.—One hundred thirty-seven 12-year-old VLBW children and a control sample of 148 matched peers were assessed for a number of psychiatric symptoms, including Attention Deficit/Hyperactivity Disorder (ADHD), depression, anxiety, and antisocial behavior. Researchers used the Child and Adolescent Psychiatric Assessment parent interview, among other child and parent questionnaires.

Results.—The major psychiatric risk in VLBW children was ADHD. Thirty-one of 136 VLBW children (23%) met clinical criteria for ADHD, compared to 9 of 148 (6%) controls. Generalized anxiety and symptoms of depression were also more common in VLBW children than in controls. Twenty-eight percent of VLBW children had a psychiatric disorder of some type, compared to 9% of controls.

Conclusion.—At 12 years, VLBW children are at increased risk for psychiatric symptoms, particularly ADHD. Predictors of these outcomes are not clearly delineated and may vary across type of psychiatric problem. Parents, teachers, and VLBW children themselves need to be aware of the importance of combating potential long-term impairment.

▶ The lack of specificity in risk factors for child and adolescent psychiatric disorders has been a persistent and perplexing finding. This article proves the exception to the rule, demonstrating that while VLBW children have an overall risk for psychiatric disorders, the most pronounced increase in risk was for development of ADHD (23% of VLBW children vs. 6% of controls).

Such findings provide critical new insights, because the determination of differential risk factors can shed light on possible etiologic mechanisms for specific conditions. Regardless, the finding that 28% of VLBW children met criteria for 1 or more psychiatric disorders should heighten our awareness of the need for early screening and intervention programs for these at-risk children.

P.S. Jensen, M.D.

Neuroendocrine Response to Fenfluramine Challenge in Boys: Associations With Aggressive Behavior and Adverse Rearing

Pine DS, Coplan JD, Wasserman GA, et al (Columbia Univ, New York)
Arch Gen Psychiatry 54:839–846, 1997   1–30

Background.—Serotonin, aggressive behavior, and a childhood history of socially adverse child-rearing conditions appear to be associated. Prolactin response to fenfluramine hydrochloride challenge was studied in young boys with clinically significant aggressive behavior or who were being raised in a social environment conducive to the development of chronic aggression.

Methods.—Thirty-four younger brothers of convicted delinquents were included in the study. Standardized psychiatric and observation-based evaluations of the boys' social environments conducted during home visits were performed. Psychiatric status was reassessed about 2 years later, and central serotonergic activity was determined using the fenfluramine challenge procedure.

Findings.—Prolactin response to fenfluramine challenge was correlated positively with increasing degrees of aggressive behavior at either assessment. Social environment conducive to the development of aggressive behavior was also positively associated with prolactin response. The latter association was independent of the correlation between aggression and the prolactin response.

Conclusions.—Aggressive behavior in young boys and social circumstances conducive to the development of aggressive behavior are associated positively with a marker of central serotonergic activity. Future researchers might perform fenfluramine challenges at different developmental stages to further elucidate the longitidunal associations among serotonin, child-rearing conditions, and childhood aggression.

▶ Although few would doubt that biology influences behavior, the hypothesis that psychosocial environments shape the human biological substrate is controversial in both scientific and policy circles. Yet this study raises this intriguing possibility by demonstrating that children's environments are related to their serotonin levels. Even though serotonin systems appear to be malleable among primates when their social status hierarchies and rearing conditions are manipulated, such strategies would obviously be unethical in children. Yet if these same environment biology relations can be demonstrated longitudinally in children, and if reductions in stressful rearing conditions can be demonstrated to reduce measures of serotonin system perturbation, dramatic implications for social policy would be suggested concerning the degree to which our society allows many young children to be exposed to moderately distressed social and rearing environments. This interesting research area will likely be the focus of great interest over the next decade.

P.S. Jensen, M.D.

Cerebrospinal Fluid Concentrations of Somatostatin and Biogenic Amines in Grown Primates Reared by Mothers Exposed to Manipulated Foraging Conditions

Coplan JD, Trost RC, Owens MJ, et al (Columbia Univ, NY; SUNY, Brooklyn; Emory Univ, Atlanta, Ga)
Arch Gen Psychiatry 55:473–477, 1998   1–31

Introduction.—Early disruptions in maternal-infant affective interaction can have long-term behavioral and biological effects on primate infants. In a previous study, infant primates were nursed by mothers randomized to variable foraging demand (VFD; food was obtained easily for 2 weeks, then with difficulty for 2 weeks) or to nonvariable foraging conditions (non-VFD). Compared with non-VFD animals, those that were VFD-reared exhibited elevations of cisternal CSF corticotropin-releasing factor (CRF) concentrations and decreased CSF cortisol levels. This study compared CSF concentrations of serotonin, dopamine, and norepinephrine metabolites and of somatostatin (SOM) between VFD-reared and non-VFD-reared animals.

Methods.—Study subjects were 30 bonnet macaques, aged 17 weeks, 15 raised under VFD conditions, 8 under high-foraging demand (HFD) conditions, and 7 under low-foraging demand (LFD) conditions. Cisternal CSF sampling was performed in the VFD condition when animals had a mean age of 4 years, a significantly younger age than that of the HFD and LFD animals. Because the 2 latter groups were similar in all CFS measures assayed, they were combined as a single non-VFD group.

Results.—Compared with the non-VFD reared group, all neurochemicals assayed (except for 3-methoxy-4-hydroxyphenethylene-glycol [MPHG]) were elevated in the VFD-reared group. The VFD group exhibited strong positive correlations of CSF, SOM, and homovanillic acid. In non-VFD animals, no significant correlations with corticotropin-releasing factors were present.

Conclusion.—Disturbances of early rearing in the nonhuman primate are associated with long-term neurobiological sequelae. Chemical changes seen in VFD-reared animals may be CRF-driven and result from disruption of the maternal-infant reaction. Another possibility is that lactation during periods of stress leads to excessive passage of glucocorticoids to the infant.

▶ This exceptionally interesting study provides evidence that apparently subtle conditions may have important effects on offspring that persist into their adulthood. In this study, investigators examined CSF somatostatin and biogenic amines in adult primates who were reared by mothers exposed to experimentally manipulated levels of stress (food availability and predictability) during rearing of the now-grown primates. This study parallels other findings that have shown relations between exposure to early stressful experiences and later behavioral sequellae reminiscent of anxiety in humans. Although the exact mechanism of action mediating these biological findings is not clear (eg, maternal rearing behaviors, corticosteroids passed through the mother's breast milk, etc.), they do illustrate the complexity of development and the range of factors that must likely be explored if we are to fully understand mental health and disorder in human populations.

P.S. Jensen, M.D.

Low Resting Heart Rate at Age 3 Years Predisposes to Aggression at Age 11 Years: Evidence From the Mauritius Child Health Project
Raine A, Venables PH, Mednick SA (Univ of Southern California, Los Angeles)
J Am Acad Child Adolesc Psychiatry 42:680–686, 1997   1–32

Introduction.—Low resting heart rate has been linked to antisocial and aggressive behavior in children. This finding has been well replicated; however, it has not been tested longitudinally, potential confounders and mediators have not been studied, and its generalizability across cultures has not been evaluated. These factors were addressed in a study to determine whether low resting heart rate at age 3 predicts aggressive behavior at age 11.

Methods.—The study included 1,795 children living on the island of Mauritius in the Indian Ocean. Resting heart rate was evaluated in all children at age 3. When the children reached age 11, the Child Behavior Checklist was used to evaluate them for antisocial behavior, both aggressive and nonaggressive.

Results.—Heart rates were significantly lower for highly aggressive children than for nonaggressive children, and children with low heart rates were more aggressive than those with high heart rates. This relationship was unaffected by gender or ethnicity. Heart rate was not related to nonaggressive antisocial behavior. The differences in heart rate could not be attributed to various mediators and confounding factors, including height, weight, and bulk; motor activity; crying; physical development; health; muscle tone; circadian effects; temperament; family discord; socioeconomic deprivation; and hyperactivity.

Conclusions.—Children with low resting heart rates at age 3 are predisposed to aggression at age 11. Low resting heart rate appears to be a specific, well-replicated, and early biologic marker of later aggressive behavior, and should be studied further in future studies. The results suggest that treatment and intervention to prevent violence should start much earlier in life.

▶ This interesting article, based on a large, prospectively-followed Mauritian sample, indicates that a lower resting heart rate is related to later risk for emergence of antisocial behavior. The study nicely illustrates the problems investigators have in trying to unravel the etiology of childhood behavior problems, and in understanding the complex mixture of environmental and biologic factors that interact to produce adaptive and maladaptive behaviors. While the finding appears robust, the potency of the heart rate variable as a risk factor does not appear to be very high—the heart rate difference between 11-year-old aggressive vs. nonaggressive children was modest, 123 vs. 129 beats/min at age 3. This fact alone likely obviates heart rate's value as a screener. Nonetheless, the finding holds up, even after controlling for all potential confounders, suggesting that biologic factors measurable at age 3 can be related to later behavior. I guess we should not be surprised, but neither should we be surprised that measurable aspects of brain functioning in early life are related to measurable aspects of brain functioning in later life! The challenge lying ahead is to determine how risk factors (both biologic and environmental) combine to yield later disturbances in behavior. We have a long way to go, and while it was not this study's original intent, the article nicely illustrates how much we have to learn about the interactions among brain development, environmental and genetic factors, and subsequent behavior. So, in the meantime, please don't start measuring heart rates to generate clinical predictions!

P.S. Jensen, M.D.

Verbal Dichotic Listening in Boys at Risk for Behavior Disorders
Pine DS, Bruder GE, Wasserman GA, et al (Columbia Univ, NY)
J Am Acad Child Adolesc Psychiatry 36:1465–1473, 1997   1–33

Introduction.—Numerous studies have shown an association between disruptive behavior in children and a deficit in verbal processing skills. Evidence for this association derives from investigations using verbal intelligence quotient (VIQ) as assessed by standardized intelligence tests. To determine the potential neural basis for the association between disruptive behavior and VIQ, researchers assessed the results of dichotic listening tests that measure lateralized brain functions.

Methods.—The 126 high-risk boys aged 6–10 years and younger brothers of adjudicated delinquents were identified for the study. These boys received an initial psychiatric, neuropsychological, and language assessment from 1992 to 1993 and follow-up assessment from 1994 to 1995. All 110 (87%) boys who could be tracked were invited to take part in an assessment of lateralized brain function; 100 (91%) participated. Thirteen boys were excluded because of hearing losses or inability to perform the listening test. Most of the remaining 87 boys who formed the study group were from low income households; 57 were African American, 27 Hispanic, and 3 white. A dichotic consonant-vowel listening test was used to assess the neural basis of language-processing ability.

Results.—Twenty-eight boys (32%) met the criteria for a disruptive behavior disorder. Twenty of these, (71%) received a diagnosis of attention-deficit hyperactivity disorder (ADHD), 17 (61%) of oppositional defiant disorder (ODD), and 6 (21%) of conduct disorder (CD); ODD and CD were combined in the data analysis. The boys exhibited the expected profile on the consonant-vowel dichotic listening test, with the percentage correct for the right ear significantly higher than for the left ear (58% vs. 44%). Signs of language delay were common in the group. Disruptive psychopathology in these boys predicted reduced right-ear accuracy for dichotic syllables, a finding indicative of a deficit in left hemisphere processing ability. A correlation was also noted between deficits in reading and language ability and right-ear accuracy for dichotic syllables.

Conclusion.—In this group of boys at risk for behavior disorders, those who did exhibit disruptive behavior were found to have a deficit in verbal processing abilities on dichotic listening tasks compared with nondisruptive boys. This deficit was also associated with low scores on tests of reading achievement and language comprehension. The precise association between lateral brain abnormalities and disruptive behavior is yet to be determined as is, likewise, the association between dichotic listening performance and disruptive behavior. Studies in larger samples of both boys and girls should be done to evaluate more accurately these associations.

▶ As our understanding of child psychopathology grows more sophisticated, we must invariably ask ourselves, "What is the specific nature of the brain-behavior linkages in children with various forms of psychopathology?" Psychopathology does not "just happen"; its emergence (although not necessarily its etiology) must be understood in the context of demonstrable changes in the neural substrate. Fortunately, our ability to ask sophisticated questions is being advanced by better theories, and by better measurement tools. Much of the challenge lies in knowing where to look if we wish to understand the neural correlates of psychopathology. Pine and colleagues have drawn upon the much replicated finding of deficits in verbal intelligence and their relations to externalizing behavior problems to demonstrate that children with externalizing behavior disorders exhibited deficits in a dichotic listening task (the ability to identify 2 different sounds presented simultaneously to both ears). In particular, these children showed greater problems in correctly identifying syllables presented to the right ear, suggesting deficits in left hemisphere verbal processing ability. Although the various subgroups with discrete disorders (e.g., ADHD only vs. ODD/CD only) were small and normal control subjects were not included, further studies of dichotic listening ability in children with disruptive disorders are indicated, including research focusing on the specificity of these findings and the plasticity and developmental emergence of hemispheric processing abnormalities.

P.S. Jensen, M.D.

Maternal Smoking During Pregnancy and the Risk of Conduct Disorder in Boys

Wakschlag LS, Lahey BB, Loeber R, et al (Univ of Chicago; Univ of Pittsburgh, Pa)
Arch Gen Psychiatry 54:670–676, 1997   1–34

Background.—Prenatal exposure to nicotine has been associated with altered neural structure and functioning, cognitive deficits, and behavior problems. Whether such behavioral problems in offspring were severe enough to qualify for *DSM-III-R* diagnoses after statistical adjustment for a broad range of correlates of maternal smoking was investigated.

Methods.—One hundred seventy-seven boys aged 7–12 years were assessed longitudinally for 6 years. All were referred by a clinic. Structured diagnostic interviews were given annually. The logistic regression analyses included correlates of maternal smoking during pregnancy and previously identified demographic, parental, perinatal, and family risk factors for the disruptive behavior disorders.

Findings.—Compared to mothers who did not smoke during pregnancy, mothers who smoked more than half a pack of cigarettes a day during pregnancy were significantly more likely to have a boy with conduct disorder, with an odds ratio of 4.4. This correlation was significant after adjustment for socioeconomic status, maternal age, parental antisocial personality, substance abuse during pregnancy, and maladaptive parenting.

Conclusions.—Maternal smoking during pregnancy appears to be a strong independent risk factor for conduct disorder in boys. It may either directly adversely affect the developing fetus or be a marker for previously undetermined maternal characteristics that are etiologically important for conduct disorder.

▶ Much of the history of psychiatric theorizing has been preoccupied with the presumed etiologic role of psychodynamic and psychosocial factors in the emergence of mental disorders, despite inadequate evidence supporting such assumptions. In no diagnostic condition has this etiologic role been more prominent than in the area of conduct disorders. Although psychosocial factors are clearly important, relatively insufficient attention has been devoted to the understanding of early risk factors, particularly the effects of prenatal toxins on brain development, even socially sanctioned toxins such as tobacco. In this study, the authors controlled for the presence of various psychosocial and parenting factors that might otherwise explain the relationships between maternal smoking during pregnancy and conduct disorder, yet the relationships persisted. Just as important, the risk factor of smoking more than half a pack of cigarettes per day during pregnancy was specifically related to the diagnosis of conduct disorder vs. other psychiatric disorders. Although the size of the etiologic role of maternal prenatal smoking on the development of conduct disorders is likely to be small, widespread, effective public educational effort devoted to the protection of the developing brain during pregancy seems likely to yield substantial public health benefits.

P.S. Jensen, M.D.

Mothers' and Fathers' Reports of Children's Reactions to Naturalistic Marital Conflict

O'Hearn HG, Margolin G, John RS (Univ of Southern California, Los Angeles)
J Am Acad Child Adolesc Psychiatry 36:1366–1373, 1997   1–35

Introduction.—Although children have been evaluated for their responses to adult strangers simulating conflict, few studies have assessed the impact on children of observing actual interparental conflict. Researchers report the results of a study in which parents kept diaries to record their children's reactions to marital conflict.

Methods.—The mothers and fathers of 110 children aged 8 to 11 participated in the study. Their marriages were categorized by conflict level: physical conflict (PHYCON, 38 families), non-physical conflict (NOPHYCON, 35 families), and low conflict (LOWCON, 37 families). For 5½ weeks, parents recorded independently how their children responded to conflict. Possible answers on the questionnaires included crying, no reaction, became angry or frightened, left the room, listened, took sides, misbehaved, or tried to make peace.

Results.—During the observation period, mothers reported a mean of 3.53 days of conflict and fathers a mean of 3.14 days. The mean number of different reactions reported by mothers was 2.62; the mean reported by fathers was 2.18. Compared with children from LOWCON and NOPHYCON homes, those from PHYCON homes were more likely to leave the room, misbehave or feel angry, and appear sad or frightened in response to witnessing their parents' marital conflict. The only significant difference between NOPHYCON and LOWCON groups was that children in the NOPHYCON group were 4.85 times more likely to try to make peace.

Conclusion.—Children in families characterized by physical violence often exhibit distress when exposed to their parents' marital conflict. Behaviors observed included tantrums, anger, and fright. Different histories of exposure to marital conflict appear to contribute to the way in which children react to parental conflict.

▶ Just as we need to gain more understanding in the area of child psychopathology by "breaking apart the phenotype"[1] similar research efforts are needed to break apart the "environtype." To wit, "What is the impact of children's exposure to various types of environment stressors, particularly when we more carefully dissect the specific nature of the environmental stressors?" Along this line of reasoning, *marital conflict* needs to be disaggregated into its component parts to understand how children respond to various permutations of this stressor. This study by O'Hearn and colleagues does just that and provides data indicating that it is exposure to *physical* marital conflict per se (as opposed to verbal conflict) that is related to children's (boys more than girls, according to the authors) symptomatic responses.

P.S. Jensen, M.D.

Reference

1. Leung PW, Connolly KJ: Test of two views of impulsivity in hyperactive and conduct-disordered children. *Dev Med Child Neurol* 39:574–582, 1997.

Youth Violence in the United States: Major Trends, Risk Factors, and Prevention Approaches
Dahlberg LL (Natl Ctr for Injury Prevention and Control, Atlanta, Ga)
Am J Prev Med 14:259–272, 1998   1–36

Background.—Violence among youths is an important problem in the United States. Homicide rates among 15–19-year-olds increased by 154% between 1985 and 1991. Major trends, risk factors, and approaches to prevention were discussed.

Discussion.—Among highly industrialized nations, the United States ranks first in homicide rates, exceeding the rates of other nations by severalfold. Young people are represented disproportionately as homocide victims in the United States. In 1995, 38% of all homicide victims were younger than 25.

Key risk factors for aggression, violence, and delinquency have been identified. Individual factors include a history of early aggression, beliefs that support violence, attributional biases, and social cognitive deficits. Family factors include problem parental behavior, low emotional attachment to parents or caregivers, poor monitoring and supervision, exposure to violence, and poor family functioning. Peer and school factors include negative peer influences, low commitment to school, academic failure, and certain other school environments and practices. Environmental and neighborhood risk factors include high concentrations of poor residents, transiency, and family disruption; low community participation; decreased economic opportunity; and access to firearms.

Identifying risk factors is an important step in the prevention of youth violence. Most U.S. intervention programs focus on changing individual attitudes, beliefs, and behavior. The more common approaches are cognitive-behavioral, behavior modification, and social-skills training. Less common are programs that attempt to change the natures of peer-group interactions, peer-group norms, and family functioning. Interventions designed to change children's daily environment include attempts to change teacher management practices, school security, and other school policies. Currently, the effectiveness of such programs is not clear.

▶ This article presents national data on the prevalence of youth homicide over the last 30 years, comparing rates with those of other age groups.

Potential contributing factors in the dramatic rise in youth violence from 1965 (5/100,000) to 1995 (30/100,000) are discussed. This area, including the study of youth violence by government agencies, is unfortunately quite controversial. Although it is not clearly and specifically related to mental disorder, the mental health consequences of violence and aggression deserve the ongoing and systematic attention of mental health professionals and researchers alike.

P.S. Jensen, M.D.

Effects of Child-rearing by Schizophrenic Mothers: A 25-Year Follow-up
Higgins J, Gore R, Gutkind D, et al (Univ of California, Santa Barbara; Univ of Southern California, Los Angeles; Inst for Preventive Medicine Copenhagen; et al)
Acta Psychiatr Scand 96:402–404, 1997   1–37

Background.—The effects of maternal schizophrenia on child rearing are unclear. A 25-year diagnostic follow-up involving 50 children of schizophrenic mothers, 25 reared at home and 25 reared by individuals with no history of psychiatric disorder, was reported.

Methods and Findings.—The psychiatric status of the adult offspring was assessed in a 3-hour structured interview. A battery of syndrome checklists and scales was used. The incidence of psychopathology, including schizophrenia-spectrum disorders, was slightly higher among the individuals who had been reared apart from their mothers. Mother-reared offspring were more likely to have obtained some college education and to have been married, possibly indicating a higher degree of psychosocial functioning. However, the mothers of this group had more severe illness; thus the greater prevalence may be attributed to a greater genetic predisposition.

Conclusions.—These data provide no evidence that being reared by a schizophrenic mother increases psychopathology in children at genetic risk. The somewhat higher level of psychiatric illness in the offspring reared apart from their mothers may be caused by a greater genetic predisposition.

▶ Extremely long-term follow-up studies are rare, but even among that rarified group, this 1 is a jewel. This study compares 25-year diagnostic follow-ups in 50 subjects of mothers with schizophrenia, half of whom had been adopted, and the other half who were raised by the ill parent. Despite the often devastating effects of schizophrenia on many aspects of parental functioning, children raised by the ill parent did not have worse outcomes than those adopted. In fact, counting all forms of psychopathology and substance dependence, almost half of individuals reared by the ill parent (12 of 25) had no mental disorder at follow-up, compared with only 7 of 25 adopted individuals.

P.S. Jensen, M.D.

Increased Nocturnal Activity and Impaired Sleep Maintenance in Abused Children

Glod CA, Teicher MH, Hartman CR, et al (Harvard Med School, Boston)
J Am Acad Child Adolesc Psychiatry 36:1236–1243, 1997   1–38

Background.—Some researchers have suggested that sleep disturbance is the hallmark of posttraumatic stress disorder (PTSD). However, several studies have found no evidence for sleep disruption in persons with PTSD. Whether intense adverse stimulation in early development (physical or sexual abuse) results in sleep disruption was further investigated.

Methods.—Nineteen abused prepubertal children were compared with 15 children who had not been abused and with 10 children with depression. A complete semistructured diagnostic interview was administered to all children. Sleep-related activity was evaluated by ambulatory activity monitoring for 3 consecutive nights.

Findings.—Abused children were twice as active at night as the normal and depressed children. Abused children also emitted a greater percentage of their total daily activity at night than did the other groups. On actigraph-derived sleep measures, abused children appeared to have prolonged sleep latency and reduced sleep efficiency. Sleep efficiency was more impaired in physically abused than in sexually abused children.

Conclusions.—Abused children have greater levels of nocturnal activity than normal or depressed children. Abused children appear to have more problems falling and staying asleep. However, physical abuse rather than PTSD seems to be the salient factor.

▶ Previous studies have suggested that depression and trauma have quite different, perhaps even diametrically opposed, neurobiological relations to the stress-responsiveness of the hypothalamic-pituitary-adrenal axis. Namely, although abuse has been hypothesized to heighten the reactivity of subjects' stress responses (with consequent hypersuppression of the adrenal cortex to cortisol), depressed subjects manifest a failure to suppress adrenal responses to cortisol challenge. This study is intriguing, because it contrasts abused children with 2 comparison groups (children with neither a history of abuse nor any psychiatric disorder, as well as a group of depressed children). Interestingly, abused children had more disturbed sleep patterns than subjects in the 2 control groups. Moreover, a subgroup of abused children who were also depressed showed more normal sleep patterns than those abused children who were not depressed. Although these findings are preliminary, they do point out that we have much to learn about the disturbed processes that underpin many of our neuropsychiatric syndromes. Better understanding is likely to emerge not from gross categories such as "depression" or "abuse," but through a clearer appreciation of the specific pertubations in neurobiological systems, and how these systemic perturbations, alone and in combination, give rise to the external manifestations of disturbed behaviors.

P.S. Jensen, M.D.

Enhanced Dexamethasone Suppression of Plasma Cortisol in Adult Women Traumatized by Childhood Sexual Abuse
Stein MB, Yehuda R, Koverola C, et al (Univ of California, San Diego; San Diego Veterans Affairs Med Ctr, Calif; Mount Sinai Med School, NY; et al)
Biol Psychiatry 42:680–686, 1997   1–39

Background.—Previous studies have shown disruptions in the function of the hypothalamic-pituitary-adrenal (HPA) axis among male patients with combat-related posttraumatic stress disorder (PTSD). Changes include enhanced cortisol suppression in response to low-dose dexamethasone, and increased density of lymphocyte glucocorticoid receptors. This study looked for similar abnormalities of the HPA axis in women with a history of childhood sexual abuse (CSA).

Methods.—The study included 19 women with a history of severe sexual abuse during childhood and/or adolescence and 21 controls with no such history. Severe abuse was defined as attempted or completed vaginal or anal penetration occurring when the victim was 14 years old or younger, with an abuser at least 5 years older than the child. All participants underwent a low-dose dexamethasone suppression test, and gave blood for measurement of lymphocyte glucocorticoid receptor binding.

Results.—Suppression of plasma cortisol in response to dexamethasone was significantly enhanced in the women with a history of CSA. The pattern of HPA axis dysfunction was similar to that noted in male combat veterans with PTSD. Though mean lymphocyte glucocorticoid receptor density was increased in the CSA group, the difference was not significant. None of the HPA axis indices was significantly related to measures of symptom severity.

Conclusions.—Childhood sexual abuse is associated with a pattern of HPA axis dysfunction similar to that noted in combat-related PTSD. This pattern, which differs from that associated with acute stress or major depressive disorder, may be characteristic of psychiatric disorders occurring after traumatic experiences. The preliminary findings require further research.

▶ Studies of victims of trauma indicate that persistent abnormalities in neurohumeral stress-reponse systems may result as a function of the trauma. This study may be the first to report abnormalities in this system (tested by dexamethasone suppression on plasma cortisol levels) among adult survivors of childhood sexual abuse. While the study numbers were too small to disentangle the effects of the abuse history from current psychiatric status (most survivors had PTSD or dissociative disorder), the findings point the way to necessary future studies, including determinations of why some childhood victims of sexual abuse recover and do well (such individuals were not included in this small sample).

P.S. Jensen, M.D.

Relationship of Childhood Abuse and Household Dysfunction to Many of the Leading Causes of Death in Adults: The Adverse Childhood Experiences (ACE) Study

Felitti VJ, Anda RF, Nordenberg D, et al (Southern California Permanente Med Group, San Diego; Ctrs for Disease Control and Prevention, Atlanta, Ga; Emory Univ, Atlanta, Ga; et al)
Am J Prev Med 14:245–258, 1998   1–40

Background.—The relationship of childhood abuse and household dysfunction to leading causes of death in adulthood has not been established. The association between health-risk behavior and disease in adulthood and breadth of childhood emotional, physical, or sexual abuse and household dysfunction was investigated.

Methods.—A questionnaire about adverse childhood experiences was mailed to 13,494 adults who had undergone a standard medical assessment at an HMO. The response rate was 70.5%. Data were elicited for 7 categories of childhood experiences: psychological, physical, or sexual abuse; violence against mother; and living with household members who were substance abusers, mentally ill or suicidal, or ever imprisoned. Measures of adult risk behavior, health status, and disease were obtained for correlation.

Findings.—More than half the respondents reported at least 1 category of adverse childhood experience. One fourth reported 2 or more. There was a graded relationship between the number of categories of childhood adverse experiences and each adult health-risk behavior and disease studied. Compared with participants reporting none of these categories, participants reporting 4 or more had a 4- to 12-fold increase in risk for alcoholism, drug abuse, depression, and suicide attempt. They also had a 2- to 4-fold increase in smoking, poor self-rated health, 50 or more sexual intercourse partners, and sexually transmitted disease. In addition, they had a 1.4- to 1.6-fold increase in physical inactivity and severe obesity. The number of categories had a graded relationship to the presence of adult disease, including ischemic heart disease, cancer, chronic disease, skeletal fractures, and liver disease. The 7 categories of adverse childhood experiences were strongly interrelated. Participants reporting many such categories were likely to have multiple health-risk factors.

Conclusions.—Breadth of exposure to abuse or family dysfunction in childhood was found to have strong, graded relationships with multiple risk factors for several leading causes of death in adults. Further research is needed to clarify how social, emotional, and medical problems are linked throughout life.

► For too long, psychiatric and psychosocial factors have been seen as peripheral to the study of medical illnesses, yet this article nicely points out the interlocking of early childhood experiences and substantial risks for adult cardiovascular, liver, and lung disease, as well as cancer. Not surprisingly, even stronger associations (12-fold increases in risk) with later alcoholism, drug abuse, depression, and suicide were found. These findings illustrate very clearly that phenomena such as child abuse and household parenting problems are not just "social ills," but also "health problems." Unfortunately, as a society we have not paid sufficient heed to such psychosocial health hazards, and interventions that are feasible (and allowable within a democratic society) and effective may be difficult to identify. Nonetheless, given that most of our current health hazards have prominent behavioral components, further research in this area, and in effective early interventions to enhance the quality of children's homes and of parenting practices, is urgently needed.

P.S. Jensen, M.D.

Physiological and Behavioral Responses to Minor Stressors in Offspring of Patients With Panic Disorder

Battaglia M, Bajo S, Ferini Strambi L, et al (Univ of Milan, Italy)
J Psychiatr Res 31:365–376, 1997   1–41

Background.—Studying the children of patients with panic disorder (PD) may provide information about neurophysiologic and behavioral indicators of liability to the disease. Physiologic and behavioral variables in a group of children born to patients with PD and a group born to nonpsychiatric subjects exposed to mildly stressful situations were compared.

Methods.—Nineteen children of patients with PD and 16 children of healthy subjects were exposed to novel, mildly stressful situations. These included visiting an unfamiliar place and watching a movie containing anxiogenic scenes. Behaviors, heart and respiratory rates, and salivary cortisol secretion were recorded.

Findings.—Children of the patients with PD had significantly longer latency of first spontaneous verbalization on arrival in the unfamiliar place, as well as fewer prosocial behaviors and increased distress and attachment behaviors. While watching the movie, the 2 groups differed in attachment, distress, and exploration behaviors. The children of patients with PD demonstrated increased behavioral inhibition and faster heart rates during the anxiogenic scenes. The 2 groups were similar in autonomic modulation, respiratory rates, and cortisol secretion.

Conclusions.—The children of patients with PD appear to differ from those of healthy subjects in several behavioral and physiologic aspects. Certain distinct psychophysiologic patterns seem to constitute early manifestations of the transmitted liability to PD.

▶ Better ability to discriminate children at risk from children who are not at risk is necessary if we are to mount effective prevention and early intervention approaches. This is particularly true for childhood anxiety, 1 area where psychiatric research has been lacking. Of interest, although many anxiety disorders identified in adults have their origins in childhood, very few children are seen in clinical settings for treatment of a primary anxiety disorder. This study's strengths relied upon multiple types of measures, use of a group of control children, and careful teasing out of the effects of concurrent anxiety disorder in the child vs. family history of PD. This study, among a small but growing cadre of others, provides further support for the importance of the construct of "behavioral inhibition" in the evolution of childhood anxiety disorders, as well as the relevance of family history of PD.

P.S. Jensen, M.D.

Magnetic Resonance Imaging of the Brain in Very Preterm Infants: Visualization of the Germinal Matrix, Early Myelination, and Cortical Folding

Battin MR, Maalouf EF, Counsell SJ, et al (Hammersmith Hosp, London)
Pediatrics 101:957–962, 1998   1–42

Background.—At the authors' center, a specially designed, dedicated MRI system has been installed in the neonatal ICU to assess preterm infants. The MR appearance of preterm infants' brains, first scanned between 25 and 32 weeks' gestation, was described.

Methods.—Seventeen infants born at a gestational age of 24–31 weeks (median, 28 weeks) were imaged a total of 53 times between delivery and term. The scanning protocol included T1-weighted conventional spin echo, inversion recovery fast spin echo, and T2-weighted fast spin echo sequences.

Findings.—In neonates aged less than 30 weeks, the germinal matrix was visualized at the margins of the lateral ventricles. The matrix had a short T1 and short T2. The bulk of it involuted at between 30 and 32 weeks' gestational age. White matter showed a relatively homogeneous low signal, except bands of altered signal, which were most evident anterolateral and posterolateral to the lateral ventricles. Myelination was noted in the posterior brainstem, cerebellum, and ventrolateral nuclei region of the thalamus. At 25 weeks' gestational age, infants had very little cortical folding, but this subsequently developed in an orderly manner.

Conclusions.—This neonatal MR system enables the safe assessment of extremely preterm infants. The images obtained showed the germinal matrix, early myelination, and early cortical folding. Serial imaging demonstrated the evolution of these features.

▶ As we increasingly appreciate the impact of early brain development on normal and abnormal forms of behavior and emotional regulation, it will be more important to determine what new imaging technologies can contribute to the clinical diagnostic and research settings. Unfortunately, MRI of very young children can be very difficult. These authors describe the implementation of a neonatal MRI system, which, through serial studies, was able to document evolution in neonatal brain structures. In the next few years, we will need information from such studies to be systematically pulled together, so that clinicians and researchers alike can determine the boundaries of normal and abnormal brain development in children and infants. With such technologies, it may be possible to increase diagnostic precision about early brain disorders, as well as to intervene earlier in children at risk for developmental disorders.

P.S. Jensen, M.D.

Psychiatric Outcomes in Low-Birth-Weight Children at Age 6 Years: Relation to Neonatal Cranial Ultrasound Abnormalities

Whitaker AH, Van Rossem R, Feldman JF, et al (Columbia Univ, New York; Univ of Delaware, Newark; City College of the City Univ of New York; et al)
Arch Gen Psychiatry 54:847–856, 1997   1–43

Introduction.—Studying the sequelae of perinatal brain injury was made possible with the introduction of ultrasonography, a noninvasive means of imaging the brain in low–birth weight (LBW) newborn infants. Little is known about the relation of cranial ultrasound abnormalities to childhood psychiatric disorders. Some have suggested a link between attention deficit–hyperactivity disorder (ADHD) and LBW. In 1997, an estimated 6.5% of children who became of school age had LBW. The relation of neonatal cranial abnormalities to psychiatric disorders at 6 years of age was examined in a group of LBW children.

Methods.—A total of 564 children were studied. The neonatal cranial ultrasound abnormalities were divided into 2 classifications: parenchymal lesions and/or ventricular enlargement (PL/VE) (suggestive of white matter injury) with or without germinal matrix–intraventricular hemorrhage, and isolated germinal matrix and/or intraventricular hemorrhage (GM/IVH) (suggestive of injury to glial precursors). A structured parent interview was used to assess psychiatric disorders at age 6 years. First, the entire sample was used for the analysis; then, only data from children with normal intelligence were analyzed.

Results.—At least 1 psychiatric disorder was seen in 22% of the cohort, the most common being ADHD (15.6%). In the entire sample, parenchymal lesions and/or ventricular enlargement increased relative risk independently of other biological and social predictors, for the category of any psychiatric disorder, ADHD, and tic disorders. Relative Risk increased for any disorder, ADHD, and separation anxiety with parenchymal lesions/ ventricular enlargement in children of normal intelligence. Female sex or social advantage did not ameliorate these effects. Psychiatric disorder at 6 years of age was not related to isolated germinal matrix/intraventricular hemorrhage.

Conclusions.—Risk for some psychiatric disorders at 6 years of age was significantly increased in LBW children if they had neonatal cranial ultrasound abnormalities suggestive of white matter injury.

▶ This study offers valuable new information from a LBW (501–2,000 g) cohort of more than 1,100 children studied with cranial ultrasound at birth.

Overall, 47% of children with evidence of white matter injury met criteria for a DSM-III-R diagnosis at age 6 years, compared with approximately 20% to 21% of PL/IVH children and children with no evidence of cranial ultrasound abnormalities. After controlling for all potentially confounding factors, PL/VE status increased psychiatric risk fourfold, compared with GM/IVH and normal ultrasound status. In addition, maternal smoking, social disadvantage, and male sex were related to increased risk for psychiatric disorder to a similar degree across all groups (PL/VE, GM/IVH, and no ultrasound abnormality). In contrast to prevailing notions of protective effects of social advantage among children with perinatal problems, this study showed simple main effects for PL/VE status on risk for later psychiatric morbidity. This important study with exceptional methodology should prove of great interest as the sample continues to age, and findings if replicated in other samples may reshape our understanding of the impact and interaction of environmental and CNS factors in the onset and persistence of psychiatric disorders.

P.S. Jensen, M.D.

Childhood-onset Schizophrenia: Progressive Ventricular Change During Adolescence

Rapoport JL, Giedd J, Kumra S, et al (Natl Inst of Mental Health, Bethesda, Md)
Arch Gen Psychiatry 54:897–903, 1997   1–44

Purpose.—Childhood-onset schizophrenia (COS) is a rare but severe condition in which symptoms of schizophrenia appear before the age of 12 years. This condition produces a unique opportunity to study the risk factors and neurodevelopmental abnormalities associated with schizophrenia. There is ongoing debate regarding the progression of brain abnormalities in patients with later-onset schizophrenia. This study examined progression brain abnormalities during adolescence in patients with treatment-refractory COS.

Methods.—The study included 16 patients with COS, defined as documented onset of psychosis by 12 years of age. Twenty-four temporally yoked healthy controls, matched for age and sex, were studied for comparison. The participants underwent anatomic brain MRI scanning at baseline and again 2 years later. All scans were performed with the same equipment and measurement techniques.

Results.—Ventricular volume increased to a significantly greater extent in the patients with COS. The COS group also showed a significant reduction in midsagittal thalamic area, whereas this value was unchanged in controls. These longitudinal brain changes were significantly correlated with each other. They were also related to prepsychotic developmental abnormality, as rated by the Premorbid Assessment Scale, and to the follow-up Brief Psychiatric Rating Scale.

Conclusions.—Patients with COS show a greater-than-normal increase in ventricular size during adolescence. The ventricular enlargement is greater than that reported for patients with adult-onset schizophrenia. The findings are consistent with those of other brain imaging studies showing early and late deviations in brain development for children with COS. The authors plan further longitudinal study of the COS patients, to gain insight into the core of the process responsible for eroding brain function in schizophrenia.

▶ Schizophrenia has been increasingly conceptualized as having its origins in neurodevelopment. Yet studies of neurodevelopment in adults with schizophrenia may be less feasible than in other patients because progressive changes in brain structure and function may have slowed or be otherwise negligible. Moreover, the patients' lifetime exposure to antipsychotic medications has largely confounded most previous studies, because traditional antipsychotic treatment has been related to enlargement of basal ganglia structures. This remarkable article by Rapoport and colleagues constitutes the first report that among patients with the very rare condition of childhood-onset schizophrenia, progressive ventricular enlargement and increasing ventricular-brain ratios are seen over a 2-year scan-rescan period. To the extent that this and related research can identify the molecular triggers for this neurodegenerative process in various forms of schizophrenia, true prevention in high-risk groups may eventually be possible.

P.S. Jensen, M.D.

Altered Serotonin Synthesis in the Dentatothalamocortical Pathway in Autistic Boys

Chugani DC, Muzik O, Rothermel R, et al (Wayne State Univ, Detroit)
Ann Neurol 42:666–669, 1997   1–45

Introduction.—Positron emission tomography (PET) has been used to develop α[¹¹C]methyl-L-tryptophan ([¹¹C]AMT) as a tracer for measuring serotonin synthesis in animals and humans. Because PET allows the measurement of regional changes in brain serotonin synthesis, this tracer is ideal for evaluating alterations of serotonin metabolism in the brains of autistic individuals. Alterations in regional brain serotonin synthesis were assessed in autistic children and nonautistic siblings, using [¹¹C]AMT PET.

Methods.—Seven and 1 autistic boys and girl, respectively, with a mean age of 6.6 years, and 4 and 1 and nonautistic brothers and sister, respectively, with a mean age of 9.9 years, underwent [¹¹C]AMT PET.

Results.—Unilateral alterations of serotonin synthesis were observed in the dentatothalamocortical pathway in autistic boys. In all 7 autistic boys, but not in the autistic girl, asymmetries of serotonin synthesis were detected in the frontal cortex, thalamus, and dentate nucleus of the cerebellum. In 5 and 2 autistic boys, respectively, decreased serotonin synthesis was seen in the left and right frontal cortex and thalamus. Elevated serotonin synthesis was observed in the contralateral dentate nucleus in all 7 boys. Significant differences were detected between autistic boys and their nonautistic siblings in asymmetry indices for frontal cortex, thalamus, and dentate nucleus combined, as well as individually for frontal cortex and thalamus.

Conclusion.—The serotonin abnormalities observed in the brain pathway are important in language production and sensory integration. These findings may explain 1 mechanism underlying the pathophysiology of autism.

▶ For understanding the causes and correlates of specific disorders such as autism, new technologies are providing us with a degree of precision. Using PET with a new radioactively labeled tracer to measure serotonin synthesis, these authors demonstrate that all (7) autistic children studied show decreases in serotonin synthesis in the frontal cortex, with associated contralateral decreases in the dentate nucleus of the cerebellum. This study may help explain why findings of serotonin metabolism in autistic children have produced somewhat divergent results (absolute increases vs. none), and it also nicely illustrates the principle that various brain regions are closely interconnected, so that changes in 1 area are often linked to changes in other areas. The brain is *not* a simple "bag of neurotransmitters"; rather, it is a complex yet coherent and interconnected set of circuits that have both facilitory and inhibitory characteristics. Perturbations in 1 area often lead to nonintuitive changes quite distal from the site of the original lesion. Thus, understanding these connections and circuits provides clues to unlock the mysteries of disorders such as autism.

P.S. Jensen, M.D.

A Clinicopathological Study of Autism

Bailey A, Luthert P, Dean A, et al (Inst of Psychiatry, London; Inst of Child Health, London)
Brain 121:889–905, 1998   1–46

Background.—Because autism is associated with epilepsy, electroencephalogram abnormalities, and mental handicap, it may have neocortical involvement. Whether neuropathologic abnormalities are more extensive than previously believed was investigated.

Methods.—Brain tissue was obtained postpartum from 6 mentally impaired patients who had had autism. Five patients had died in early adulthood, and 1 had died at age 4 years. Data from clinical and educational records were analyzed. In addition, standardized diagnostic interviews were conducted with the parents of patients who had not been seen before death.

Findings.—Four of the 6 brains were megalencephalic. Areas of cortical abnormality were also identified in 4. Developmental abnormalities of the brainstem were observed, especially in the inferior olives. The 5 adults had a decreased number of Purkinje cells, sometimes accompanied by gliosis.

Conclusions.—These data do not support the possibility of any single, specific, or localized neurodevelopmental abnormalities in patients with autism. However, the cerebral cortex is likely to be involved.

▶ Neuroimaging studies of children and adults with autism have been inconclusive, characterized by disagreements concerning the extent to which specific vs. global brain regions can be implicated in autism. Postmortem studies have been exceptionally rare, so this article fills an important void. This article documents the increased brain weight and size in persons with autism (more than 2.5 standard deviations above the mean). The authors also document abnormal neuronal migration in the brainstem and cerebellum, and provide evidence of other disturbances, including neuronal number, survival, and orientation in the cerebral cortex. We have come a long distance from old notions of "refrigerator parenting"!

P.S. Jensen, M.D.

Emerging Treatments

INTRODUCTION

The articles in this section cover the gamut of interventions, both clinical and preventive. In addition, factors related to the successful employment of interventions, such as effectiveness and services research, are also described here.

Unfortunately, this section is not nearly as long as it should be, given the urgent public health need for safe and effective interventions. For example, prescription of psychotropic medications to children and adolescents has risen dramatically in the last decade, but other than for stimulant treatments of attention deficit-hyperactivity disorder, there are only a handful of well-controlled studies examining the safety and efficacy of most psychoactive agents for children with psychiatric disorders. Given the well-known problems with uncontrolled studies, I have generally avoided them here. Nor have I chosen "same-old, same-old" studies that merely replicate well-established findings from the literature. So you may find it interesting (or sobering?) to count the number of well-controlled pharmacologic studies cited here.

Given the current and rising concerns about youth violence, child abuse, and other social ills, prevention/early intervention studies have been sought out and selected for this section. Again, whenever possible, only well-controlled studies are included.

One area worth special note: there is an increasing literature on the effectiveness of cognitive behavior therapies for a range of conditions. Yet I worry that most of us (myself included) did not receive adequate training in these methods in residency programs. Given the increasing literature that indicates that they are effective, but only when given with appropriate skill, there is a real need for most of us to get up to speed on these new treatments. Unfortunately, the eclectic psychotherapies that most of us use have never been rigorously tested. According to most meta-analytic studies, these treatments that we implicitly trust appear to be not much better than the "tincture of time." "Evidence-based medicine" is the applicable term here, I believe.

Peter S. Jensen, M.D.

Early Intervention in Adoptive Families: Supporting Maternal Sensitive Responsiveness, Infant–Mother Attachment, and Infant Competence
Juffer F, Hoksbergen RAC, Riksen-Walraven JM, et al (Utrecht Univ, The Netherlands; Nijmegen Univ, The Netherlands; Leiden Univ, The Netherlands)
J Child Psychol Psychiatry 38:1039–1050, 1997   1–47

Introduction.—In The Netherlands, 22,000 internationally adopted children have been placed in Dutch families since intercountry adoption was initiated in the late 1960s. Adoptive families (always a married couple) typically are middle-class, have higher educational levels, and are older than other parents. Several trials have suggested that the socioemotional development of the large majority of internationally, interracially adopted children does not differ from that of their nonadoptive peers. Yet, adoptive parents are confronted with behavioral problems and out-of-home placement of their internationally adoptive child more frequently than nonadoptive parents. Reported are outcomes of 2 early intervention programs designed to support families in The Netherlands with an internationally adopted child.

Methods.—The intervention programs were based on attachment theory, with focus on promoting maternal sensitive responsiveness, secure infant-mother attachment relationships, and infant exploratory competence. All children were adopted before age 5 months. Of 90 families with an interracially adoptive child, 71 children were from Sri Lanka and 19 were from Korea. Thirty families each were assigned to either a control group or an intervention group. The first intervention group received a personal book on sensitive parenting. The second intervention group was given the book and 3 video-feedback sessions presented during a home visit. Controls received no intervention.

Results.—Change in mothers or infants was not observed in the control or personal-book intervention group. The group that received the book and video feedback experienced intervention effects based on maternal sensitive responsiveness, infant competence, and infant-mother attachment.

Conclusion.—The personal book alone did not yield significant effects of intervention. The personal book plus video intervention may prove to be a promising approach for adoptive families of internationally adopted children.

▶ One of the major challenges facing mental health professionals in the next decade is to identify and provide interventions that have demonstrated efficacy with selected groups at risk for or with full-blown disorder. Of particular interest to professionals working with children are the impact of various risk factors and the extent to which critical, well-timed early interventions might shape (and ultimately benefit) later outcomes. This article nicely demonstrates that children at risk for problematic outcomes (in this case, children from adoptive families) can be benefitted, as can their parents, by systematic training procedures. While the therapy which used a video-feedback session delivered in the home resulted in increased maternal responsiveness and infant competence, such therapies are not known or readily provided by most mental health practitioners. We have a lot of work to do, both in applying what we know and in studying areas where not enough is known!

P.S. Jensen, M.D.

Early Intervention and Mediating Processes in Cognitive Performance of Children of Low-Income African American Families
Burchinal MR, Campbell FA, Bryant DM, et al (Univ of North Carolina, Chapel Hill)
Child Dev 68:935–954, 1997   1–48

Background.—In the United States, children raised in poverty are most at risk for below-average cognitive performance and academic failure. Poverty and ethnicity are confounded, with nearly half of black children living in economic hardship. In this longitudinal study of low-income black children, influences such as early childhood interventions and characteristics of the child and family on patterns of children's cognitive performance were determined.

Methods and Findings.—One hundred sixty-one black children were followed up from 6 months to 8 years of age. Factors associated with better patterns of cognitive development were intensive early educational child care, responsive stimulating care at home, and higher maternal intelligence quotient (IQ). Consistent with a general systems model, child care experiences were apparently associated with better cognitive performance, partly through enhancing infants' responsiveness to their environment.

Conclusions.—This analysis demonstrated developmental diversity among low-income black children, and related alternative developmental pathways to environmental effects. Maternal IQ had both direct and indirect effects on cognitive performance in early childhood, the latter through its influence on the family environment.

▶ Previous research has generally indicated that low-income children are at risk for declining cognitive and behavioral profiles over time, despite the fact that such children score within average ranges during infancy. In our continuing search for "environtypes," data from this longitudinal study combines samples from 2 randomized clinical trials of early childhood interventions: the Abecedarian Project and Project CARE (Carolina Approach to

Responsive Education). Children receiving some form of center-based, enriched child care in the 2 studies had consistently higher IQs over multiple time points from 12 months through 96 months, compared with no-intervention controls and families receiving less intensive home-based services. Above and beyond intervention effects, however, factors related to better outcomes (less cognitive decline) included the presence of 2 parents in the home, higher maternal IQ, quality of the home environment, and increased infant responsiveness as a function of the center-based care. Somewhat different than the interpretations derived from the infamous 1995 book, *The Bell Curve*, don't you think?

P.S. Jensen, M.D.

School Violence Reduction: A Model Jamaican Secondary School Program
Sacco FC, Twemlow SW (Community Services Inst, Springfield, Mass; Univ of Kansas, Wichita)
Community Ment Health J 33:229–234, 1997   1–49

Background.—The primary community mental health response to violence in schools is to deal with the victims or perpetrators, with mental health workers' roles being an extension of the clinical role, providing mediation, awareness training, anger management, and group work. An alternative is for mental health workers to form new partnerships with police and teachers in the schools to decrease school violence.

A Model Jamaican Secondary School Program to Reduce School Violence.—At Montego Bay Secondary School, a several-phase intervention was carried out. First, the program focused on 1 discipline issue: tucking in shirts. Any students leaving their shirts untucked quickly got a verbal response from the Jamaican Constabulary Force officer. This officer also led a clubhouse for the students at the school. Activities included a formal meeting focused on preventing violence and on life skills as well as recreational sports. The officer used the clubhouse to develop a core group of students who became an active information and support network, the group composed mostly of unruly boys called an "honor group." The Jamaican Constabulary Force officer also clearly communicated to the student body that weapons would not be tolerated. Random classroom searches were conducted, and weapons immediately confiscated. This officer succeeded in creating a mythical protective figure, who became known as "Mr. Bruno"—a fierce, protective guard dog (not an attack dog) in Jamaican folklore. He also assumed the community mental health worker role of outreach therapist, working with students' parents on school violence issues. The officer routinely spent his own money on shoes and other essentials for the students, despite his low salary, highlighting his deep personal commitment to the job.

Outcomes and Conclusions.—The "Bruno Effect" resulted in a marked decrease in the number of physical attacks, from 5 fights per day to 1 per week. When "Bruno" left the school, the violence rate returned to its former level. The initial positive outcomes can be explained by the unique personality of the adult protector and a combination of the special role of the police and outside intervention team.

▶ The federal government and private foundations spend a lot of money on prevention trials. The results of many of these expensive efforts are often disappointing, in terms of the effects on children's real world outcomes. I found this study both intriguing and heartening, because it involved a common-sense, "real-world" feasible approach of placing a friendly but stern police officer ("Bruno") in a school setting where a high degree of physical violence had become a daily fact of life. And should we be too surprised that the levels of violence returned to their previous high levels after Bruno left? Does that mean that the intervention did not work, or rather, that children in distressed environments need heightened levels of support on an ongoing basis? You be the judge.

P.S. Jensen, M.D.

Short-term Effects of Coping Skills Training as Adjunct to Intensive Therapy in Adolescents
Grey M, Yu C, Boland EA, et al (Yale Univ, New Haven, Conn)
Diabetes Care 21:902–908, 1998   1–50

Background.—Effective programs to improve diabetic adolescents' ability to achieve metabolic control are urgently needed. The efficacy of coping-skills training (CST) combined with intensive diabetes management in improving metabolic control and quality of life among adolescents beginning intensive therapy regimens was determined.

Methods.—Sixty-five patients, aged 13–20, who elected to begin intensive insulin treatment were assigned randomly to intensive management with or without CST. In the CST group, the patients were taught the coping skills of problem-solving, social skills training, cognitive behavior modification, and conflict resolution in a series of small-group efforts. Before and 3 months after the intervention, the patients were assessed using the Self-Efficacy for Diabetes Scale, Children's Depression Inventory, Issues in Coping with IDDM scale, and the Diabetes Quality of Life Youth Scale. Clinical data were recorded monthly.

Findings.—At baseline, the 2 groups were comparable in all measures. Patients in the CST group had lower HbA_{1c} and higher diabetes self-efficacy after therapy. The CST group also found it easier to cope with diabetes and felt less of a negative impact of diabetes on the quality of their lives.

Conclusions.—Coping skills training appears to be useful for improving both metabolic control and quality of life among adolescents with diabetes. Adding this behavioral intervention may help adolescents to achieve metabolic and life goals.

▶ Psychotherapy studies have been increasingly documenting the role of cognitive-behavioral therapies in treating adolescent psychiatric disorders. So it should not be surprising that investigators are now applying similar techniques and therapies to adolescents with other conditions that have pronounced behavioral components. In this randomized clinical trial, the authors showed that diabetic adolescents provided with up to 8 sessions of a specific coping-skills training and intensive clinical management showed better diabetic outcomes and improved quality of life, compared to those receiving intensive clinical management alone.

P.S. Jensen, M.D.

Prevention and Early Intervention for Anxiety Disorders: A Controlled Trial
Dadds MR, Spence SH, Holland DE, et al (Griffith Univ, Queensland, Australia; Univ of Queensland, Australia)
J Consult Clin Psychol 65:627–635, 1997   1–51

Introduction.—Anxiety problems develop in a significant number of children and, if untreated, may result in long-term impairment. Psychosocial interventions can be effective for anxiety disorders in late childhood and early adolescence. The Queensland (Australia) Early Intervention and Prevention of Anxiety Project (QEIPAP) evaluated the benefits of a cognitive-behavioral and family-based group intervention for preventing the onset and development of anxiety problems in children.

Methods.—The initial participants were a cohort of 1,786 children (1,056 girls and 730 boys) in grades 3–7 of 8 preselected primary schools. Children ranged in age from 7–14 years and represented a variety of socioeconomic levels. Most were white, Anglo-Saxon, Catholic or Protestant Christian, and from working to middle-class families. Those at risk for anxiety disorders were identified by a screening procedure that employed both children's and teachers' reports. After diagnostic interviews with parents of those identified through screening, 128 children were assigned to psychosocial intervention or to a monitoring group.

Results.—Boys were overrepresented in the externalizing disorder categories, and girls in all of the anxiety disorders (generalized anxiety, separation anxiety, and simple phobia) except social phobia. The treated group took part in a 10-week school-based child- and parent-focused psychosocial intervention. Both intervention and monitoring groups exhibited improvements immediately after the 10-week period, but only the intervention group maintained improvement at 6-month follow-up. The rate of existing anxiety disorder was reduced in the intervention group, and the onset of new anxiety disorders was prevented.

Conclusion.—Results of the QEIPAP were promising. The intervention was successful in reducing rates of disorder in children with mild to moderate anxiety disorders and in preventing the onset of such disorders in children with early features of anxiety disorders. In more than half of the at-risk children in the monitoring group, a formal anxiety disorder developed.

▶ At a time when we are seeing increasing pressures for demonstrably effective treatments for child conditions, controlled evidence of the efficacy of psychological interventions is much needed, though hard to find. This study is a valuable extension of earlier studies of cognitive-behavioral treatments for children with anxiety disorders by Kendall and Southam-Gerow.[1] In contrast to this earlier work, Dadds and colleagues employed cognitive-behavioral intervention in parent- and child-group settings with a high-risk, screened school population.[1] Though many of us have not been extensively trained in cognitive-behavioral treatment approaches, these methods deserve much more emphasis in clinical training, given the consistency of the accumulating evidence, the time-limited yet cost-effective nature of the interventions, ready availability of training manuals, and its applicability across prevention, early intervention, and clinical treatment settings.

P.S. Jensen, M.D.

References

1. Kendall PC, Southam-Gerow MA: Long-term follow-up of a cognitive-behavioral therapy for anxiety-disordered youth. *J Consult Clin Psychol* 64:724–730, 1996.

Brief Treatment to Mild-to-Moderate Child Depression Using Primary and Secondary Control Enhancement Training

Weisz JR, Thurber CA, Sweeney L, et al (Univ of California, Los Angeles; Univ of Sydney, New South Wales, Australia; Univ of North Carolina, Chapel Hill)

J Consult Clin Psychol 65:703–707, 1997   1–52

Introduction.—Current recommendations for treatment programs designed for children with depression often involve 12 or more sessions (range 12–27). Most referred children, however, drop out before completing 10 sessions. Given this lack of compliance and cost considerations, it is important to examine whether brief interventions can produce significant benefit. An 8-session child depression treatment program was evaluated in a group of school children with mild to moderate depressive symptoms.

Methods.—Children were identified through a 3-step selection procedure. Those children for whom consent was obtained completed the Children's Depression Inventory (CDI). Teachers and counselors were asked to identify children thought to have significant problems involving depression. The third step was an individual Revised Children's Depression

Rating Scale (CDRS-R) interview with those nominated by teachers or counselors or who scored greater than 10 on the CDI. Included in the final sample were 26 boys and 22 girls with a mean age of 9.6 years; 30 were white, and 18 were ethnic minority (primarily black). Children were randomly assigned to either the depression treatment program or to a no-treatment control group. Children were treated during school hours, meeting with 2 therapists in groups of fewer than 6.

Results.—The 8-session program focused on primary control (changing objective conditions to fit one's wishes) and secondary control (changing oneself to buffer the impact of objective conditions). Compared with controls, children assigned to the intervention group showed greater reductions in depressive symptoms as measured by the CDI and the CDRS-R. The improvements in the intervention group were apparent both immediately posttreatment and at 9-month follow-up. More treated children shifted from above to within the normal range on both measures of depression.

Conclusion.—The short-term treatment used in this group of elementary school children with mild to moderate depressive symptoms was successful in reducing their symptoms. Additional research is needed to determine the effect of short-term, school-based intervention in children with more severe depression.

▶ The authors combine several known effective components of cognitive-behavioral treatment strategies to fashion an integrated, time-limited intervention for childhood depression. "Primary" control strategies taught and encouraged in the children included identifying and engaging in mood-enhancing activities, and skill-building and practice in valued activities. "Secondary" control strategies included the children's learning to identify and modify depressogenic cognitions, cognitive reframing, and relaxation and imagery. The intervention improved children's self-reported depression ratings, both immediately posttreatment and after long-term follow up. Clearly, we have accumulating evidence that a number of treatments are effective for depression, both in high-risk screened school samples (as seen here) as well as in clinical samples, and in individual and group-based formats. This evidence, coupled with new data demonstrating the effectiveness of selective serotonin reuptake inhibitors for adolescent depression points the way for a new generation of studies: Which treatment is most effective? Which children need which treatment, and who needs both in combination?

P.S. Jensen, M.D.

A Clinical Psychotherapy Trial for Adolescent Depression Comparing Cognitive, Family, and Supportive Therapy

Brent DA, Holder D, Kolko D, et al (Univ of Pittsburgh, Pa)
Arch Gen Psychiatry 54:877–885, 1997   1–53

Background.—In nonclinical samples, psychosocial treatments of adolescent depression have been found effective. However, few psychotherapy studies involve clinically referred, depressed adolescents.

Methods.—One hundred seven teenaged patients with major depressive disorder (MDD) were assigned randomly to individual cognitive behavior treatment, systemic behavior family therapy (SBFT), or individual nondirective supportive therapy (NST). The patients attended 12–16 sessions, conducted once a week.

Findings.—Seventy-eight patients (72.9%) completed the study. At the end of treatment, the rate of MDD was lower after cognitive behavior therapy than after NST (17.1% and 42.4%, respectively). Cognitive behavior therapy also resulted in a greater remission rate than SBFT or NST (64.7%, 37.9%, and 39.4%, respectively.) In addition, cognitive behavior therapy was associated with more rapid relief in interviewer-rated and self-reported depression. All treatment resulted in significant and comparable decreases in suicidality and functional impairment. Parents' views of the credibility of treatment were greater with cognitive behavior therapy than with SBFT or NST.

Summary.—In this group of clinically referred adolescents with MDD, cognitive behavior therapy was more effective than SBFT or NST. Treatment responses to cognitive behavior therapy were more rapid and complete than with the latter 2 methods.

▶ Given all that we don't know about effective psychotherapies for depression in children and adolescents, this is a very welcome study. Its findings may surprise you, as they did me. Although a number of the study findings did not quite reach significance, others did, and the overall patterns were quite consistent. Family therapy and nonspecific supportive therapy appeared inferior to cognitive behavior therapy (CBT), and did not result in as rapid improvement. Further, over time CBT was more credible to parents than SBFT. This is a very important and useful set of findings that can be further strengthened by studies which demonstrate just how many sessions are needed to achieve clinical benefit. We can expect that such studies will eventually translate to clinical guidelines in managed care settings. So how many of us have been rigorously trained in CBT, as compared to nonspecific supportive therapies?

P.S. Jensen, M.D.

A Double-blind, Randomized, Placebo-controlled Trial of Fluoxetine in Children and Adolescents With Depression

Emslie GJ, Rush AJ, Weinberg WA, et al (Univ of Texas, Dallas)
Arch Gen Psychiatry 54:1031–1037, 1997   1–54

Introduction.—Depression is a major cause of morbidity and mortality among children and adolescents, with school failure and school dropout as common outcomes. There is an increased interest in selective serotonin reuptake inhibitors, particularly fluoxetine, for the treatment of depression. The efficacy of antidepressant medications for major depressive disorder is well established for adults, but little is known about the medications' effectiveness for children. In child and adolescent outpatients with nonpsychotic major depressive disorder, the efficacy, safety, and tolerability of fluoxetine treatment were compared with placebo.

Methods.—There were 96 child and adolescent outpatients, aged 7–17 years, who had a nonpsychotic major depressive disorder. They were randomized into groups receiving 20 mg of fluoxetine (48 patients) or placebo (48 patients) and seen every week for 8 consecutive weeks. Before patients were randomized into treatment, they had 3 evaluation visits with structured diagnostic interviews during 2 weeks. Global improvement on the clinical Global Impressions scale and the Children's Depression Rating scale were the primary outcome measurements.

Results.—There was much or very much improvement on the clinical Global Impressions scale at study exit in 56% of those receiving fluoxetine and 33% of those receiving placebo. There were also significant differences in weekly ratings of the Children's Depression Rating Scale. In 31% of fluoxetine-treatment patients and in 23% of placebo patients, complete symptom remission occurred.

Conclusion.—In child and adolescent outpatients with severe, persistent depression, fluoxetine was superior to placebo in the acute phase treatment of major depressive disorder. It was rare to have complete remission of symptoms.

▶ Many clinicians have been troubled by the persistent difficulty of demonstrating any efficacy of the traditional tricyclic antidepressants in treating child and adolescent depression. In part, some of the lack of these agents' demonstrable efficacy could be due to the fact that most child and adolescent studies have generally been "underpowered" (i.e., with sample sizes too small to find what may be only a modest effect). Child and adolescent depression also may have different neurobiologic characteristics, at least in terms of its treatment responsivity. Emslie and colleagues wisely examined the lessons learned from previous studies in the design of their study. Thus, they obtained an adequate sample size, used an extensive (3-week) evaluation period and a 1-week single-blind placebo treatment phase prior to randomization, and avoided use of participants recruited through the media. This article appears to break the streak of "no difference" findings, and is welcome news to clinicians who treat depression in children and adolescents. This study lends credence to clinicians' impressions that selective serotonin reuptake inhibitors as a class seem to be effective in younger patients. Not surprisingly, a number of pharmaceutical companies are now supporting studies with these newer agents in juvenile populations, so we should witness a new generation of research results to guide depression treatment practices in the next several years.

P.S. Jensen, M.D.

Double-blind and Placebo-controlled Study of Lithium for Adolescent Bipolar Disorders With Secondary Substance Dependency

Geller B, Cooper TB, Sun K, et al (Washington Univ, St Louis; Columbia Univ, New York)

J Am Acad Child Adolesc Psychiatry 37:171–178, 1998   1–55

Introduction.—There are more than 400 published articles about the use of lithium for mood disorders in adults. However, no double-blind, placebo-controlled trials on lithium use for bipolar disorders (BP) in children or adolescents have been reported. Controlled investigations of lithium or any other psychopharmacological agent for substance dependency disorders (SDD) during adolescence are also nonexistent. The use of lithium in adolescents with BP and temporary secondary SDD was assessed in a 6-week random-assignment, parallel-group, pharmacokinetically-dosed, double-blind, and placebo-controlled trial.

Methods.—Mean age of 25 adolescents with BP and SDD was 16.3 years. Patients were randomized to lithium treatment or placebo. During twice-weekly visits, 1 scheduled and 1 at random, evaluations included: mood and SDD, lithium side effects, random weekly lithium levels and urine drug assays, pregnancy tests, and pill counts.

Results.—Data were available for 21 of 25 participants. For both intent-to-treat and completer analyses, there were significant differences, in continuous and categorical measures, between the active and placebo groups for psychopathology and weekly urine drug assays. Mean serum lithium level in treated patients was 0.9 mEq/L. The most common SDD abuses were alcohol and marijuana. Mean ages for onset of BP and SDD were 9.6 and 15.3 years, respectively. Multigenerational mood disorders and multigenerational SDD were observed in 96% and 56% of families, respectively.

Conclusion.—Lithium was efficacious in treating BP with secondary SDD in adolescents. The mean 6-year interval between BP onset and SDD onset presents a definite argument for earliest recognition of BP. Long-term follow-up of adolescents with BP and secondary SDD is warranted.

▶ Although the effectiveness of lithium treatment for bipolar disorder has been well established in adults, this article is, amazingly, the first to document lithium's effectiveness in adolescents. Moreover, the study is a "two-fer": it is also the first to report a beneficial effect of a well-controlled treatment, using double-blind and placebo-control methodology, for adolescent substance use. The article, overdue and more than welcome, illustrates the important problem that many of the treatments in use and likely efficacious for adults are prescribed with a much more meager knowledge base for children and adolescents. Additional courageous and difficult-to-conduct studies are very much needed.

P.S. Jensen, M.D.

Effects of Electroconvulsive Therapy in Adolescents With Severe Endogenous Depression Resistant to Pharmacotherapy
Strober M, Rao U, DeAntonio M, et al (Univ of California, Los Angeles; Duke Univ Med Ctr, Durham, NC)
Biol Psychiatry 43:335–338, 1998   1–56

Background.—Several recent, primarily retrospective studies suggest that electroconvulsive therapy (ECT) may be beneficial in adolescents with severe endogenous depression resistant to pharmacotherapy. The current prospective, longitudinal study further investigated the value of ECT in such patients.

Methods.—Ten adolescents with primary, endogenous, psychotic depression resistant to antidepressant medications were enrolled. Changes in symptom severity were noted weekly on the Hamilton Depression Rating Scale. Outcome was determined at 1 month and at 1 year after ECT administration.

Findings.—Improvement was dramatic in 9 of the 10 patients. Significant reductions in mean Hamilton Depression Rating Scale scores were noted after the first week of treatment. The benefits of treatment were maintained in all responders. Of the 9 patients available for follow-up at 1 year, 7 had had no relapses. In the other 2 patients, relapses into full major depression occurred at 9 and 11 months, respectively.

Conclusions.—The serious morbidity associated with delusional depression among adolescents justifies the sensible use of somatic treatments that are effective in adults. Electroconvulsive therapy was effective in adolescents with phenomenological characteristics that predict ECT response in adults.

▶ Very little research has demonstrated the effectiveness, under controlled conditions, of treatments for depression. Although a few studies now offer evidence for the serotonin reuptake inhibitors and cognitive behavioral therapy, such treatments are not invariably effective. This study is a first, and potentially quite important, because it shows that adolescents with severe, unremitting major depression can respond to electroconvulsive therapy. In this case series, 9 of 10 patients showed dramatic improvements. Controlled studies of ECT in adolescents with major depression may not be ethical or feasible, but the fact that these adolescents generally showed dramatic responses within the first week of treatment, despite previous treatments with tricyclic and serotonergic antidepressants, bolsters confidence in the potential value of ECT in selected, treatment-resistant adolescents with major depression.

P.S. Jensen, M.D.

Side Effects of Methylphenidate and Dexamphetamine in Children With Attention Deficit Hyperactivity Disorder: A Double-blind, Crossover Trial

Efron D, Jarman F, Barker M, et al (Royal Children's Hosp, Melbourne, Victoria, Australia)
Pediatrics 100:662–666, 1997   1–57

Introduction.—Stimulant medications have been used for more than 50 years to treat attention-deficit hyperactivity disorder (ADHD), and these agents remain the most effective therapy for children with ADHD. Side effects, which include insomnia, headaches, irritability, and anxiousness, tend to be dose-dependent and of mild to moderate severity. Behavioral symptoms need to be assessed before the start of treatment so that true side effects can be distinguished from a child's preexisting behavioral profile. A study of 125 children with ADHD compared the severity and prevalence of side effects of 2 stimulants, methylphenidate (MPH) and dexamphetamine (DEX).

Methods.—The children were participants in a double-blind crossover trial that examined the relative efficacy of MPH and DEX. Mean age of the study group was 104.8 months. Children received DEX (0.15 mg/kg/dose) and MPH (0.3 mg/kg/dose) twice a day for 2 weeks, each in a randomized order. Outcome was measured by the Barkley Side Effects Rating Scale, completed by parents at baseline and after each medication regimen.

Results.—All children met diagnostic criteria for ADHD. The mean IQ of the group was estimated to be 98.9. Common findings on the Child Behavior Checklist were attention problems (75.9%) and aggressive behavior (73.4%). Parents rated most children as being improved overall, both with DEX and MPH. The mean severity of side effects was greater with DEX than MPH, with more severe insomnia and appetite suppression with DEX, compared with baseline. Appetite suppression was the only item rated more severe with MPH than at baseline. Compared with MPH, 6 side effects were significantly more severe with DEX: insomnia, irritability, proneness to crying, anxiousness, sadness/unhappiness, and nightmares. Overall tolerance of the 2 stimulants was good; only 4 children (2 receiving each stimulant) discontinued the trial period because of severe adverse effects.

Conclusion.—Most children with ADHD appear to tolerate both DEX and MPH, although DEX was associated with more side effects in this group. A child's symptoms should be evaluated before any stimulant medication is started, in order that treatment-related side effects can be distinguished from preexisting behavioral features.

▶ This important finding supports the nature of current clinical practices. Methylphenidate has been the most widely prescribed medication treatment for ADHD, far exceeding dextroamphetamine, pemoline, and the trycyclics combined. This practice seems to have grown more by tradition and the original assumption (incorrect, as it turned out) that MPH was not likely to be abused, compared with prescribed amphetamine medications. Nonetheless, this study nicely demonstrates that, although both medications are quite safe and relatively benign apart from "nuisance" side effects, lower side effects were seen with MPH. Moreover, it is intriguing to note that many so-called side effects are just as likely to be symptoms of the ADHD clinical profile, since many of these symptoms were manifested during the baseline condition.

P.S. Jensen, MD

Long-term Stimulant Treatment of Children With Attention-Deficit Hyperactivity Disorder Symptoms: A Randomized, Double-blind, Placebo-controlled Trial
Gillberg C, Melander H, von Knorring A-L, et al (Univ of Göteborg, Sweden; Univ of Uppsala, Sweden; Univ of Lund, Sweden; et al)
Arch Gen Psychiatry 54:857–864, 1997   1–58

Background.—The short-term efficacy of stimulants used to treat childhood attention deficits and hyperactivity has been demonstrated. The long-term effects of amphetamine on behavior and cognition as well as the adverse effects of such treatment were studied.

Methods.—Sixty-two children aged 6–11 years were enrolled in a randomized, double-blind, placebo-controlled study. All met *DSM-III-R* symptom criteria for attention-deficit hyperactivity disorder. Some children had comorbid diagnoses. Children in the active treatment group were given amphetamines for 15 months.

Findings.—Amphetamine treatment was clearly better than placebo in decreasing inattention, hyperactivity, and other disruptive behavior problems. Active treatment also tended to result in improved results on the Wechsler Intelligence Scale for Children-Revised. Time-to-treatment failure was longer among children given amphetamines. Few adverse effects were documented during active treatment. Adverse effects were considered relatively mild.

Conclusions.—The long-term results of amphetamine treatment for attention-deficit hyperactivity disorder are promising. Further research is needed to verify these findings.

▶ This double-blind, placebo-controlled trial for children with attention-deficit hyperactivity disorder is unusual on 2 accounts: first, 1 group was randomly assigned to placebo and maintained for up to 12 *months*, while a second group was assigned to and maintained with stimulants. This was ethically possible only because parents could request active treatment at any time, should they become concerned about their child's well-being. The second unusual feature was other aspects of the design, which allowed the difficult question of treatment persistence to be addressed. Both arms included an initial 3-month period during which the child was given maintenance doses of stimulants under single-blind conditions, followed by 12 months of the randomly assigned 2 treatments, and culminating in a final 3-month single-blind placebo period. This design allowed investigators to determine whether gains that emerged after initial and sustained use of stimulants persisted. Indeed, treatment gains appeared to persist, even under placebo withdrawal conditions during months 15–18. Moreover, stimulant-treated subjects showed gains in Wechsler Intelligence Scale for Children-Revised scores, compared to placebo-treated subjects. This study is unique in the literature, in that it shows effects of stimulants compared to placebo over a longer period than the typical 12–16 weeks of treatment.

P.S. Jensen, M.D.

Racial Disparity in Psychotropic Medications Prescribed for Youths With Medicaid Insurance in Maryland

Zito JM, Safer DJ, dosReis S, et al (Univ of Maryland, Baltimore; Johns Hopkins Univ, Baltimore, Md)
J Am Acad Child Adolesc Psychiatry 37:179–184, 1998   1–59

Background.—Studies from the 1980s to the present show that black children visit physicians less often than white children, and are given fewer drug prescriptions even when they receive equivalent medical services. It is unclear if this disparity also applies to psychotropic drugs. This may be an important issue because of the growing emphasis on psychopharmacological treatment for mental or emotional disorders.

Methods.—A retrospective analysis was performed of state Medicaid drug reimbursement claims for psychotropic and nonpsychotropic drugs prescribed to children 5–14 years old. The rate of prescription recipients per 100 eligible enrollees, relative prescription use ratios according to black or white race, and the interrelation of race and geographic region to prescription prevalence were determined.

Results.—There were 5 major findings: the rate of prescriptions for psychotropic medication among black children with Medicaid insurance was 39% to 52% of the rate for white children with Medicaid insurance; the rate of prescriptions for nonpsychotropic medication for black children was 60% to 87% of the rate for white children; the greatest difference in prescription rates between black and white children was for stimulants, mainly methylphenidate; the racial disparity in prescriptions for psychotropic medication was unchanged by partial eligibility status; and racial differences were reduced but not eliminated by geographic variation.

Discussion.—These findings show that black children 5–14 years old with Medicaid insurance have a lower rate of treatment with psychotropic medication than their white counterparts. In spite of the availability of free, comprehensive medical services through the Medicaid insurance program, differences in treatment with psychotropic medication do occur, according to race.

▶ Despite the recent hoopla concerning presumed overprescribing of methylphenidate and other stimulant medications in children and adolescents, it is likely that still only 1 in 2–3 children with attention deficit hyperactivity disorder is treated with psychostimulants or other medications. The risk for undertreatment or lack of access to services is not uniformly distributed, however, as this article illustrates. Black children with Medicaid were less likely to receive psychotropic medications than white children with Medicaid. While the absolute of under- vs. over-prescribing cannot be determined by this study, it demonstrates the lack of access to services experienced by substantial portions of the nation's children, as well as the potential impact of cultural attitudes and concerns on help-seeking, particularly for populations that already face other stigmatizing situations.

P.S. Jensen, M.D.

Barriers to Treatment Participation Scale: Evaluation and Validation in the Context of Child Outpatient Treatment
Kazdin AE, Holland L, Crowley M, et al (Yale Univ, New Haven, Conn)
J Child Psychol Psychiatry 38:1051–1062, 1997   1–60

Background.—Retaining children and adolescents in outpatient treatment is difficult: 40% to 60% of those entering such treatment leave early and against the advice of providers. Families' experiences and perceptions that predict dropping out, and other indices of participation in treatment, were reported.

Methods.—Two hundred sixty children, aged 3–13 years, and their families were included. All children had been referred for outpatient treatment. The Barriers to Treatment Participation Scale was developed and administered.

Findings.—The scale showed high levels of internal consistency. Experience of barriers to participation, rated by parents or therapists, predicted greater drop-out rates, fewer weeks in therapy, and higher rates of cancelled appointments and of not showing up for sessions. Perception of barriers could be differentiated from family, parent, and child characteristics assessed at intake and from the experience of critical life events during treatment. Perceived barriers contributed important information enabling better prediction of poor participation.

Conclusions.—Barriers to treatment participation can be identified on the scale described. The information provided may be used to identify patients at risk for dropping out and to design interventions to improve retention.

▶ One of the great challenges clinicians face is how to overcome obstacles that interfere with treatment, factors which lead patients to terminate treatment prematurely, to fail to implement recommended treatment strategies, or even never to seek help. Too often we have attributed the cause to some fault of the patient. But other factors, often unappreciated by the therapist, can and do interfere: transportation problems, scheduling conflicts, family illness, difficulties getting time off from work, problems finding child care, noncompliance on the part of the child, costs, and lack of family control in the focus and type of treatment. This article provides a new tool that systematically assesses these barriers. Importantly, the authors show that the instrument independently predicted subsequent compliance, over and above variables which have been traditionally invoked to explain lack of treatment participation (socioeconomic status, etc.). If we are to be most effective as therapists, we will have to not only assess such barriers, but also design our treatments so that they take such obstacles into account, to ensure maximum likelihood of effectiveness and subsequent "uptake" by families and treatment participants.

P.S. Jensen, M.D.

A Treatment Study for Sexually Abused Preschool Children: Outcome During a One-year Follow-up
Cohen JA, Mannarino AP (Allegheny Univ, Pittsburgh, Pa)
J Am Acad Child Adolesc Psychiatry 36:1228–1235, 1997   1–61

Introduction.—Few studies of treatment for sexually abused children have employed a control treatment design, included an adequate sample, or been continued through a follow-up period. To address this issue, researchers compared 2 distinct treatment methods for sexually abused preschool children during a 1-year follow-up period.

Methods.—Children eligible for the study had experienced sexual abuse, with the most recent episode occurring no more than 6 months before referral. Other requirements were that the abuse be substantiated by an independent source and that the child had reached a minimal level of symptomatology. The final study sample included 43 children with a mean age of 5 years and 9 months. Treatment models were the Cognitive-Behavioral Therapy for Sexually Abused Preschoolers (CBT-SAP) in 28 cases and nondirective supportive therapy (NST) in 15 cases. After randomization, each child received 12 treatment sessions. Parents completed standard behavior checklists to measure symptoms in their children.

Results.—The 2 treatment groups were similar at study entry with respect to symptomatology. Significant differences were noted at the end of treatment, with the CBT-SAP group being less symptomatic than the NST group on the Child Sexual Behavior Inventory, the Weekly Behavior Report total behavior score, and 2 of the 4 broad-band Child Behavior Checklist scales. The superiority of CBT-SAP over NST persisted at 6-month and 12-month follow-ups. Twelve children in the NST group, but none in the CBT-SAP group, were removed from the study at some point because of persistent sexual behavior problems.

Conclusion.—A structured, time-limited, cognitive-behavioral intervention for sexually abused preschool children and their nonoffending parents was found to be superior to nondirective treatment. Sexually inappropriate behaviors in such children respond more readily to behavioral interventions than to nondirective therapy.

▶ A recent report by the National Academy of Sciences indicates that studies of the effectiveness of interventions in children exposed to child abuse and neglect are desperately needed. Even more lacking (if that is possible!) are longitudinal outcome studies comparing results of different interventions over time. This study accomplishes both and is a very welcome addition to the sparse literature in this area. Using randomized clinical trial methodologies, Cohen and Mannarino compared a 16-session cognitive behavior therapy intervention targeted to sexually abused preschoolers and their nonoffending parent with 16 sessions of a nonspecific supportive therapy. Another nail in the coffin of nonspecific therapies? One point I take from this is that for many situations where psychotherapy is warranted, we need to be very clear about the specific ingredients of our therapies, clearly identify the targets of behavioral change, and then set about accomplishing this in a straightforward fashion that is interpretable to children and families.

P.S. Jensen, M.D.

Factors That Mediate Treatment Outcome of Sexually Abused Preschool Children: Six- and 12-Month Follow-up
Cohen JA, Mannarino AP (Allegheny Univ, Pittsburgh, Pa)
J Am Acad Child Adolesc Psychiatry 37:44–51, 1998   1–62

Introduction.—Sexually abused children experience a wide variety of symptoms. Some children do not exhibit any significant psychological symptoms. Predictors of symptomatology in children include levels of stressful parental reaction to the sexual abuse, the child's own abuse-related attributions and perceptions, and locus of control. Only 1 controlled treatment outcome trial of sexually abused children has assessed the impact of demographic, developmental, and familial factors on treatment outcome. It revealed that parental emotional distress related to the child's abuse was predictive of the child's posttreatment symptomatology, regardless of type of treatment. The impact of developmental, demographic, and familial factors on the psychological outcome of sexually abused preschool children 6 and 12 months after completion of treatment was assessed.

Methods.—Forty-three sexually abused preschool children and their parents were assigned to either cognitive-behavioral therapy or supportive counseling. Children were evaluated at baseline, posttreatment, and 6 and 12 months after treatment using the Child Behavior Checklist, the Child Sexual Behavior Inventory, and the Weekly Behavior Report to measure several emotional and behavioral symptoms in the children. Other measures included the Beck Depression Inventory, Family Adaptability and Cohesion Evaluation Scales-III, Parent Emotional Reaction Questionnaire, Parental Support Questionnaire, and Mental Social Support Index. The Battelle Developmental Inventory and Peabody Picture Vocabulary were used at pretreatment assessment.

Results.—The Parental Emotional Reaction Questionnaire was the strongest familial predictor of treatment outcome. At 6- and 12-month follow-up, parental support was a strong predictor of outcome. The strongest overall predictor of outcome at posttreatment and 12-month follow-up was treatment group. Cognitive-behavioral therapy was more effective than supportive counseling. Outcome was not strongly predicted by demographic or developmental factors.

Conclusion.—Findings show the strong impact of parental support and parental emotional reaction to abuse in sexually abused preschool children over a 12-month follow-up period. Cognitive-behavioral therapy was superior to supportive counseling in treating sexually abused children.

▶ One down side of our fairly exclusive Diagnostic and Statistical Manual focus in recent years is the lack of sufficient attention to the environmental factors shaping children's outcomes. This article nicely illustrates that to achieve the best outcomes in children who have been sexually abused, careful and systematic attention to mediating variables, in particular family support, is needed. Emotional support given to the parent was related to children's 6- and 12-month outcomes, above and beyond the effectiveness of the cognitive behavioral therapy itself. Such findings illustrate that families must be partners in the treatment process, and that our most effective efforts, in the long run, will be to assist those persons who spend most of each day with the child to increase the quality of their interactions. However, the strongest factor predicting positive child outcomes was related to treatment group assignment, clearly indicating that a good relationship between parents and children (or between therapist and parent) alone is not sufficient. For example, were I to have a brain tumor, I would certainly hope to find a compassionate, empathic, and personable neurosurgeon, but I would also want to ensure that his technical treatment skills were top-notch. So maybe some of our newly emerging therapies are more than just "psychosocial support"?

P.S. Jensen, M.D.

Abstinence and Safer Sex HIV Risk-reduction Interventions for African American Adolescents: A Randomized Controlled Trial

Jemmott JB III, Jemmott LS, Fong GT (Princeton Univ, NJ; Univ of Pennsylvania, Philadelphia; Univ of Waterloo, Ont, Canada)
JAMA 279:1529–1536, 1998

1–63

Background.—Black adolescents are at high risk for contracting sexually transmitted HIV infection. The most effective approach to behavioral interventions to reduce this risk is not known.

Methods.—Six hundred fifty-nine black adolescents from 3 middle schools in Philadelphia were recruited for a Saturday program. Mean age was 11.8 years. The trial was randomized and controlled, with follow-up at 3, 6, and 12 months. Interventions were based on cognitive-behavioral theories and elicitation research. Eight 1-hour sessions were implemented by adult facilitators or peer cofacilitators. The abstinence intervention emphasized delaying sexual intercourse or reducing its frequency. The safer-sex intervention stressed condom use. The control intervention focused on health issues unrelated to sexual behavior. The main outcome measures were self-reported sexual intercourse, condom use, and unprotected sexual intercourse.

Findings.—Ninety-three percent of the group were available for the 12-month follow-up. Compared with the control group participants, those in the abstinence intervention group were less likely to report, at 3 months after the intervention, having sexual intercourse, but were not less likely at 6 or 12 months. Compared with the control group, the safer-sex intervention group reported, at 3 months, significantly more consistent condom use, and also reported, at all follow-up assessments, greater frequency of condom use. Among participants who had had sexual experiences at baseline, those in the safer-sex intervention group reported less sexual intercourse, in the previous 3 months, at the 6- and 12-month follow-up than did those in the control and abstinence intervention groups, as well as less unprotected intercourse at all follow-ups. Intervention effects did not differ between the adult facilitator and peer cofacilitator conditions.

Conclusions.—Interventional programs designed to emphasize abstinence and safer sex can decrease HIV sexual risk behaviors. The safer-sex emphasis may be especially effective with sexually experienced adolescents and may have longer-lasting effects.

▶ A good deal of attention has focused on sex education of adolescents to stop the spread of sexually transmitted diseases, but this area has been marked by controversies concerning family values and whether sexual abstinence or "safer sex" is the appropriate goal for teaching, and the relative effectiveness of each approach. Results indicated that both approaches have merit, but only the "safer sex" approach reduced rates of unprotected sexual intercourse, including persisting effects seen at 12 months postintervention. This article nicely illustrates the conflict between societal values and scientific data: even though the evidence indicates greater reductions in unprotected sexual intercourse with the "safer sex" intervention, implementing such an intervention on a large scale would likely have enormous political fallout. What should be our approach, as health professionals, when values and data collide? How can we empower our communities and families to make sensible choices, while still respecting that the choices are indeed *theirs* to make?

P.S. Jensen, M.D.

2 Psychotherapy

Introduction

Concerns about managed care notwithstanding, psychotherapy practice flourishes, and the realm of psychotherapy research continues to expand. Particularly gratifying are the emerging attempts to operationalize psychoanalytic concepts so that they can be studied in a research setting. A number of articles in this edition illustrate this evolving area of research, including a number of interesting articles on group therapy which, is an undertaught and underutilized effective treatment modality in psychotherapy. As in previous years, a large number of studies here investigate the use of cognitive behavioral therapies in a variety of illnesses. Included for the first time are several articles investigating eye movement desensitization research. This controversial therapy still has not been adequately studied, and the jury is out regarding its ultimate utility in the psychotherapy field.

As always, a number of articles discuss psychotherapy training and supervision. I have little doubt that psychotherapeutic interventions will remain a key part of psychiatric practice. The need for a cadre of well-trained clinicians within psychiatry and the mental health fields demands that we continue to improve our educational approaches to psychotherapy education. I hope readers of this section will be stimulated to think about this in more depth.

The role of the therapeutic alliance as a curative factor in psychotherapy and the nature of the relationship between patient and therapist is still largely unexplored territory. Because of the importance of this area, this year's section begins with a number of interesting articles on this topic. The need for studies of both patients with comorbid illnesses and patients in whom combined psychotherapeutic and psychopharmacologic interventions are prescribed is also important for the future of psychotherapy research. As the field of psychotherapy research becomes more sophisticated in its methodologies, I have little doubt that we will begin to see more and more articles reporting results of such studies.

Allan Tasman, M.D.

Therapeutic Alliance and Relationship

The Therapeutic Alliance in Psychodynamic-Interpersonal and Cognitive-Behavioral Therapy

Raue PJ, Goldfried MR, Barkham M (The New York Hosp–Cornell Med Ctr, White Plains; State Univ of New York at Stony Brook; Univ of Leeds, England)
J Consult Clin Psychol 65:582–587, 1997   2–1

Background.—The therapeutic alliance plays a crucial role in all types of psychotherapy from psychodynamic-interpersonal to cognitive-behavioral therapy. The Working Alliance Inventory (WAI) was developed as a means of assessing the therapeutic alliance—the client-therapist agreement as to the tasks and goals of therapy and the development of a therapeutic bond—in all types of therapy. The quality of the therapeutic alliance in psychodynamic-interpersonal and cognitive-behavioral therapy was compared using the WAI.

Methods.—The study was part of the larger Sheffield Psychotherapy Project 2, a randomized comparison of the 2 psychotherapeutic approaches. The analysis included 57 clients with major depression who underwent 16 sessions of psychodynamic-interpersonal or cognitive-behavioral therapy. High- and low-impact sessions were identified for each client, and the therapeutic alliance for these sessions was rated by coders using the WAI. The quality of the alliance was compared between types of therapy and between high- and low-impact sessions. The relationship between alliance ratings and the depth and smoothness of sessions were analyzed as well.

Results.—Cognitive-behavioral therapy was associated with significantly greater alliance scores than psychodynamic-interpersonal therapy. However, the difference was small, and there was no significant difference between high-impact sessions of the 2 forms of therapy. Alliance scores were also greater for high-impact sessions than for low-impact sessions. In addition, alliance ratings were positively rated to therapist ratings of session depth and smoothness, and to clients' ratings of mood.

Conclusions.—The quality of the therapeutic alliance differs between cognitive-behavioral and psychodynamic-interpersonal therapy. Alliance scores are higher for cognitive-behavioral vs. psychodynamic-interpersonal therapy, and for high-impact vs. low-impact sessions. However, the difference between types of psychotherapy is relatively small, and is not present for high-impact sessions. Other postsession evaluations should be assessed for their effects on the therapeutic alliance.

▶ The difference in therapeutic alliance between cognitive-behavior and psychodynamic-interpersonal psychotherapy situations was relatively small here even though statistical significance between the two was reached. Interestingly, rating of alliance tended to be higher when therapists and patients thought the session had a positive impact and was helpful. Also, the mood of the patient after the session contributed to the ratings of alliance. This study raises important questions regarding assessment of therapeutic alliance and whether it is influenced by factors specific to the psychotherapy or events which transpire within a particular therapy session.

A. Tasman, M.D.

Expectancy, the Therapeutic Alliance, and Treatment Outcome in Short-term Individual Psychotherapy

Joyce AS, Piper WE (Univ of Alberta, Edmonton, Canada)
J Psychother Prac Res 7:236–248, 1998

2–2

Introduction.—Patients' expectations about psychotherapy may have an important impact on the process and outcomes of treatment. However, little research has been done in this area, and the only consistent finding has been a direct relationship between the expected and actual duration of therapy. The effects of patient and therapist expectations on the therapeutic alliance and outcomes of psychotherapy were evaluated.

Methods.—The analysis was based on a controlled trial of time-limited interpretive therapy. A sample of 64 patients, balanced for quality of object relations (QOR), immediate vs. delayed treatment, and therapist, was selected. Patient and therapist expectancy variables were measured on the basis of a "typical" session. These expectancy ratings were assessed for their relationship to measures of therapeutic alliance and treatment outcome. The relationships were tested in the presence of a competing predictor variable, i.e., severity of depressive symptoms before therapy or QOR.

Results.—Strong associations were noted between expectancies and the quality of the therapeutic alliance. Expectancies were less strongly related to therapy outcome, although the relationship was still significant. On multivariate analysis, expectancy variables often combined additively to account for variances in therapeutic alliance and outcome. Quality of object relations, therapeutic alliance, and patient expectancy all made independent contributions to the benefit of therapy.

Conclusions.—Patient expectations appear to be strongly related to the outcomes of psychotherapy, whereas therapist expectancies are not. The patient's ability to form a good relationship, the expectation that sessions will be comfortable, and the experience of a strong therapeutic alliance have a strong effect on the likelihood of therapeutic benefit. Ensuring early on that sessions can be productive and comfortable may aid the patient and therapist in forming a good working relationship, the experience of which forms the basis for a good treatment outcome.

▶ In this study of alliance, disappointment when high expectations are not met (however unrealistic the expectation) often accounted for low ratings in the therapeutic alliance. In addition, expectancies regarding the comfort the patient would feel within the session also played a role in ratings of alliance.

These findings demonstrate that education of patients about the nature of the transactions within psychotherapy might have a beneficial effect on outcome. Furthermore, this variable should be taken into account when studies of alliance are conducted.

A. Tasman, M.D.

A Match Made in Heaven? A Pilot Study of Patient-Therapist Match
Dolinsky A, Vaughan SC, Luber B, et al (Columbia Univ, New York)
J Psychother Prac Res 7:119–125, 1998   2–3

Objective.—Patient-therapist match refers to the concept of "goodness of fit," as applied to the psychotherapeutic relationship. Match is generally regarded as distinct from other concepts such as therapeutic alliance, transference, and countertransference; however, the boundaries between these entities remain unclear. Most studies of patient-therapist match have focused on the initial selection of a therapist. The patient-therapist match and its correlation with other variables were examined.

Methods.—The pilot study included 50 dyads of patients and therapists participating in psychodynamic therapy. Therapy sessions were held twice weekly for an average of 1 year. The patients and therapists gave simultaneous assessments of each other, the psychotherapeutic process, and the patient-therapist match. Patient and therapist agreement about the quality of the match was assessed. The relationship between a positive match and other variables was evaluated, as was patient-therapist agreement on questions related to perceived similarities and differences.

Results.—Fifty-eight percent of patients and 56% of therapists reported a positive match. In two thirds of cases, the therapist and patient agreed about the quality of the match. A positive match was significantly related to positive assessments of the progress and process of therapy by both patients and therapists. However, positive match was unrelated to the perceived similarity of personal characteristics between patients and therapists. There was no relationship between patients' and therapists' perceived similarities and differences from each other.

Conclusions.—This pilot study suggests that a positive patient-therapist match is significantly related to therapeutic alliance, therapeutic process, and outcome. Match does not appear to be related to the perception of shared personal characteristics between patient and therapist. In studying patient-therapist match, it is feasible and necessary to collect data from both parties. Future studies of this issue should concentrate on defining and operationalizing the concept of matching, and on studying longitudinal data collected from both members of the dyad.

▶ This study of the "match" between patient and therapist builds on earlier discussions that a significant variable in predicting outcome is the patient-therapist match. The results here add to the body of evidence supporting a correlation between match and outcome and demonstrate that this issue is worthy of much greater in-depth study. Furthermore, the study demonstrates that data can be gathered from both patient and therapist without having an adverse impact on the nature of the therapeutic experience.

A. Tasman, M.D.

Therapist Responsiveness to Client Interpersonal Styles During Time-limited Treatments for Depression
Hardy GE, Stiles WB, Barkham M, et al (Univ of Leeds, England; Miami Univ, Fla; Univ of Wales, Bangor)
J Consult Clin Psychol 66:304–312, 1998   2–4

Objective.—Several authors have examined the characteristic styles by which adults with depression relate to others. One style is characterized by an ongoing pattern of overinvolvement in interpersonal relationships; the other, characterized by autonomy and extreme independence, may be termed underinvolvement in relationships. These competing styles may affect the response of depressed clients to psychotherapy. Responding to each style with an appropriate mixture of interventions should lead to a strong therapeutic alliance and a good outcome for both groups. The effects of clients' interpersonal styles on the processes and outcomes of psychodynamic-interpersonal (PI) and cognitive-behavioral (CB) therapy for depression were assessed.

Methods.—A total of 117 patients receiving manualized, time-limited PI or CB therapy for depression were studied. With use of the Inventory of Interpersonal Problems, the clients' predominant interpersonal styles were classified into 3 groups: underinvolved (20.5% of clients), overinvolved (44.4%), and balanced (32.5%). This information was not provided to therapists. The effects of clients' interpersonal style on therapist interventions, session impact, therapeutic alliance, and therapeutic outcome were analyzed.

Results.—Interpersonal style had a significant effect on the type of interventions used by the therapists. Clients with an overinvolved style—particularly those receiving PI therapy—tended to receive more affective and relationship-oriented interventions. In contrast, clients with an underinvolved style, particularly those in CB therapy, tended to receive more cognitive treatment methods. There were no significant differences in the therapeutic alliance or in the treatment outcomes of the various style groups. At baseline, both the overinvolved and underinvolved groups had lower self-esteem scores than the balanced group. For the overinvolved group, 8-session PI therapy appeared particularly powerful and valuable; for underinvolved clients, 16-session CB treatment appeared to be more engaging.

Conclusions.—Differences in clients' interpersonal styles are associated with differences in the implementation of psychotherapy, suggesting that therapists are appropriately responsive to differences in client style. Clients with different interpersonal styles can receive different versions of treatments but still achieve similar therapeutic alliances and outcomes. The results suggest that manualized therapies can be individualized to meet the differing needs of clients.

▶ It is not surprising, as this study demonstrates, that a good psychotherapist intuitively responds to the PI style of the patient, even without this issue being assessed before the onset of therapy. The results argue for flexibility of approach when dealing with various patients in either an PI or CB type of psychotherapy.

A. Tasman, M.D.

Anonymity, Neutrality, and Confidentiality in the Actual Methods of Sigmund Freud: A Review of 43 Cases, 1907–1939
Lynn DJ, Vaillant GE (Brigham and Women's Hosp, Boston; St. Francis Med Center, Pittsburgh, Pa)
Am J Psychiatry 155:163–171, 1998   2–5

Purpose.—A growing body of information is available on how Sigmund Freud actually conducted psychotherapy. Several previous reports have suggested that the methods used by Freud did not always match his recommendations. Freud's psychoanalytic methods were compared with his published recommendations regarding anonymity, neutrality, and confidentiality.

Methods and Findings.—Information provided by Freud's analysands, including reports, letters, and interviews, as well as Freud's writings and clinical records, were reviewed. Cases conducted during Freud's mature years, from 1907 to 1939, were analyzed. Information on the actual methods used was available for 43 cases: 10 clinical psychoanalyses, 198 didactic analyses, and 14 combined clinical and didactic cases. The cases probably accounted for most of Freud's clinical hours during the historical period studied, although not necessarily most of his cases. In every case, Freud diverged from his own recommendation regarding strict confidentiality. In 72%, he took part in extra-analytic relations with analysands, and/or chose analysands to whom he already had significant connections. Freud departed from his recommendation for neutrality in 86% of cases, and his recommendation for confidentiality in 53%. In nearly half of cases, Freud gave analysands information about other analysands.

Conclusions.—Sigmund Freud's actual practice of psychotherapy varied greatly from his published recommendations on the subject. The consistent and logical recommendations recommended by Freud were not used or tested in his practice. He never explicitly described his methods in writing, and therefore they can never be replicated.

▶ Modern psychoanalysts are still influenced by Sigmund Freud's writings about the recommended nature of the interactions between therapist and patient. This review of a number of Freud's cases, although small and not "scientific," demonstrates that it is not possible to separate the outcome in Freud's work in psychoanalysis with his psychotherapeutic interpersonal style. His style differs from his writings that indicate the therapist should not overtly demonstrate warmth, support, acceptance, or trust in interactions with the patient. In fact, Freud's actual style seems to be consistent with what is now being learned about the role of the therapeutic relationship in positive psychotherapy outcome.

A. Tasman, M.D.

Psychodynamic Issues

Reconsidering the Transference Paradigm in Treatment With the Bereaved
Rubin SS (Univ of Haifa, Israel)
Am J Psychother 52:215–228, 1998

2–6

Background.—Psychodynamic therapy has offered great insight and sensitivity into the treatment of bereaved clients. However, in many cases, the client's therapy has been made secondary to theoretical constraints, resulting in loss of sensitivity to the client's needs. Elements of psychodynamic theory that are helpful in work with the bereaved were reviewed, and some modifications that may increase their efficacy were suggested.

The Transference Paradigm in Bereavement Work.—The psychodynamic model includes the real relationship between client and therapist, including the therapeutic alliance; the relationship of client to therapist, which the client constructs out of transference and parts of the real relationship; and the relationship of the therapist to the client, which the therapist constructs out of the countertransference and the real relationship. In clients receiving therapy for dysfunctional bereavement, the client may be unable to become heavily involved with anyone but the deceased individual. In such cases, the author believes that it is sometimes appropriate to shift to the deceased individual as the central relationship of the therapy. The transference phenomena typically directed toward the therapist may have more meaning and potential for change when directed toward the client's relationship to the bereaved figure.

In many cases, the therapy can maintain a joint focus on the relationship with the deceased and the relationship with the therapist. After a while, it may be appropriate to shift the focus from the deceased to the client-therapist relationship. Until then, putting too much emphasis on the transference relationship may interfere with the work of bereavement therapy. If the goal of such therapy is to loosen the bond to the deceased individual and permit it to take a new form, transference to the therapist may be a secondary focus for most if not all of the treatment.

Discussion.—The author suggests that, in psychodynamic therapy with the bereaved, it is sometimes appropriate to shift the central relationship of therapy away from the transference relationship to the relationship with the bereaved. This strategy may allow the work of mourning to reach a satisfactory conclusion. The approach is illustrated in the case report of a widower whose attachment to his deceased wife interfered with his attempts to form new relationships with women.

▶ For many years, dynamically-oriented therapists have addressed the role of transference and how it should be dealt with in psychotherapy. In this case report, Rubin suggests that a non-transferential focus is particularly appropriate with bereaved patients. This does not suggest that therapists should not attend to transference manifestations, but, rather, they should focus the work and interventions around matters of more immediate importance to this group of patients.

A. Tasman, M.D.

Transference and Countertransference Interpretations: Harmful or Helpful in Short-term Dynamic Therapy?
Schaeffer JA (Franciscan Family Wellness Program, Inc, Colorado Springs, Colo)
Am J Psychother 52:1–17, 1998   2–7

Introduction.—Short-term dynamic therapy (STDT) is essential to the survival of psychotherapy under the pressures of health care reform. However, there are persistent questions about specific short-term interventions, including transference interpretations (TRIs) and countertransference interpretations (CTRIs). Some theorists maintain that both transference and countertransference have important diagnostic use, but proscribe the use of TRIs and CTRIs in therapy. Others permit TRIs under stringent rules but do not allow CTRIs, whereas still others maintain that both TRIs and CTRIs are essential to positive outcomes. Key issues relevant to the use of TRIs and CTRIs in STDT were reviewed.

Transference Interpretations and CTRIs in STDT.—These 3 views regarding TRIs and CTRIs were reviewed, as well as the empirical basis for each. There have been few reliable studies of this issue, but the available data suggest some tentative conclusions. Used properly, TRIs appear to promote successful outcomes by positively influencing rapport, therapeutic alliance, and continuance in therapy. They can promote good outcomes for patients with mild-to-moderate Axis I and II disorders, as well as for those with no specific diagnosis. However, TRIs must reflect the unique therapeutic situation, must be sensitive to the client's pathology, and must have relatively low usage. Used with similar care, CTRIs can also promote good outcomes by maintaining the working alliance and preventing acting-out behaviors by the therapist. These interpretations may help patients to gain the insight necessary for change, and may perform a useful modeling function.

On the other hand, both types of interpretations may interfere with positive outcomes or even prove harmful. This occurs when the patient is highly resistant or has severe psychopathology that interferes with functioning, blurs boundaries, or encourages damaging acting out. They may also be harmful if the patient needs verification and processing of events denied by significant others. Although TRIs and CTRIs may play a role in successful outcomes, there is no evidence to show that they are required to achieve such outcomes.

Discussion.—The limited available data suggest that TRIs and CTRIs can be helpful in STDT. If appropriate to specific patient characteristics and presenting problems, these interpretations can have positive effects on alliance building, perseverance in therapy, and goal attainment. If not used carefully, however, they can lead to premature termination of therapy and other negative effects. There is no support for the position that TRIs and CTRIs are essential to positive outcomes.

▶ Schaeffer appropriately cautions that clinicians, especially those conducting brief psychotherapy, should be careful in making TRIs or CTRIs. She points out the limitations of present research and highlights the fact that further research is necessary to demonstrate the appropriate role and effective use of transference and countertransference in STDT.

A. Tasman, M.D.

Object Relations as a Predictor of Treatment Outcome With Chronic Posttraumatic Stress Disorder

Ford JD, Fisher P, Larson L (Nat Ctr for PTSD, White River Junction, Vt; Oregon Social Learning Ctr, Eugene; Portland Veterans Affairs Med Ctr, Ore)
J Consult Clin Psychol 65:547–559, 1997   2–8

Background.—Chronic posttraumatic stress disorder (PTSD) does not respond well to treatment. It has been suggested that an aptitude-treatment interaction approach could help in differentiating between patients who are likely to respond to existing treatment programs and those who should receive alternative treatment approaches. Chronic PTSD can be associated with profound characterologic deficits and problems with regulation of affect, consciousness, and bodily functioning. Thus, object relations was evaluated as a key aptitude and predictor of treatment outcome in patients with chronic PTSD.

Methods.—Seventy-four male patients admitted to a VA inpatient PTSD residential rehabilitation program were studied. These veterans all had chronic and severe psychosocial impairments linked to war trauma. Ninety percent were Vietnam veterans, and their mean age was 48. All were abstinent from alcohol and substance abuse at the start of treatment. The patients received intensive multimodal care during a 3-month inpatient stay, including individual and group psychotherapy, various psychoeducational classes, and in vivo experiences. The effects of treatment on psychometric and service utilization outcome measures were assessed. Object relations were assessed using Westen's social cognition object relations system.

Results.—At discharge, the patients showed mixed results on psychometric indices, suggesting little clinically significant change, with only 12% of cases moving into the "functional" range. There was a significant reduction in utilization of inpatient psychiatric services, from 45% to 12% in the years before and after treatment. Utilization of homeless domiciliary services also decreased significantly. Moderate levels of object relations—as opposed to low levels—were significantly associated with reliable change outcomes, including symptoms of PTSD, anxiety, internalized anger, and global distress, as well as quality of life and perceived self-control. This relationship was independent of demographic variables, presence of an axis II diagnosis, symptom severity, or trauma exposure during childhood or in combat.

Conclusions.—In patients with chronic PTSD, clinician-related object relations level appears to be a consistent predictor of the outcomes of inpatient treatment. Patients with moderate-level object relations have reliable gains in key symptom and adjustment measures, compared with those with low-level object relations. Patients in the latter group might benefit from treatments aimed at basic social support connections and life management competencies.

▶ This study adds to the literature on the role of the patient's capacity for object relations in therapeutic outcome. Especially with patients with PTSD, who as a group are well known to be difficult to treat and whose clinical outcomes are not always optimal, the capacity for the development of object relations seems to be correlated with a positive outcome. Thus, screening for this variable before acceptance into treatment would seem to be particularly important with these patients. The role of the patient's capacity for a relationship with the therapist has been discussed for years as an important factor in therapeutic outcome, and this study builds on the research literature in this area and highlights the need for much more research.

A. Tasman, M.D.

Conceptualization and Measurement of Insight

Baier M, Murray RLE, McSweeney M (Southern Illinois Univ at Edwardsville; Saint Louis Univ, Mo; Univ of Missouri, St. Louis)
Arch Psychiatr Nurs 12:32–40, 1998   2–9

Introduction.—Insight plays an important role in the treatment of schizophrenia, and measurement of insight is essential for comparison and clinical application of research findings. However, definitions of insight have varied widely, making it difficult to correlate insight with treatment outcomes in patients with schizophrenia. The conceptual and methodological problems associated with the study of insight in schizophrenia were reviewed, and some recommendations as to its definition and measurement were made.

Definitions of Insight.—Insight is sometimes used synonymously with "awareness of illness." Other authors suggest that insight implies "correct judgment of all the symptoms and the illness as a whole." Still others suggest that insight is a symptom of schizophrenia, which can be assessed only as present or absent. More recent reports describe insight as a multidimensional phenomenon including acknowledgment of schizophrenia and the need for treatment, the risk of relapse, and the effects of psychosocial stressors. In psychiatry, some authors have suggested that insight is by definition impaired in psychotic disorders. Three concepts of the source of insight have been described: a neurologic model, in which lack of insight is attributed to a brain dysfunction; a cognitive model, in which insight is a set of beliefs about mental symptoms; and a psychological model, which defines insight in psychoanalytic terms. The lack of insight present in schizophrenia can be viewed as an integration of these 3 models. The choice of measurement tool would depend on the purpose of the study and the definition of insight used.

Measurement of Insight.—Several different insight measurement tools have been described. Problematic issues raised by these instruments include lack of agreement on definitions, lack of instrument validity, and arbitrary categorization of data. From a statistical standpoint, these instruments have had problems with small samples of patients with schizophrenia, inappropriate statistical techniques, and failure to correct the level of significance. Nonparametric tests have reduced sensitivity and may sometimes give nonsignificant results. On the other hand, parametric tests may be used in inappropriate situations, and thus give misleading results.

Recommendations.—These findings underscore the need for further research to clarify the concept of insight. The concept of insight needs to be assessed conceptually and empirically by means of techniques such as factor analysis. Concurrent validity and construct validity need to be assessed, and the simplification (dichotomization or trichotomization) of insight scales needs to be rationalized. Nonparametric analyses may be appropriate for small samples of non-normal distribution. The authors encourage further work from the viewpoint of insight as a dynamic process, including input from patients. Qualitative exploratory studies may help in clarifying the construct of insight and in developing instruments to measure it.

▶ The patient's capacity for insight into his or her illness has long been thought to play a role in treatment outcome. Unfortunately, the body of research literature is difficult to interpret because of the statistical difficulties and lack of common definitions when comparing samples. Because previous studies have indicated that the presence of insight is positively correlated with treatment outcome, it would seem prudent that further research be done in this area.

A. Tasman, M.D.

A Comparative Analysis of the Therapeutic Focus in Cognitive-Behavioral and Psychodynamic-Interpersonal Sessions
Goldfried MR, Castonguay LG, Hayes AM, et al (State Univ of New York at Stony Brook; Pennsylvania State Univ; Univ of Miami, Fla; et al)
J Consult Clin Psychol 65:740–748, 1997   2–10

Introduction.—There is growing clinical interest in psychotherapy integration, but few studies have compared integrated interventions with "pure form" treatments. In an effort to gain a clearer understanding of different intervention procedures, researchers compared therapeutic foci in a sampling of 30 cognitive-behavioral and 27 psychodynamic-interpersonal manual-driven treatments for depression.

Methods.—The therapy sessions used were from a 1994 study (Shapiro et al.) in which half of the clients received 16 weekly sessions. Clients were stratified according to level of depression (high, medium, low), but all had a diagnosis of major depressive disorder and were adversely affected in their occupational functioning. Five therapists conducted both treatments and used high- and low-impact sessions within each course. Therapists rated the impact of the therapy (7 = greatly helpful; 1 = greatly hindering) after each session. Sessions were coded using the Coding System of Therapeutic Focus.

Results.—Nine analyses were conducted for specific components of the client's functioning. Only 2 components—emotion and situation—had statistically significant main effects for treatment orientations. In contrast to cognitive-behavioral sessions, which were more likely to focus on external circumstances in the client's life, psychodynamic-interpersonal interventions placed twice as much emphasis on emotion. In addition, the cognitive-behavioral sessions stressed the client's ability to make decisions and to focus on the future. The psychodynamic-interpersonal sessions focused on the impact that clients made on others, including clients' parents and the therapists themselves.

Conclusion.—In general, psychodynamic-interpersonal therapy underscores the importance of "insight," whereas cognitive-behavioral therapy emphasizes the importance of "action." The first form of therapy provides insights into what has not worked in the past; the second focuses on what can be done to deal with events in the future. In certain aspects of therapeutic focus, however, the 2 orientations did not differ.

▶ Clinicians often agree that the broad aims of psychodynamic psychotherapy and cognitive behavior therapy are similar, although the methods to attain positive therapeutic change are quite different. This study highlights the differences in therapeutic focus between these 2 types of psychotherapy and suggests that flexibility in focus might be of benefit to therapists practicing either treatment modality. How this could be accomplished has yet to be described, but would be important to more appropriately match not only the aims but the techniques of the therapy to the patient's individual needs.

A. Tasman, M.D.

Interpretive and Supportive Forms of Psychotherapy and Patient Personality Variables
Piper WE, Joyce AS, McCallum M, et al (Univ of Alberta, Edmonton, Canada; Lions Gate Hosp, North Vancouver, British Columbia, Canada)
J Consult Clin Psychol 66:558–567, 1998   2–11

Introduction.—Supportive psychodynamic psychotherapy has been promoted in recent years as an effective treatment for a variety of disorders. Supportive therapy emphasizes improving the patient's immediate adaptation, whereas interpretive therapy stresses enhancing the patient's insight about underlying conflicts and trauma. A randomized clinical trial examined the efficacy of interpretive and supportive forms of short-term individual psychotherapy. In addition, the interaction of 2 personality characteristics, quality of object relations (QOR) and psychological mindedness (PM), was investigated.

Methods.—A total of 258 patients were referred; 144 completed therapy. The research coordinator matched patients in pairs on the basis of their QOR score, PM score, use of medication, and, when possible, gender and age. One patient from each pair was randomized to supportive therapy and 1 to interpretive therapy; assignment to therapist was also randomized. Patients had an average age of 34.3 years; 61% were women, 94% were white, and 67% were educated beyond high school. Outcome was assessed by a comprehensive battery of tests.

Results.—When the entire set of matching demographic, diagnostic, and initial-disturbance variables was considered, the 2 patient samples proved to be well balanced. Of 27 dropouts, 81.5% were from the supportive therapy group and 18.5% from the interpretive group, a significant difference. Patients in both therapy groups showed improvement, and outcome did not differ between the 2 groups. There appeared to be a direct relation between QOR and outcome for interpretive therapy, but almost no relation for supportive therapy. For both forms of therapy, a multivariate main effect indicated a direct relation between PM and outcome.

Conclusion.—Patients in both interpretive and supportive therapies experienced substantial improvement in a range of outcome variables. Greatest improvements were seen in target objectives, life satisfaction, and symptomatology. The dropout rate in supportive therapy was unusually low.

▶ For decades, dynamically-oriented therapists have debated whether the curative factors were more related to the interpretive aspects or the supportive aspects of psychotherapy. This study categorized psychotherapy as either supportive or interpretative and studied differences in outcome.

Although the results are preliminary, there is interesting support for the notion that both interpretative and supportive work play important roles in therapeutic outcome. Another aspect of this study, in support of other work, is that the patient's capacity for a relationship with the therapist is a key variable when assessing the utility and efficacy of interpretative interventions.

A. Tasman, M.D.

Psychodynamic Psychotherapy for Cancer Patients
Straker N (Cornell Univ, New York)
J Psychother Prac Res 7:1–9, 1998   2–12

Introduction.—Psychodynamic psychotherapy offers an approach that can help patients to understand the psychological conflicts and the psychiatric symptoms associated with cancer. The approach is also useful for planning psychological interventions. In a discussion of psychodynamic psychotherapy, the author reviews findings on the effects of psychosocial factors and psychotherapy on medical outcome, disease recurrence, and survival.

Background.—A number of studies have shown the following factors to be associated with improved survival among patients with cancer: emotional expression, social supports, lower levels of emotional distress, and a fighting spirit. Most controlled studies have also shown that psychotherapeutic intervention can reduce psychological stress, and some reports indicate a direct benefit of social support on survival.

Approaches to the Cancer Patient.—Patients who come for psychotherapy at any disease stage require a flexible approach because of the shifting nature of cancer phases. Crisis intervention may be needed, and quality-of-life issues should remain in focus. Clinicians must recognize the power of an empathetic relationship and of the transference, especially in terminally ill patients.

Phases of Cancer.—Four phases are identified: diagnosis, follow-up, recurrence, and the terminal stage. Each phase is discussed in general terms and illustrated with clinical examples. Most patients handle diagnosis surprisingly well, and the psychotherapeutic efforts are directed toward adapting to the crisis and toward choosing treatment. After initial therapy, patients may be particularly vulnerable despite being physically well. Some may become dysfunctional, whereas others may seek to address unaccomplished life goals. Anger, depression, anxiety, and distrust often appear with recurrence, especially among patients who have relied on denial. The terminal palliative phase is the most difficult, and psychiatric consultation in this phase is quite common. Patients, however, are sometimes more realistic than their physicians about prognosis.

Conclusion.—Dynamic psychotherapy involving patients with cancer can be emotionally challenging, intellectually stimulating, and highly rewarding. The patient and therapist are extremely motivated to work productively and rapidly toward resolving long-standing conflicts.

▶ Over the last several decades, there has been a great deal of change in psychiatrists' willingness to engage in psychotherapeutic work with patients who have cancer. This article reinforces clinical wisdom that, while difficult and fraught with potential countertransference difficulties, psychotherapeutic work with cancer patients can be gratifying and beneficial to the patient. The importance of supervision or some other opportunity to reflect on the work being done is highlighted here. This is significant because therapists often practice in isolation without adequate support for their own work. Especially with cancer patients, such support is essential.

A. Tasman, M.D.

Group Therapy

Promoting Group Psychotherapy in Managed Care: Basic Economic Principles for the Clinical Practitioner
Gross JM (La Canada, Calif)
Int J Group Psychother 47:499–507, 1997

2–13

Introduction.—Group psychotherapy is a cost- and outcome-effective intervention, but the belief that patients are unwilling to participate in a public form of therapy has led to resistance to its use. Under managed care, however, more patients are being referred to group psychotherapy and psychoeducational intervention. The author introduces a model of the managed-care marketplace, discusses the interaction of medical necessity and patient copayment, and explains the significance of demand-management economics.

The Marketplace Model.—The 4 categories of participants in the model are purchasers (usually employers or governmental bodies), patients, providers, and payers (managed-care organizations). This model has inside and outside relationships that differ considerably in their missions, goals, and operations. The outside system involves the business transactions between payers and purchasers, whereas the inner system concerns itself with the relationships between patients and providers. Increasingly, the MCO rather than the patient selects the treatment type and the service provider. Mental health practitioners need to actively lobby and educate the managed care organization with which they do business to maintain practice standards. Purchasers, patients, providers, and payers would all benefit from systems that promote restoration of the traditional mental health treatment team and the development of policies that pay for group therapy and psychoeducational intervention.

Outlook.—Patients need choices about price and duration of treatment, and providers must be able to diagnose and treat patients based on clinical data. Purchasers need to be satisfied that their employees have mental health insurance benefits, and payers should be able to promote cost-effective group-based psychological interventions. Development of facilitative and cooperative relationships among all 4 categories of participants is the most important factor in improving patient care and the economics of third-party payment.

▶ What a shame that, as this article points out, managed care companies don't reimburse for group therapy. It's too bad that such a cost-effective and clinically-effective modality for so many patients in so many different diagnostic categories is so under appreciated by managed care administrators. My guess is that perhaps, like so many mental health professionals, those individuals have not been well trained in group therapy, and therefore don't appreciate its utility.

A. Tasman, M.D.

The Contribution of Group Cohesion and Group Alliance to the Outcome of Group Psychotherapy
Marziali E, Munroe-Blum H, McCleary L (Univ of Toronto)
Int J Group Psychother 47:475–497, 1997   2–14

Introduction.—The contributions of group cohesion and group alliance to the outcome of group psychotherapy were examined in a randomized, controlled treatment trial that included patients with borderline personality disorder (BPD). There is currently little consensus about the dimensions that best describe the complex phenomena of group cohesiveness, and group alliance, which shows some overlap with group cohesiveness, also requires definition.

Methods.—In the context of a 30-session therapy, group members from 4 time-limited groups of an experimental model of group psychotherapy completed measures of both group cohesion and group alliance. The treatment strategy used in the model of group psychotherapy (Interpersonal Group Psychotherapy) was designed to address personality traits typical of BPD. The BPD client seeks to resolve instability and ambiguity in the context of interpersonal relationships. The 79 clients in the study were randomized to Interpersonal Group Psychotherapy, the experimental treatment model; or to the comparison model, Individual Dynamic Psychotherapy. Outcome was measured in terms of psychiatric symptoms, social adaptation, and indicators of behavioral dysfunction.

Results.—Both treatment groups experienced significant improvements, as reflected on each of the outcome indicators. Cohesion and alliance were correlated significantly and separately contributed to outcome on most of the dependent variables. When compared with cohesion, however, alliance accounted for more outcome variance on the dependent measures.

Discussion.—The process factors of group cohesion and group alliance are related conceptually and in terms of measurement focus, but the 2 factors also differ. Each captures a different dimension of group process. The focus is member-to-member transactions in group coherence vs. member-to-therapist transactions in group alliance.

▶ This is an interesting study that operationalizes, in a research environment, 2 process factors that have always been thought to be related to positive outcome in group therapy. Those factors are group cohesion and group therapeutic alliance. Although this is only a preliminary study of a complex phenomenon, the findings here support the role of these 2 factors in therapeutic outcome. One clearly hopes for further research in this area and for more study regarding how group cohesion and group therapeutic alliance can be fostered.

A. Tasman, M.D.

The Rationale and Foundations of Group Psychotherapy for Women With Metastatic Breast Cancer
Leszcz M, Goodwin PJ (Univ of Toronto)
Int J Group Psychother 48:245–273, 1998   2–15

Introduction.—The diagnosis of metastatic breast cancer usually means an average life expectancy of 2–3 years. This article reviews and describes the rationale and foundations for group psychotherapy, which has become an important intervention in psycho-oncology, for women with metastatic breast cancer.

Methods.—An earlier study showed that women with metastatic breast cancer who participated in structured group psychotherapy had improved psychosocial adjustment and significantly longer survival than similar women who were not involved in group psychotherapy. The 86 women in Spiegel's[1] study were treated for 1 year with weekly, supportive-expressive group therapy. Some more recent studies of patients with other cancers have had similar outcomes. The authors of the present study are engaged in a multicenter randomized controlled trial, the Breast Expressive-Supportive Therapy study, designed to evaluate the effectiveness of group supportive-expressive therapy in women with metastatic breast cancer.

After completing a battery of psychological questionnaires, women are randomized in a ratio of 2:1 to a weekly support group with educational materials or to a control arm given educational materials only. Follow-up and outcome data are collected every 4 months. Case examples are presented to illustrate the benefits of group supportive-expressive therapy at the various stages of disease.

Discussion.—Cancer patients are often faced with a range of psychological and emotional challenges that affect quality of life. The burgeoning field of psycho-oncology focuses on mind-body interactions, and the reach of group psychotherapy is now expanding into this clinical area. There is a need for research that involves prospective, randomized controlled studies of psychosocial interventions for patients with cancer.

▶ Since David Spiegel's 1989 study, support groups have nearly become a required component in comprehensive breast cancer treatment. This review thoughtfully discusses the role of group support in this patient population.

One would hope that greater use of group therapy for patients with other severe medical illnesses would grow as rapidly as has its use in oncology.

A. Tasman, M.D.

Reference

1. Spiegel D, Bloom JR, Kraemer HC, et al: Effect of psychosocial treatment on survival of patients with metastatic breast cancer. *Lancet* 2:888–891, 1989.

Conflict and Aggression in Group Psychotherapy: A Self Psychological Vantage Point
Livingston MS, Livingston LR (New York Inst for Psychoanalytic Self Psychology)
Int J Group Psychother 48:381–391, 1998   2–16

Introduction.—The emphasis of self psychology is on listening and understanding from a patient's vantage point. This characterization has led to the view that self psychology ignores conflict and aggression, a misconception that the authors intend to correct.

Basic Concepts.—Self psychology does not ignore conflict and aggression. Experiences of conflict are best understood from the patient's subjective viewpoint, and in the group setting this means that the leader must balance multiple sensitivities. With empathetic attunement, the group leader can create a sense of safety. Promotion of safety, however, does not imply avoiding conflict and aggression as they occur in a group, but rather viewing these events as an opportunity to address underlying issues.

A Self Psychological Understanding of Rage and Aggression.—The group leader's role is to accept, understand, and interpret conflict and aggression as inevitable reactions to actual or imaginary slights within the multiple transferential context of the group. The angry response is understood in the patient's subjective context and is legitimized. Thus, the rage can shift to the broader contexts of the experience from which it arose, the functions it serves, and the childhood roots of the experiences. A case example is presented that illustrates the development of conflict and aggression in a small group with little history of conflict among its members.

Discussion.—Group psychotherapy provides an unusually potent medium for working through self-pathology that arises as conflict, aggression, and rage. The focus of a self psychological attempt at cure is on the underlying self-pathology, not the rage itself. Thus, it is not the aggression that is affected, but the underlying structure. With the underlying vulnerability expressed and explored, a curative process can be reached.

▶ Soon after Kohut's groundbreaking work in the '70s,[1] which forms the basis for that body of theoretical and clinical work that has come to be known as "self psychology," theorists and clinicians began applying the principals of self psychology to an understanding of group process. One of the criticisms of Kohut's work is of Kohut's assumption that most (if not all) anger and rage flows from narcissistic injury and the resultant experience of vulnerability. However, this has been an extremely useful concept in psychotherapeutic work with many patients. These authors apply this formulation to understanding conflict and aggression in group therapy in a way that is clinically valuable for every group therapist.

A. Tasman, M.D.

Reference

1. Kohut H: Thoughts on narcissism and narcissistic rage, in Ornstein PH (ed): *The Search for the Self*, vol 2. New York, International Universities Press, 1978, pp 615–658.

Empirically Supported Individual and Group Psychological Treatments for Adult Mental Disorders
DeRubeis RJ, Crits-Christoph P (Univ of Pennsylvania, Philadelphia)
J Consult Clin Psychol 66:37–52, 1998   2–17

Introduction.—This article attempts to provide a comprehensive, annotated list of therapeutic approaches that are of confirmed efficacy for adult, nongeriatric patients with the following diagnoses or problems: major depressive disorder, generalized anxiety disorder, social phobia, obsessive-compulsive disorder, agoraphobia, panic disorder (with or without agoraphobia), posttraumatic stress disorder, schizophrenia, substance abuse and dependence, and alcohol abuse and dependence. Interventions not included are often ones that have not been subjected to clinical trials.

Approaches of Efficacy.—Cognitive therapy is perhaps the most widely respected psychological intervention for serious mental disorders. There has been skepticism about its use for depression, but overall data indicate that cognitive therapy for depression is an efficacious treatment with relapse prevention effects. Other treatments of value are behavioral therapy and interpersonal therapy. Cognitive-behavioral therapy and applied relaxation are efficacious treatments for generalized anxiety disorder, and the former is a specific treatment. In cases of social phobia, exposure therapy (alone or with cognitive-behavioral therapy) has been effective. The addition of cognitive restructuring procedures appears to be of little benefit, however.

Exposure and response prevention therapy is able to extinguish obsessive fears and can reduce obsessive-compulsive symptoms more than relaxation training can. Treatment of agoraphobia also involves exposure therapy, which has been effective. One study found systematic desensitization therapy to be equally beneficial. Cognitive therapy has proved successful in cases of panic disorder, and 2 distinct behavioral therapy approaches—exposure-based treatments and applied relaxation—also did well in outcome research. Patients with posttraumatic stress disorder benefit from exposure (behavioral therapy), and stress inoculation therapy and eye movement desensitization and reprocessing are considered possibly efficacious.

Psychological treatment of schizophrenia is usually examined as an adjunct to antipsychotic medications. A possibly efficacious treatment is social skills training, shown in some studies to lower the relapse rate. Treatments for alcohol abuse/dependence and substance abuse/dependence are possibly efficacious and include, for the former, social skills training and urge coping skills, and, for the latter, cognitive therapy, relapse prevention therapy, and reinforcement for abstinence.

Discussion.—For every adult disorder in this review, there are psychological treatments that are promising. Most such treatments are behavioral or cognitive-behavioral. All of the treatments have led to a reduction or remission of the disorder or have outperformed an alternative active therapy.

▶ This is a thorough review of the present psychotherapy research literature for various psychological treatments for psychiatric disorders in adults. Clearly, the research literature to date has been skewed towards projects involving cognitive behavioral approaches, and this produces a somewhat skewed report compared with clinical experience. However, the authors correctly note that for future utility we need to develop more specificity in matching treatment recommendations to patient characteristics.

A. Tasman, M.D.

Working With Spiritual and Religious Themes in Group Therapy
Jacques JR (Portsmouth, NH)
Int J Group Psychother 48:69–83, 1998   2–18

Introduction.—Some patients come to group treatment with unresolved spiritual or religious conflicts in addition to the usual indications of psychopathology. The analytic therapy group can provide the transitional space for exploring and working through members' spiritual or religious themes. When such themes are explored, it is possible to reveal rich data about patients' intrapsychic conflicts, interpersonal relationships, and sense of self.

Religion and Psychology.—Freud viewed religion as a form of transference and a dangerous illusion, whereas Jung saw God as an archetype and religion as the traditional route to the process of integration. A religious category is contained in the Diagnostic and Statistical Manual of Mental Disorders (IV): Religious or Spiritual Problems. Examples of the disorder include a questioning of spiritual values, conversion to a new faith, and distressing experiences involving a loss of faith. The analytic therapy group can be seen as a spiritual community that can deepen the implications of group transference. In a clinical illustration, members of a midphase group discuss childhood religious experiences and how these are related to family conflicts.

Discussion.—Spiritual or religious themes can provide an additional lens for understanding group members' transferences, projective identifications, and object relationships. Confession offers an opportunity for repairing the breaks between good and bad self and between self and God. Group members grieve the losses and failures of parental figures, then begin to create new objects and relationships. Patients most likely to benefit from such discussions have the capacity to think symbolically and to tolerate diversity, ambiguity, and the unknown.

▶ The last several decades have been marked by renewed interest in spiritual and religious themes within psychotherapeutic practice. Ms. Jacques presents a rich clinical view of the importance of these themes in a variety of psychiatric symptomatology. Her work emphasizes the value of viewing religious and spiritual concerns as valid in their own right and not as manifestations of maladaptive psychological processes.

A. Tasman, M.D.

Group Therapy for Somatization Disorders in General Practice: Effectiveness of a Short Cognitive-Behavioural Treatment Model
Lidbeck J (Lund Univ, Malmö, Sweden)
Acta Psychiatr Scand 96:14–24, 1997   2–19

Introduction.—Somatization disorders are commonly seen in general practice and somatizing patients are high-level consumers of medical care services. Research on treatment for such patients, however, has been a neglected area. A study was designed to evaluate the effect of a short cognitive-behavioral group therapy program in primary care for somatization disorder.

Methods.—Patients eligible for the study were aged 30–60 years, had somatization disorder in accordance with the definition of functional somatic symptoms, and 1 or more symptoms fulfilling the criteria of specific functional disorders as outlined in the International Classification of Health Problems in Primary Care. As defined by Kellner, functional somatic symptoms are "somatic symptoms not caused by physical disease or tissue damage, although specific physiological changes can be detected in some of these symptoms by special techniques." The treatment model focused on patient education and stress relaxation. Fifty patients, 42 women and 8 men, were included in the final sample. Approximately two thirds had a low level of education and low occupational status. The 3 most frequently reported complaints were headache, myalgia, and abdominal dysfunction. Mean duration of illness was 8.3 years.

Results.—The group treatment sessions were held weekly over a 2-month period. Patients were assessed before and after treatment and at 6-month follow-up. Thirty-three had been randomized to the stress reduction intervention and 17 to a control waiting list. Patients in the treatment group were moderately but significantly improved in measures of physical illness and somatic preoccupation, hypochondriasis, and medication usage. No such improvements were seen in the control group. There was a high level of satisfaction with the treatment program; 95% of patients in this group experienced some benefit of relaxation training and 90% reported improvement in self-knowledge.

Conclusion.—The short treatment program provided to these patients with somatization disorders proved beneficial. Although depression, anxiety, and quality of sleep were unchanged, improvements were reported in perception of illness, somatic preoccupation, hypochondriasis, and use of medication.

▶ Group therapy has much to contribute to the care of the medically ill patient. This study demonstrates the benefit of a cognitive behavioral group program for somatizing patients in a general medical setting. Because these patients are both notoriously difficult to treat and high utilizers of health care, such an approach is worth investigating in more depth for implementation on a broader scale.

A. Tasman, M.D.

Staff Support Groups for High-stress Medical Environments
Lederberg MS (Mem Sloan-Kettering Cancer Ctr, New York)
Int J Group Psychother 48:275–304, 1998   2–20

Objective.—Staff support groups have long been used in health care settings. Such groups are popular and achieve positive results, though there have been few rigorous outcome studies. With the increasing demands placed on medical staff, the need for such support groups is more apparent than ever. Drawing on her personal experience, the author discusses a conceptual approach to staff support groups in health care environments, including the goals, techniques, and developmental stages of these groups.

The Concept of Staff Support Groups.—Medical staff support groups improve staff well-being in ways that lead to improved patient care and unit functioning. The support group is intended to address the "work self," and does not encompass the usual therapy techniques used to reveal the inner self. The group must have realistic goals, based on a knowledge of what is and is not changeable. Because of difficulties with continuity of attendance, it becomes the group facilitator's job to provide continuity of process. The focus on the support group must include why the group was requested, the suspected underlying issue, and the role of the support group within the parent group and institution. In most cases, the unit leader does not attend the group; this increases group spontaneity, but may require a period of scapegoating of the leader. The group facilitator must prove insight if she is from outside the institution, and loyalty if she is from inside.

Staff Psychologic Responses.—The adaptation of staff members reflects the professional ego-ideal and underlying past contradictory attitudes, which may be conscious or unconscious. Caregivers often believe they are alone in their feelings, both inside and outside the workplace. Dysfunctional responses, including reactive anxiety and depression, or even clinical psychiatric disorders, can occur at any point in a caregiver's career.

Staff Support Group Approach.—Staff support groups have many important effects on the individual, group, and professional levels. A growing body of evidence underscores the positive effects of support groups, particularly the protective effects of social support and recognition. Though group facilitators do not use the techniques of psychodynamic psychotherapy, they do use the insights. Support groups differ from therapy groups in almost every important regard, except in the need for authenticity and the provision of reality checks for members.

Group Development.—The author reviews the development of staff support groups, from definition of initial boundaries through termination. In early meetings, the group complains about being overworked and exploited. Ventilation must be followed by analysis of emotionally difficult issues. With growing trust, the facilitator helps members to acknowledge the universality of emotions, and helps to prevent members from feeling vulnerable because of their openness. At this stage, the facilitator evaluates whether the group is becoming more cohesive, and if not, why not. Feedback to the unit leader at this time may lead to changes in the ward culture. In the late stage, reduced staff isolation and anxiety lead to better self-esteem and communication, and thus to better morale and patient care. Termination should consist of a review of the experience, a discussion of the availability of future groups, and a debriefing of the unit leader. Some relevant clinical examples of staff support groups, as well as discussions of leadership and countertransference issues, are offered.

Conclusion.—With ongoing changes in health care delivery, the need for staff support groups seems to be greater than ever. This article presents a conceptual approach to staff support groups, including the relevant systems issues. Support groups provide a way for caregivers to experience themselves as complete human beings, within the setting of their vocation.

Cognitive and Behavioral Therapies

Behaviour Therapy for Obsessive-Compulsive Disorder: A Decade of Progress

Marks I (Inst of Psychiatry, London)
Can J Psychiatry 42:1021–1027, 1997   2–21

Introduction.—This article reviews research in behavior therapy for obsessive-compulsive disorder.

Methods.—The most salient research in obsessive-compulsive disorder was identified and analyzed.

Results.—Research in the last 10 years has confirmed that exposure and ritual prevention can reduce compulsive rituals and obsessive thoughts in most patients across age groups. Studies in several countries have shown that improvements persist for 2–6 years. Improvement after exposure and ritual prevention is associated with improvements in commonly associated abnormal beliefs, as well as in work and social disability. Gains are accompanied by evidence of decreased cerebral blood flow in the right caudate nucleus. Recurrence is reduced by teaching patients how to prevent relapse. Exposure and ritual prevention is somewhat more effective than antidepressant medication and is associated with less relapse after the end of treatment. Therefore, exposure and ritual prevention may be more cost-effective long-term. In cases of obsessive-compulsive disorder and comorbid depression, antidepressant medication in addition to exposure and ritual prevention can be useful. Currently, therapists teach patients how to carry out self-exposure and self-imposed ritual prevention, but do not impose therapist-administered exposure and ritual prevention on them. Pilot studies have reported success with self-help manuals and computer aids in teaching patients exposure and ritual prevention. Studies have shown that cognitive therapy without exposure and ritual prevention is as effective as exposure and ritual prevention alone.

Discussion.—Exposure and ritual prevention is valuable for treating individuals with obsessive-compulsive disorder. Future studies should address the long-term cost-effectiveness of self-administered exposure and ritual prevention compared to that of cognitive therapy and of medication. Studies should also address brief psychological treatment for obsessive-compulsive disorder with comorbid depression. A small number of patients with obsessive-compulsive disorder do not improve with any treatment.

▶ As Dr. Marks clearly presents, the use of the behavioral approaches of exposure and response prevention has been 1 of the most dramatic success stories in psychotherapy practice in the last decade. New approaches to this modality are suggested by Marks, and 1 of these—the use of computers—is of great interest for future practice.

A. Tasman, M.D.

Impact of a Mandatory Behavioral Consultation on Seclusion/Restraint Utilization in a Psychiatric Hospital

Donat DC (Western State Hosp, Staunton, Va)
J Behav Ther Exp Psychiatry 29:13–19, 1998   2–22

Background.—Although it has been shown that behavioral techniques for treating individuals with psychiatric impairments can be useful as well as cost-effective, such techniques are rarely used successfully for inpatients. The effectiveness of an administrative procedure designed to initiate a behavioral consultation for inpatients requiring high seclusion or restraint was determined.

Methods.—The use of high seclusion/restraint for 53 psychiatric inpatients was reviewed for a period of 6 months before and 6 months after a behavioral treatment plan was implemented in a psychiatric hospital.

Results.—After the approved plan was put into practice, a 62% reduction in use of seclusion/restraint occurred. Also, there was a trend of increasing use of seclusion/restraint in the 6 months before development of the plan, and a trend of decreasing use in the 6 months after development of the plan.

Discussion.—This administrative procedure designed to initiate a formal behavioral consultation for psychiatric inpatients likely to require seclusion or restraint is described. Implications of these results for health care workers in psychiatric inpatient facilities are discussed.

▶ One of the most difficult aspects of psychiatric inpatient work is the implementation of procedures for secluding patients. Donat clearly demonstrates that when a mandatory behavioral consultation was required after seclusion or restraint was ordered, and when a behavioral treatment plan resulted from such a consultation, there was a significant reduction in the need for seclusion and restraint. With increasingly short lengths of inpatient stay and increasingly disturbed inpatients, such an approach is to be recommended to all those doing a significant amount of inpatient work.

A. Tasman, M.D.

Comorbid Panic Disorder and Major Depression: Implications for Cognitive-Behavioral Therapy
McLean PD, Woody S, Taylor S, et al (Univ of British Columbia, Canada; Yale Univ, New Haven, Conn; Vancouver Hosp and Health Science Centre, British Columbia, Canada)
J Consult Clin Psychol 66:240–247, 1998   2–23

Background.—Cognitive-behavioral treatment has been shown to be effective for panic disorder and for major depression. There have been few studies of comorbid panic disorder and major depression, though these 2 conditions often occur together. Individuals with these coexisting disorders are reported to have more severe symptoms than individuals with a single disorder. The effect of preexisting comorbidity of major depression on the outcome of cognitive-behavioral treatment for panic disorder was evaluated.

Methods.—There were 37 patients with comorbid panic disorder and major depression who attended 10 sessions of individual cognitive-behavioral therapy for panic disorder. The outcome was compared to the outcome of 53 individuals with panic disorder only who also attended 10 sessions of individual cognitive-behavioral therapy.

Results.—Analysis showed that the outcome of cognitive-behavioral treatment for panic disorder was not adversely affected by the co-occurrence of major depression. Improvements were similar in patients with comorbid depression and those with panic disorder alone on all measures of anxiety. Depression did not become worse during treatment for panic disorder.

Discussion.—These findings may have implications for treatment planning for patients with comorbid panic disorder and major depression, though clinicians should be careful about generalizing these results. Future research should address the number of sessions that may be required to bring patients with single and comorbid diagnoses into remission.

▶ Thus far, there has been little in the literature about treatment for comorbid disorders, yet it is well known that panic disorder and depression coexist in a significant number of patients. The findings of this study, that cognitive-behavioral therapy for panic did not improve depressive symptoms, is well worth noting. As the relationship between depression and panic is not yet clarified on biological nor psychological grounds, it is important for the clinician to be aware that treatment geared toward relieving panic symptoms will likely have little impact on improvement of depressive symptomatology.

A. Tasman, M.D.

Cognitive-Behavioral Treatment for Depression: Relapse Prevention
Gortner ET, Gollan JK, Dobson KS, et al (Univ of Washington, Seattle; Univ of Calgary, Alta, Canada)
J Consult Clin Psychol 66:377–384, 1998   2–24

Introduction.—Two-year follow-up data of a comparative study of complete cognitive-behavioral treatment of depression, and of behavioral activation and behavioral activation with automatic thought modification, are presented. The potential of each of these 3 treatments for preventing relapse was determined.

Methods.—There were 137 participants assigned to 1 of 3 treatments for a maximum of 20 sessions with a cognitive-behavioral therapist. Relapse rates, number of asymptomatic or minimally symptomatic weeks, and survival time to first relapse were evaluated at 6, 12, 18, and 24 months.

Results.—There were no significant differences in relapse rates among treatment groups at 24 months. The number of well weeks was also similar among the 3 groups, as were survival times to first relapse.

Discussion.—The long-term outcomes of cognitive-behavioral treatment, behavioral activation, and behavioral activation with automatic thought modification for depression are similar. Patients with the 3 treatment conditions were nearly identical on measures of recovery, relapse rates, number of well weeks, and survival time to first relapse. Comprehensive cognitive-behavioral treatment of depression was no more effective in preventing relapse than its component parts. The implications of these findings for clinicians are discussed.

► This is an interesting study in which the authors attempted to isolate 2 components of cognitive-behavioral therapy in an attempt to discern whether or not the therapeutic action of this kind of treatment could be explained by either component. They found that comprehensive cognitive-behavioral therapy was no more effective in preventing relapse than either of the components tested. However, there was no control group, and this raises concerns about the ability to generalize the results of this study. The more important issue—how to minimize relapse even further—was not addressed in great detail by this study.

A. Tasman, M.D.

Cognitive-Behavioral Treatment for Depression in Alcoholism
Brown RA, Evans DM, Miller IW, et al (Butler Hosp–Brown Univ, Providence, RI)
J Consult Clin Psychol 65:715–726, 1997　　　　　　　　　　　　　2–25

Background.—Community and clinical data have shown a strong association between depression and alcoholism. Comorbid depression has been associated with poorer outcome after treatment for alcoholism. Depressed mood may also be a significant cause of alcoholic relapse. There is little information on the use of cognitive-behavioral treatment for depression in alcoholism.

Methods.—There were 35 patients with alcoholism and a depressive symptoms score of 10 or higher on the Beck Depression Inventory. Ten of the patients were women, and the mean age of all patients was 38 years. Nineteen patients were assigned to 8 individual sessions of cognitive-behavioral treatment for depression, and 16 patients were assigned to relaxation training control. All patients received standard alcohol treatment.

Results.—During treatment, patients who had cognitive-behavioral treatment showed greater reductions in somatic depressive symptoms, as well as in depressed and anxious mood, than did patients who had relaxation training control. The percentage of days abstinent was greater in patients who received cognitive-behavioral treatment than in those who had relaxation training control, but overall abstinence or fewer drinks per day at 3 months was not. Between 3 and 6 months, the patients who received cognitive-behavioral treatment had significantly better alcohol-use outcomes on measures of total abstinence, percentage of days abstinent, and drinks per day than the other group.

Discussion.—These results show that the combination of standard alcohol treatment and cognitive-behavioral treatment for depression was more effective than relaxation training control in reducing depressive symptoms and improving drinking outcome in individuals with alcoholism and increased depressive symptoms. The patients gained a better understanding of their depression and factors affecting their mood, and saw the depression coping skills they learned as useful to their recovery from alcoholism. Clinical implications of using cognitive-behavioral treatment for depression in individuals with alcoholism are discussed.

▶ Here is another study that looks at the use of cognitive-behavioral therapy in comorbidity. In this case, the comorbidity is between alcoholism and depression. The authors found that the use of cognitive-behavioral treatment was correlated with significantly better ability of patients to abstain from alcohol and stay abstinent. In addition, when cognitive-behavior therapy for depression was used, there was improvement in the symptoms of depression as well as in long-term follow-up success regarding the alcoholism. Although further study is needed, cognitive-behavioral therapy for comorbid alcohol and depression seems to be useful in treating the symptoms of both illnesses.

A. Tasman, M.D.

Prediction of Outcome and Early vs. Late Improvement in OCD Patients Treated With Cognitive Behaviour Therapy and Pharmacotherapy
de Haan E, van Oppen P, van Balkom AJLM, et al (Reinier de Graafgasthuis, Delft, The Netherlands; Vrije Universiteit Amsterdam; Leiden Univ, The Netherlands; et al)
Acta Psychiatr Scand 96:354–361, 1997   2–26

Introduction.—In the treatment of obsessive-compulsive disorders, numerous studies have shown that behavior therapy and serotonergic antidepressants are effective; however, about half of the patients do not respond. It would be useful to find the factors that could predict who are the nonresponders. Factors that can predict results of cognitive-behavior therapy and a combination of cognitive-behavior therapy with a serotonergic antidepressant were examined.

Methods.—Ninety-nine patients were treated for 16 weeks and followed up 6 months later. The patients had obsessive-compulsive disorders for at least 1 year and were between the ages of 18 and 65 years. Treatment was completed by 70 patients, and 61 were available for follow-up. Treatment consisted of cognitive therapy, exposure and response prevention, and fluvoxamine with either cognitive therapy or exposure and response prevention.

Results.—At both posttreatment measurements and at follow-up, significant time effects were found on all outcome measures. The efficacy of the 2 treatment modalities did not differ. Follow-up success appeared to be predicted by effectiveness at posttreatment measurement. At the posttreatment measurement, there were 45 nonresponders; of these, 17 had turned into responders by the 6-month follow-up. Treatment outcome appeared to be predicted by the severity of symptoms, motivation for treatment, and the dimensional score on the PDQ-R for cluster A personality disorder. Predictors that were related specifically to combined treatment or to cognitive-behavior treatment could not be found.

Conclusions.—The effectiveness of combination cognitive-behavior therapy and fluvoxamine or of cognitive-behavior therapy alone was maintained at follow-up. At posttreatment, nonresponse does not always mean there will not be a response by the 6-month follow-up. For patients with more severe symptoms, a longer period of therapy was needed for them to become responders. No evidence was found to determine which treatment modality would be successful, but predictors for treatment success were found.

▶ The next important themes of psychotherapy research will include studies such as this, which investigate the interaction between psychotherapeutic and psychopharmacologic interventions in a number of disorders. Another important finding in this study, although not intended, was the need for long-term treatment in patients with obsessive-compulsive disorder. A number of patients who did not respond at the end of the 16-week course of treatment responded when further treatment was prescribed. We need many more studies of the impact of long-term treatment to complement the many studies of short-term therapy now in the literature.

A. Tasman, M.D.

Controlled Acute and Follow-up Trial of Cognitive Therapy and Pharmacotherapy in Out-patients With Recurrent Depression
Blackburn IM, Moore RG (Newcastle Cognitive and Behavioural Therapies Centre, England; Univ of Cambridge, England)
Br J Psychiatry 171:328–334, 1997   2–27

Introduction.—Many previous studies have shown that (1) cognitive therapy is at least as effective as antidepressant medication in the treatment of outpatients with major unipolar depression; (2) the relative efficacy of cognitive therapy and medication for more severe depression is controvertible; (3) the combination of antidepressants and cognitive therapy may be somewhat superior to either treatment on its own; and (4) cognitive therapy has a long-term or prophylactic effect. The role of cognitive therapy was examined in the prevention of relapse and recurrence of depression. The acute and maintenance stages of treatment were examined.

Methods.—A total of 75 outpatients with recurrent major depression were randomly assigned to 1 of 3 treatment groups: 16 weeks of acute treatment and 2 years of maintenance treatment with antidepressants; cognitive therapy and maintenance cognitive therapy; and antidepressants and maintenance cognitive therapy.

Results.—All patients improved significantly in the acute phase of treatment, with no significant difference among the treatments. No difference was found in the pattern of improvement over time. In all 3 groups, patients kept improving over time in the maintenance stage of treatment.

Among the treatments, there was no significant difference. Medication was consistently inferior to cognitive therapy.

Conclusions.—In these depressed patients, maintenance medication and maintenance cognitive therapy had similar prophylactic effects. For maintenance after acute treatment with medication, cognitive therapy is a viable option. In addition, short-term cognitive therapy was as effective as antidepressants prescribed at therapeutic doses. These results were based on relatively small numbers. Compliance with medication was not objectively measured. There was a wide variation in the number of recurring episodes, and more restricted criteria of recurrence may be more informative.

▶ As noted in the previous comments, the need for studies of maintenance or long-term treatment are much needed. This report of patients followed for 2 years of maintenance treatment following a 4-month acute treatment phase demonstrated the therapeutic effectiveness of maintenance cognitive therapy in preventing depression relapse. The study suggests that cognitive therapy may be an important maintenance treatment, making the need for long-term medication use lower in some patients. Clearly, this is an important issue that needs much further study, but these preliminary results are interesting.

A. Tasman, M.D.

Effects of Adding Behavioral Treatment to Opioid Detoxification With Buprenorphine

Bickel WK, Amass L, Higgins ST, et al (Univ of Vermont, Burlington)
J Consult Clin Psychol 65:803–810, 1997   2–28

Introduction.—The prevalence of heroin and other opioid dependencies appears to be escalating, which has led to calls for expansion of treatment services. Detoxification, however, has a documented lack of efficacy. Buprenorphine is a partial µ-opioid agonist that has been investigated as a replacement medication for opioid dependence, but it has also resulted in a poor outcome. It has been suggested that outpatient opioid detoxification is more than a function of pharmacotherapy and that efficacy can be improved by combining pharmacotherapy with psychosocial interventions. Whether behavioral treatment improves outcome was determined during a 26-week outpatient opioid detoxification.

Methods.—A total of 39 opioid-dependent adults were randomly assigned to 1 of 2 groups: buprenorphine dose-taper combined with either behavioral treatment or standard treatment. The behavioral treatment included the community reinforcement approach, a multicomponent behavior treatment, and a voucher incentive program for providing opioid-free urine samples and engaging in verifiable therapeutic activities. Lifestyle counseling comprised the standard treatment.

Results.—Treatment was completed by 53% of patients receiving behavioral treatment compared with 20% of those receiving standard treatment. For the behavioral group, 4 weeks of continuous opioid abstinence was achieved by 68%; 8 weeks of abstinence was achieved by 47%; 12 weeks of abstinence was achieved by 26%; and 16 weeks of abstinence was achieved by 11%. For the standard group, 4 weeks of continuous opioid abstinence was achieved by 55%; 8 weeks, by 15%; 12 weeks, by 5%; and none of the patients achieved 16 weeks of abstinence.

Conclusions.—During outpatient detoxification, behavioral treatment improved outcomes. Detoxification outcomes can be modified, although the magnitude of the effect was modest. For the development of a comprehensive approach to drug abuse treatment, the pursuit of combined behavioral and pharmacologic interventions is important.

▶ Here is another study that looks at the impact of combined psychotherapeutic and pharmacologic treatment. In this case, the authors look at patients who are undergoing opioid detoxification with medication. The addition of behavior treatment clearly improved outcomes on several parameters during the course of treatment. This study lends support to a comprehensive approach that includes both psychosocial and psychopharmacologic interventions in patients with substance abuse. This will probably not come as much of a surprise to those who work a great deal with substance-abusing patients.

A. Tasman, M.D.

Eye Movement Desensitization

Flooding Versus Eye Movement Desensitization and Reprocessing Therapy: Relative Efficacy Has Yet to Be Investigated: Comment on Pitman et al. (1996)
Cahill SP, Frueh BC (State Univ of New York, Binghamton; Med Univ of South Carolina, Charleston; Veterans Affairs Med Ctr, Charleston, SC)
Compr Psychiatry 38:300–303, 1997   2–29

Introduction.—The relationship between indicators of emotional processing and outcome for therapist-directed imaginal flooding and eye movement desensitization and reprocessing therapy (EMDR) in the treatment of combat-related posttraumatic stress disorder (PTSD) was studied in a pair of companion studies by Pitman et al. In the treatment of chronic combat-related PTSD, they argued for the use of EMDR in a second study.

Assertions.—They argued that EMDR was less anxiety provoking for patients and therapists, was better tolerated, and produced fewer adverse consequences than flooding. They also asserted that it was at least as effective as flooding.

Reservations.—There was a nonrandom assignment of participants to treatment conditions. Between the 2 studies, several significant procedural differences existed, as well as the specific treatments under investigation. There were different inclusion and exclusion criteria. There were differences in assessment procedures and confounding of psychological treatment with psychiatric medication status. Because the 2 treatments were not compared in a single head-to-head controlled trial, their relative efficacy has yet to be investigated.

Conclusions.—If Pitman et al. had not attempted to establish the effectiveness of 1 treatment over the other, none of this criticism would be warranted. For evaluating the relationship between indicators of emotional processing and outcome after treatment, their studies are appropriately designed and well executed and produced interesting results.

▶ EMDR has been controversial since its introduction. This article suggests that previous work asserting the effectiveness of EMDR therapy for patients with PTSD is not warranted because of methodologic concerns. One would hope that the authors of the previous study (Abstract 2–28) would address these.

A. Tasman, M.D.

Eye Movement Desensitization and Reprocessing Treatment for Panic Disorder: A Controlled Outcome and Partial Dismantling Study
Feske U, Goldstein AJ (Agoraphobia and Anxiety Treatment Ctr, Bala Cynwyd, Pa; Temple Univ, Philadelphia)
J Consult Clin Psychol 65:1026–1035, 1997   2–30

Introduction.—Although eye movement desensitization and reprocessing (EMDR) was developed initially as a treatment for traumatic memories, it has since been used for various disorders, especially anxiety disorders other than posttraumatic stress disorder. In previous studies, EMDR was more beneficial than a no-treatment control. The importance of the eye movement was examined in a randomized controlled trial with a larger treatment dose than in previous studies, by comparing the effectiveness of EMDR with that of the same treatment but without the eye movement—otherwise known as eye fixation exposure and reprocessing.

Methods.—There were 43 patients with a *Diagnostic and Statistical Manual of Mental Disorders* III-R diagnosis of primary panic disorder. They were randomly assigned to receive 6 sessions of EMDR, to a waiting list, or to eye fixation exposure and reprocessing. The outcome measures were the Agoraphobic Cognitions Questionnaire and Body Sensations Questionnaire to assess thoughts concerning catastrophic consequences of anxiety and fear of physical sensations; the Mobility Inventory for Agoraphobia to assess avoidance of situations; the Beck Anxiety Inventory to assess clinical anxiety; and the Panic Appraisal Inventory to assess panic attacks in agoraphobic situations.

Results.—Eye movement desensitization and reprocessing was more effective than the waiting-list procedure in alleviating panic and panic-related symptoms. It also led to greater improvement on 2 of 5 primary outcome measures at posttest than eye fixation exposure and reprocessing. Three months after treatment, eye movement's advantages had dissipated.

Conclusions.—The usefulness of the eye movement component in this type of therapy was not firmly supported for treating panic disorder. There is initial support for EMDR in treating panic disorder with agoraphobia. However, it should not be the first-line treatment for this severe anxiety disorder until it is shown to be as effective as exposure and cognitive-behavior therapy.

▶ This study shows that in a short-term follow-up, after EMDR therapy use for patients with panic disorder, any treatment benefit seems to disappear. This study raises significant questions about the long-term benefits of this treatment approach in these patients.

A. Tasman, M.D.

Fifteen-month Follow-up of Eye Movement Desensitization and Reprocessing (EMDR) Treatment for Posttraumatic Stress Disorder and Psychological Trauma
Wilson SA, Becker LA, Tinker RH (The Spencer-Curtis Found, Colorado Springs, Colo; Univ of Colorado, Colorado Springs)
J Consult Clin Psychol 65:1047–1056, 1997   2–31

Introduction.—Limited information is available about the long-term effectiveness of eye movement desensitization and reprocessing (EMDR) or other psychological interventions for posttraumatic stress disorder (PTSD). Maintenance of treatment effects has been found with follow-up periods of 1–3 months. In using interventions other than EMDR for PTSD, the controlled outcome research has shown maintenance of treatment effects for up to 6 months. The effects of EMDR was investigated at 15 months after treatment on the functioning of participants with PTSD.

Methods.—Of the 66 participants, 32 had received a diagnosis of PTSD. They received EMDR therapy. The outcome measures were impact of event scale; state-trait anxiety inventory; symptom checklist; PTSD interview; and subjective units of disturbance scale, a self-report measure of the degree of disturbance experienced while thinking about a particular traumatic event. They received three 90-minute sessions of EMDR.

Results.—There was equal improvement among those with PTSD and those without the disorder. The gains were maintained by both groups at 15 months. There was an 84% reduction of PTSD diagnosis and a 68% reduction in PTSD symptoms at the 15-month follow-up. None of the participants were reliably worsened by this therapy.

Conclusions.—There was an average treatment effect size of 1.59, and an average reliable change index of 3.37. The study results provide encouraging evidence of the durability of EMDR effects on a civilian sample of chronically traumatized adults. Eye movement therapy may be less aversive than exposure therapies, but for some individuals, eye movement therapy did not result in complete treatment.

▶ In contrast to the previous study (Abstract 2–30), this research project showed a remarkably positive response when EMDR therapy was used in patients with PTSD. Unfortunately, because the findings in the few research projects that have been published in EMDR are so disparate, it is difficult to make clinical recommendations regarding the use of EMDR until further research clarifies matters.

A. Tasman, M.D.

Schizophrenia

Effectiveness of Attention Training in Schizophrenia

Medalia A, Aluma M, Tryon W, et al (Montefiore Med Ctr, Bronx, New York; Fordham Univ, Bronx, New York)
Schizophr Bull 24:147–152, 1998
2–32

Introduction.—On tasks that require vigilance, quick responses, or sustained attention, patients with schizophrenia have been shown to perform poorly. During episodes of active psychosis as well as during periods of remission, these deficits are evident. Maladaptive functioning correlates with attention impairments. Treatment efforts should be directed toward the rehabilitation of these deficits, given the impact of attention deficits on psychosocial adjustment and cognitive functioning. The impact of attention training on information processing in schizophrenia was assessed.

Methods.—After baseline assessment with the Continuous Performance Test, 54 inpatients with chronic schizophrenia, aged 20–45, were randomly assigned to 1 of 2 groups. The control group participated in individual sessions during which they viewed video documentaries. The experimental group participated in individual sessions of computerized attention remediation. The computer program contained 5 modules: attention reaction conditioner, zeroing accuracy conditioner, visual discrimination conditioner, time estimates, and rhythm synchrony conditioner.

Results.—Patients in the experimental group made significantly more improvement than the control group after 18 sessions, according to reassessment with the Continuous Performance Test. The control group made no significant change. Both groups improved on the total score of Psychiatric Rating Scale Assessments that were made before and after the study phase. Significantly more improvement, however, was made by the experimental group.

Conclusions.—To remediate a core attention deficit in chronic schizophrenia, it is feasible to use practice and behavioral learning. More research is needed to determine whether significant changes on tests of attention are paralleled by changes in ability to sustain focus on vocational tasks. Systematic cognitive rehabilitation may become a cardinal aspect of treatment of schizophrenia, much like it is in treating traumatic brain injury.

▶ For several years authors have suggested the use of attention training for patients with schizophrenia as an attempt to deal with what has been hypothesized to be a core deficit related to the pathophysiology of schizophrenia. This is another study demonstrating that attention training can be used with positive benefit in patients with schizophrenia.

A. Tasman, M.D.

Comprehensive Countertransference and Comprehensive Treatment for the Schizophrenic Patient: The Psychotherapeutic Heart of Mutative Treatment
Feinsilver DB (Chesnut Lodge Hosp, Rockville, Md)
Psychiatry 60:248–261, 1997   2–33

Introduction.—Therapists can get caught up in a schizophrenic patient's confusing, emotionally fragmenting dichotomizing process. They must see patients as people who can benefit from interpretation of underlying conflict and from medication, rather than from just 1 of these treatments. Therapists must be on guard against viewing any treatment of the patient as the "be-all-and-end-all" answer. By attending to the therapist's countertransference in the comprehensive sense, an awareness of this parallel will be created. For schizophrenic patients, this can serve as a guide to comprehensive, mutative treatment.

Clinical Vignette.—A patient with a sleeping problem was about to move from an inpatient unit to a supervised living situation. She called the therapist for something to help her sleep. The therapist noticed he was angry that his prescription of medications was not the "be-all-and-end-all" solution for the patient. The patient previously confessed that she could not sleep because she wished she were married to a man who would always be with her, and it seemed she was hinting that she wished the therapist would play that role. When the therapist recognized his anger, he was able to call her back and curb his tendency to react angrily. Subsequent sessions were dedicated to addressing this separation anxiety.

Results.—Because the therapist did not react with a further fragmenting, dichotomized response, siding either with the medication or interpretation, the patient benefited. The therapist responded by encouraging both aspects to survive integratively as enduring aspects of the treatment. By recognizing a patient's need for a perfect solution, the therapist can use this identification to rise to the occasion and overcome the frustration and deliver the combination of support and clarification of conflict that the patient needs.

Conclusions.—Awareness of comprehensive countertransference can illuminate a therapist's counteridentification with what is frustrating the patient at the moment of great urgency. This recognition would enable the therapist to target interventions that would integrate various aspects of treatment to benefit the patient.

► This article and the 1 that follows (Abstracts 2–33 and 2–34) review the role of fairly traditional psychoanalytic psychotherapeutic approaches in the treatment of patients with schizophrenia. Since the advent of psychopharmacologic interventions and the rise of rehabilitative psychosocial treatment approaches, the use of psychoanalytic psychotherapy has drastically declined in treatment of patients with schizophrenia. This decline was reinforced by studies that showed that a traditional psychoanalytic approach often produced a worsening of symptoms in schizophrenic patients. Dr. Feinsilver presents a view based on significant clinical wisdom that may be useful in a small, well-selected subgroup of patients with schizophrenia.

A. Tasman, M.D.

Romantic and Classic Visions in the Therapy of Psychosis: A Personal Perspective and Evolving Theory of Schizophrenia
Kafka JS (George Washington Univ, DC)
Psychiatry 60:262–274, 1997   2–34

Introduction.—Psychoanalytic visions and literary and philosophical romantic and classic visions have autonomy as a common value, with autonomy being an individual's recognition that he is an aspect of the general structure of reality and in submission to the laws of the whole. It has also been defined as an individual's ability to attain his own subjective truth. A romantic vision of therapists is that no human being is so different from us as to be inaccessible, incomprehensible, permanently isolated, and unresponsive, so if only a therapist's efforts to make contact are heroic enough, the patient's suffering and isolation would be alleviated.

Narrow Focus.—A patient was viewed not as a victim in the family drama but as an actor in its transactions. The romantic-classic framework sees the individual with a longitudinal life-history approach, whereas the cross-sectional view focuses on a patient's symptoms at a given moment, which can lead to the disorder being diagnosed differently at various cross-sectional points. When the focus is too narrow, the heterogeneity of schizophrenia may be ignored and may discourage inference, formulation of theory, and abstract conceptualization.

Theories.—In some European countries, interpersonal therapeutic approaches to schizophrenia are currently widely practiced. There is a great tendency among therapists to negate or minimize the differences between themselves and those of the patient, which must be recognized. There are dangers in overextending and underextending theories in treating schizophrenics. The unitary theory, which is congruent with a romantic vision, asserts a continuity between schizophrenic and neurotic behaviors and considers intrapsychic conflict and defense as primary determiners of schizophrenic behavior. The specific theory focuses on a deficiency in mental representation.

Conclusion.—In this age of cost-effectiveness, many hospitals are using new antipsychotic medications. There is less focus on individual psychotherapy now, as medication, residential care, social therapies, and rehabilitation are increasingly emphasized. The development of a tolerance of the ambiguity inherent in the tension of "experiencing ourselves from within and to reflect about ourselves from without" is a treatment goal. A central issue in schizophrenia was described as the need for and the fear of closeness. It also addresses extreme individualism that cuts off contacts with others or that leads to total merging and dissolution of the self.

▶ Dr. Kafka, like Feinsilver, (Abstract 2–33), argues that there is still a role in selected situations for a psychoanalytic psychotherapeutic approach in the care of patients with schizophrenia. Whether one believes that such a psychotherapeutic approach should be a part of a treatment plan, Dr. Kafka's insights regarding the nature of the psychological struggles experienced by patients with schizophrenia are well worth reading and considering.

A. Tasman, M.D.

Treatment Research

Toward a More Clinically Valid Approach to Therapy Research
Goldfried MR, Wolfe BE (State Univ of New York, Stony Brook; American Schools of Professional Psychology, Virgina Campus)
J Consult Clin Psychol 66:143–150, 1998   2–35

Introduction.—The current state of the art for conducting psychotherapy outcome research and conclusions about intervention procedures are presented. There has been controversy surrounding the attempt to arrive at a consensus by which therapies have been validated or supported. In light of current pressures for the accountability of psychotherapy, research designs must have external or clinical validity, particularly because insurance companies are interested in the effectiveness of intervention methods. Concerns are expressed about medicalization of outcome research, use of random assignment of clients to treatment conditions, use of a fixed number of sessions, the nature of the therapy manuals used, and the use of theoretically pure therapies.

Medicalization.—The National Institute of Mental Health required that the same standards used in pharmacotherapy research be used in the evaluation of psychotherapies. The use of *Diagnostic and Statistical Manual of Mental Disorders* diagnoses became required in outcome studies, which provided the field with consistency. Drug therapies were also providing evidence of symptomatic benefits for a number of specific disorders. Mental illness began to be viewed from the biologic perspective. By focusing on *Diagnostic and Statistical Manual of Mental Disorders* diagnoses, constraints were felt in questions concerning clinical problems, such as examination anxiety and unassertiveness.

Other therapies.—The practice of randomly assigning patients to the different therapy conditions became commonplace in research. There are problems with the heterogeneity of some of the diagnostic categories, such as depression, which may have a variety of causes. A fixed number of sessions is another methodologic advance that accommodates practical and financial concerns, but the danger always exists that the length of the intervention may not be enough to solve the clinical problem. The use of treatment manuals is another feature in the current state of the art in psychotherapy outcome, but following a manual does not guarantee the quality of therapy provided and may at times constrain clinical practice. The use of theoretically pure therapies is at odds with clinicians who often use different theoretical approaches to increase clinical effectiveness.

Conclusion.—Steps should be taken to foster a more productive collaboration between clinician and researcher, study theoretically integrated interventions, make greater use of replicated clinical case studies, use process research findings to improve therapy manuals, find a better way of disseminating research findings to the practicing clinician, and focus on less heterogeneous, dimensionalized clinical problems.

▶ One of the ongoing frustrations in all areas of research is the difficulty in translating research advances into clinical practice. Nowhere has this been more an issue than in psychotherapy research. These authors review a number of factors that contribute to this problem, including the understandable emphasis, within research, on standardizing treatments so they can be studied. Obviously, when dealing with individuals in the clinical situation, such constraints do not often hold sway when the clinical needs of the patient demand flexibility. Goldfried and Wolfe outline a number of approaches that, if implemented, would help remedy the present situation.

A. Tasman, M.D.

Behavioral Self-control Program for Windows: Results of a Controlled Clinical Trial
Hester RK, Delaney HD (Univ of New Mexico)
J Consult Clin Psychol 65:686–693, 1997   2–36

Background.—Behavioral self-control training (BSCT) is a well-established treatment for alcohol problems, particularly in patients with less severe drinking-related problems of a shorter duration. Instructional methods based on personal computers have been effective in treating agoraphobia, simple phobias, mild depression, and smoking. This study examined whether a computer-based program of BSCT would have an effect on moderating drinking behaviors of early-stage problem drinkers.

Methods.—The study involved 40 heavy drinkers (24 men and 16 women; mean age, 36.3) who were not alcoholics (8 or more on the Alcohol Use Disorders Identification Test but 19 or less on the Michigan Alcoholism Screening Test) and who completed at least 3 treatment sessions. A BSCT program was developed for Windows that taught goal setting, self-monitoring, how to control the rate of drinking, how to refuse drinks, behavioral contracting with rewards and penalties, how to evaluate and resolve triggers for overdrinking, how to prevent relapse, and the functional analysis of drinking.

The program gave each user feedback and allowed the patient to set drinking goals and to monitor drinking behaviors. The program appeared to be easy to learn and required 5–15 minutes of instruction. The patients were evenly divided into 1 group that received immediate computer instruction for 10 weeks and 1 group that received delayed computer instruction during weeks 11 to 20 of the study. Their status, including blood alcohol concentrations, was assessed before treatment and at 10, 20, and 52 weeks thereafter.

Findings.—At 10 weeks, patients receiving immediate instruction drank significantly fewer drinks and had significantly greater declines in blood alcohol content than the patients who had not yet received instruction. At 20 weeks, the patients in the immediate instruction group had not changed their new behavior significantly. However, patients who received delayed instruction had significantly fewer drinks and significantly greater declines in blood alcohol content compared with the immediate instruction group. The significant improvements in both groups were also evident at 12 months. At 1 year, 24 of 37 patients (65%) consumed less than 14 drinks/week, and 28 of 37 (76%) had a blood alcohol content of less than 80 mg per week. Gender and ethnicity had no effect on treatment outcomes. Patients who were using other drugs to a moderate extent tended to decrease this use as their alcohol consumption decreased; however, 2 patients with heavy marijuana and methamphetamine use, respectively, either relapsed to heavy drinking or increased drug use after treatment.

Conclusion.—A computer-based BSCT program can significantly influence drinking behaviors in heavy drinkers at 1 year after its completion. Consumption decreased from the equivalent of 6 beers/day before treatment to 3 beers/day afterward. The poor outcomes in patients who used other drugs heavily suggest that self-control training may have limited benefit in such patients.

▶ The field of psychiatry, and most of medicine, is still in its infancy in terms of using computers in designing and implementing treatment programs. Because of psychiatry's emphasis on psychotherapy, our discipline is more likely to take advantage of interactive aspects of computer programs in therapeutic interventions. This small, interesting study showed that such an approach could be useful and is worthy of further inquiry.

A. Tasman, M.D.

Internal Validity of Project MATCH Treatments: Discriminability and Integrity
Carroll KM, Connors GJ, Cooney NL, et al (Yale Univ, New Haven, Conn; Research Inst on Addiction, Buffalo, NY; Univ of Maryland Baltimore County; et al)
J Consult Clin Psychol 66:290–303, 1998   2–37

Background.—Project MATCH (Matching Alcoholism Treatments to Client Heterogeneity) was a multisite clinical trial that treated 1,726 patients (both hospitalized and outpatients) with alcoholism via 12-step facilitation (TSF), cognitive-behavioral coping skills training (CBT), or motivational enhancement therapy (MET). The discriminability and integrity of these treatments and whether other factors confounded results was examined.

Methods.—Treatment manuals were developed for each of the 3 treatment regimens. Manuals focused on each treatment's main mechanism(s) of action and were designed to avoid overlap in those areas. The goals of all 3 treatments were the same: to attain abstinence and to maintain sobriety. To minimize overlap across treatments, the 80 therapists (mean posttraining experience, 6.3 ± 4.5 years) participated in only 1 type of treatment. Therapists underwent a mean of 26 training sessions before they were certified; their performance after training was monitored to keep it constant. Discriminability was measured by numerous factors, including a MATCH Tape Rating Scale (MTRS) that measured the reliability of the items. Exposure to other treatments was assessed by a structured interview. Therapist skillfulness was evaluated by general skill, empathy, and nonverbal behaviors. The therapeutic alliance was assessed by the Working Alliance Inventory. The 19 raters for the MTRS and therapist skillfulness had an average of 9.8 ± 6.6 years of clinical experience.

Findings.—Therapists used the techniques associated with their treatment manual; they used few techniques associated with the other 2 treatments. The main treatment effect accounted for most of the variance in treatment effect in the 3 groups (θ = .94 or .85) and in the outpatient-vs.-inpatient arms of the study (θ = 0.82). Furthermore, MTRS scales for each treatment were significantly higher for that treatment group than for the other 2 groups (e.g., patients in the CBT group had significantly higher CBT scores than patients in the TSF or MET groups). Exposure to non–study interventions was very low and did not differ significantly in the 3 treatment groups, although patients in the TSF group were significantly more likely to attend Alcoholic Anonymous meetings than patients in the CBT or MET groups. Therapist skillfulness was rated "good" across the groups and did not account for much variation in treatment differences; nor did the therapeutic alliance.

Conclusion.—The treatments were discriminable, distinct, and implemented consistently across the study sites. The expected differences between treatment groups were seen (e.g., more patients in the MET group set goals). Other aspects of treatment did not account for much of the variance in treatment effects. Thus, high levels of discriminability and integrity can be obtained in large, multisite trials in which highly trained, skilled therapists dutifully use training manuals developed specifically for the therapeutic intervention used.

▶ Carrying out large scale research that involves matching treatments to specific patient characteristics is difficult. One significant factor is that the need for large patient populations requires the projects to be carried out across multiple sites. This introduces the potential for variability in the way the study is carried out, which would contaminate the results. A long-term project to match alcoholism treatments to patient characteristics has been carried out under the auspices of substance abuse research at Yale University. This study demonstrates that such a multisite study can be carried out and that, although some variability across sites might exist, it does not necessarily interfere with the aims of the ongoing research project. Those exploring the option of setting up multisite psychotherapy research could benefit from an awareness of the issues raised in this article.

A. Tasman, M.D.

When and How Perfectionism Impedes the Brief Treatment of Depression: Further Analyses of the National Institute of Mental Health Treatment of Depression Collaborative Research Program
Blatt SJ, Zuroff DC, Bondi CM, et al (Yale Univ, New Haven, Conn; McGill Univ, Montreal; Univ of Pittsburgh, Pa)
J Consult Clin Psychol 66:423–428, 1998   2–38

Background.—The National Institute of Mental Health's Treatment of Depression Collaborative Research Program (TDCRP) studied 239 patients with severe depression. Results revealed that outcome was significantly associated with the pretreatment levels of perfectionism or self-criticism. A review of the TDCRP data was conducted to examine how perfectionism influences therapy for depression and when, in the course of treatment, perfectionism impedes therapeutic gain.

Methods.—Of the 239 patients (30% men and 70% women; average age, 35 years) with major depressive disorder, 162 completed the TDCRP study with 12 or more treatments over 15 weeks or more. Each patient was interviewed using the Hamilton Rating Scale for Depression and gave a self-report of depression quantified by the Beck Depression Inventory. The patient's general clinical functioning was self-assessed through the Global Adjustment Scale and assessed by the therapist through the Hopkins Symptom Checklist. The therapist also assessed the patient's social functioning by the Social Adjustment Scale. Patients completed the Dysfunctional Attitudes Scale to determine their extent of perfectionism and need for approval. These parameters were assessed at admission and regularly during 18 months of follow-up. Furthermore, both patients and therapists regularly evaluated the success of treatment and the extent of therapeutic gain.

Findings.—The pretreatment need for approval did not correlate significantly with patients', therapists', or clinical evaluators' ratings of clinical condition and therapeutic gain at study termination. However, all 3 assessors reported significantly less therapeutic gain for patients with a high pretreatment perfectionism level, and therapists and clinical evaluators rated the success of treatment significantly lower in patients with high pretreatment levels of perfectionism (P less than 0.10 for patient self-ratings). Furthermore, patients with high pretreatment perfectionism scores were judged by clinical evaluators to be significantly less satisfied with the treatment ($P = 1.17$ for therapist ratings). This association between significantly less satisfaction for perfectionist patients was also evident at 18 months as rated by clinical evaluators and the patients themselves. Perfectionist patients also reported significantly less therapeutic gain at 18 months. Perfectionism × time interactions revealed that pretreatment perfectionism had significant impact on therapeutic gain and success of treatment after 8 weeks of treatment.

Conclusion.—At the end of treatment and after 18 months of follow-up, high pretreatment perfectionism scores were significantly associated with less therapeutic gain, less successful treatment, and less satisfaction with treatment. Perfectionism began to have a negative impact on treatment outcome as early as 8 weeks into the 16-week regimen. Why these negative attitudes developed at that time needs more examination, but the timing may be related to the imminent termination of the study, in that research indicates greater therapeutic gain and satisfaction when treatments are open ended.

▶ This is a retrospective review of data from the National Institute of Mental Health's TDCRP. Blatt and his colleagues attempted to use a patient characteristic as a discriminator in treatment outcome. The variable chosen was perfectionism in the patient. As I mentioned elsewhere in this volume, the quest to develop good treatment-matching protocols, which would match specific treatment interventions with patient characteristics, relies on this type of research being conducted. One would hope for an expansion of these efforts in coming years.

A. Tasman, M.D.

The Benefit of an Insight-oriented and Experiential Approach on Panic and Agoraphobia Symptoms: Results of a Controlled Comparison of Client-centered Therapy Alone and in Combination With Behavioral Exposure
Teusch L, Böhme H, Gastpar M (Univ of Essen, Germany)
Psychother Psychosom 66:293–301, 1997   2–39

Background.—Researchers currently believe that psychodynamic methods are of little benefit in patients with agoraphobia and panic disorder. These authors compared a client-centered treatment (CCT) approach alone and in combination with behavioral exposure to see whether either method proved effective in patients with agoraphobia and panic.

Methods.—Forty inpatients (16 men and 24 women; mean age, 33) with severe panic disorder and agoraphobia were enrolled. Those with psychotic disorders and drug or alcohol dependence were excluded, although subjects did have other anxiety disorders (social phobia, depression, personality disorders). Most had been treated unsuccessfully by antidepressives or neuroleptics; their anxiety had existed for 6–7 years.

Patients were evenly divided for receiving CCT alone or CCT plus exposure therapy (EXP). Patients in the CCT-alone group received individual (once a week) and group (4 times a week) therapy that avoided direct advice, prescriptive interventions, and homework, but did include psychogymnastics or creative elements. Patients in the combined group received CCT in individual (once a week) and group (3 times a week) sessions that also included psychogymnastics and creative elements. They also received exposure training for agoraphobia, including homework. Patients were treated in-hospital over 10–14 weeks, with an option of moving to a day clinic for the last 4 weeks. The Structured Clinical Interview for the *Diagnostic and Statistical Manual of Mental Disorders*, third edition, revised (SCID) (to measure panic), the Hamilton Anxiety Scale (anxiety), the SCID-Fear Survey Schedule (for agoraphobia), and the Hamilton Depression Scale (for depression) were administered at admission; at discharge; and at 3, 6, and 12 months after discharge.

Findings.—All the patients had significant improvements in severity of panic disorder, severity of agoraphobia, anxiety, and depression at discharge. Furthermore, these improvements were significantly greater at 1 year. In patients with severe panic or severe agoraphobia at discharge, these symptoms had disappeared almost completely by 1 year. Changes in effect sizes (mean pretreatment score minus mean posttreatment or follow-up score divided by pretreatment standard deviation) for the 4 symptoms were all at least moderate. Compared with patients receiving CCT alone, patients receiving CCT plus EXP experienced significantly improved agoraphobia at 3 months and a readiness to submit to exposure to phobic situations at discharge and at 6 months. However, there were no statistically significant differences in the change in effect size between the 2 groups at 1 year.

Conclusion.—Although behavioral exposure improved anxiety and agoraphobic symptoms more quickly than CCT alone, by 1 year symptoms of panic, agoraphobia, anxiety, or depression did not differ in the 2 groups. However, CCT produced significant improvements at discharge and even more improvement at 1 year. Thus, a client-centered treatment program can be effective in treating patients with severe panic disorder and agoraphobia.

▶ Clinicians skilled in psychodynamic psychotherapy have been concerned at the paucity of data in the literature using dynamic approaches. The ease of conducting cognitive-behavioral therapy using manualized approaches has led to an explosion of research using this type of therapy. Some have interpreted the lack of similar research using psychodynamic approaches as an indication of a lack of efficacy. These authors attempted to address this issue by comparing psychodynamic approaches with behavioral approaches in patients with panic and agoraphobia. They found no differences in results on long-term follow-up when the 2 treatment groups were compared, indicating that a dynamic approach was just as effective as the other. To adequately compare the utility of dynamic approaches with cognitive-behavioral approaches in a variety of disorders, much more research of this type must be conducted.

A. Tasman, M.D.

Assessment and Treatment of Social Phobia
Antony MM (Univ of Toronto)
Can J Psychiatry 42:826–834, 1997   2–40

Background.—Social phobia affects about 13% of adults at some point in their lives, usually causing moderate to severe functional impairment. It often occurs concomitantly with anxiety disorders, substance abuse, and depression. This makes identification and treatment challenging. The diagnostic approach to social phobia and the pharmacologic and other therapies used to treat this disorder were reviewed.

Diagnosis and Assessment.—The person with social phobia recognizes that fear of embarrassment or anxiety in social situations is excessive and, thus, tends to avoid such situations. This causes substantial distress, functional interference, or both. Social phobia must be distinguished from shyness or performance anxiety, from other mental disorders in which a person avoids social situations (e.g., depression, schizoid personality), and from other disorders that could be causing the anxiety (e.g., eating disorders, or Parkinson's disease in which a person does not shake hands because of a fear that hands that shook would be noticed). The clinical interview, self-report measures such as questionnaires and diaries, and behavioral assessment are the best tools for distinguishing social phobia from other co-morbidities.

Treatments of Social Phobia.—There are 2 approaches to the treatment of social phobia: pharmacotherapy and psychological approaches. The most effective drugs include monoamine oxidase inhibitors (such as phenelzine), reversible inhibitors of monoamine oxidase type A (such as moclobemide and brofaromine), selective serotonin reuptake inhibitors (such as paroxetine, fluoxetine, and sertraline), benzodiazepines (such as alprazolam and clonazepam), β-blockers (such as atenolol), and perhaps buspirone. Moclobemide, one of the most-studied drugs, has been shown to be as effective as phenelzine but with fewer side effects. However, large doses (600 mg/day) of moclobemide are needed, and relapses after the end of treatment are common (up to 88%). Current thinking is that tricyclic and heterocyclic antidepressants such as venlafaxine and nefazodone are not useful in social phobia, but more research is needed.

Cognitive behavior therapy (CBT) has also been used successfully with patients with social phobia. Cognitive behavior therapy usually takes place in a group environment for periods of between 10 and 15 weeks. Cognitive therapy can help these patients create a variety of strategies to change their anxious beliefs. Behavioral therapy involves exposure to a feared situation until the patient no longer feels fear. The least difficult situations are conquered first, then the most difficult ones, and exposures should be prolonged, predictable, and repeated frequently. Furthermore, social skills training can be useful in people whose social phobia has prevented them from developing adequate social skills. Relaxation training can also be useful. Pharmacotherapy and CBT seem to be equally effective in treating social phobia, but studies are underway to determine whether one approach is superior to the other, or whether their combination is superior to each alone.

▶ Antony reviews the literature on treatment approaches for social phobia. He concludes that there is a significant need for research investigating combined psychotherapeutic and pharmacologic treatments to more accurately assess the optimal interventions with social phobia.

A. Tasman, M.D.

Empirically Supported Couple and Family Interventions for Marital Distress and Adult Mental Health Problems
Baucom DH, Shoham V, Mueser KT, et al (Univ of North Carolina, Chapel Hill; Univ of Arizona, Tucson; Dartmouth Univ, Hanover, NH)
J Consult Clin Psychol 66:53–88, 1998   2–41

Introduction.—The past 2 decades have seen an increasing focus on the effectiveness of couples- and family-based interventions for adult mental health problems. The empirical evidence in support of such interventions for the treatment of martial distress and individual adult mental health disorders was reviewed.

Couples' Therapy for Relationship Distress.—Outcome studies suggest that behavioral marital therapy (BMT) and emotion-focused therapy are both efficacious for marital distress. Possibly efficacious treatments include insight-oriented marital therapy, cognitive-behavioral marital therapy, cognitive therapy for couples, and couples' systemic therapy. Providing treatment for distressed couples appears to be a worthwhile activity; comparative studies suggest that insight-oriented approaches may be superior to behavioral interventions at follow-up. For some couples, good long-term results may depend on gaining insight into the reasons for their destructive pattern of interactions. There is currently no way to tell which will be the most appropriate intervention for a specific couple; regardless of treatment, a certain proportion of couples will remain distressed.

Couples-based Interventions for Adult Individual Disorders.—Involving the partner or family in exposure treatment for adult patients with obsessive-compulsive disorder appears to be feasible and effective. This approach may be especially beneficial for patients who need home reinforcement to follow through with prescribed treatment. For patients with agoraphobia, involving the partner in care appears to enhance the benefits of therapy. Measures aimed at improving relationship function may be helpful even when the couple is in no overt relationship distress. There are few data on the relative benefits of marital intervention vs. individual psychotherapy for patients with depression. Some studies suggest that marital therapy may be preferable when the wife is depressed and the couple is maritally distressed. When marital distress is not present, BMT may be preferred.

A number of different interventions may be efficacious for the treatment of female sexual dysfunction: sexual skills training for primary female orgasmic disorders, Masters and Johnson's program for primary and secondary female orgasmic disorders, BMT plus Masters and Johnson's treatment for mixed (secondary) female sexual dysfunctions, and general martial therapy plus orgasm consistency training for hypoactive sexual desire disorders. However, many questions remain unanswered about treatment of sexual dysfunctions, and few studies have examined psychosocial interventions for male sexual dysfunction. There is promising evidence that involving spouses or significant others improves the outcomes of alcoholism treatment. Questions remain about how comprehensive alcoholism treatment programs need to be, and what type of treatment is best for what type of patient. It seems clinically important to address marital patterns related to problem drinking. Several studies have suggested that family treatment approaches can improve the outcomes of schizophrenia. However, few patients have access to such programs.

Discussion.—The empirical evidence regarding couples and family interventions for marital distress and individual adult mental health disorders was reviewed. Many different theoretical approaches have been studied, along with different ways of including the partner or family in treatment: partner-family–assisted interventions, disorder-specific partner-family interventions, and general couples-family therapy. Cross-diagnostic group findings and issues raised in applying efficacy criteria to the various patient populations were specifically reviewed.

▶ This study is worth highlighting because it addresses research in couples and family interventions across a variety of psychiatric disorders. Individual psychotherapy research is difficult enough, but adding a couple or a family to the mix adds variables that have made this type of research much harder. Again, the field could benefit from more research into couples and family therapy in a number of psychiatric disorders.

A. Tasman, M.D.

Education and Supervision

Structuring Training Goals for Psychodynamic Psychotherapy
Goldberg DA (Univ of Connecticut, Farmington)
J Psychother Prac Res 7:10–22, 1998   2–42

Objective.—Despite the extensive literature on education in psychodynamic psychotherapy, there is no concise framework for organizing psychotherapy training programs. A curriculum approach to psychotherapy training will promote more consistent and effective educational methods, defined goals and objects, and concisely described areas and skills. A multiaxial model providing structured educational goals for psychodynamic psychotherapy was described.

The Model.—The model assumes that structured training goals for dynamic psychotherapy will enhance the educational process, and organizes these goals into "developmental categories." The student's educational progression is outlined in discrete "phases of learning." At the same time, the model acknowledges the interaction between and individual variation in skills, knowledge, and behaviors. It is built on a traditional analytic approach, allowing for advances in psychodynamic psychotherapy or connections with approaches such as cognitive or interpersonal therapy. The phases of learning are plotted along a horizontal axis and the developmental categories along a vertical axis. The learning process is successive; the student achieves basic competence in areas within one phase before moving onto the next.

Phases of Learning.—The proposed learning sequence moves from directly observable phenomena to concepts more difficult to understand and integrate. The first phase is observation and description, emphasizing skills basic to psychotherapy: the student's capacity to observe, collect clinical data, and describe his findings. This phase emphasizes consensual validation by teachers and peers over theoretical framework. The second phase is conceptualization, which provides a framework to explain the process of psychotherapy and to help make intervention decisions. This phase, which includes analytic therapy and a psychodynamic view of behavior, promotes a shift from observable phenomena to abstract understanding. The third phase is synthesis, focusing on more complete integration of previously learned skills, knowledge, and behaviors. The student learns to view recurrent behaviors and themes in terms of the therapeutic relationship, psychodynamic formations, and the patient's life history, with an increasing focus on interactions between resistance, transference, and thematic interpretations and their role in interventions.

Developmental Categories.—Five developmental categories are identified, consistent with accepted fundamentals of psychotherapy. Specific learning tasks related to the phases of learning apply to each of the categories. The first category is boundaries, roles, and goals, which define the framework, expectations, and purposes of psychotherapy. The second category, participants, includes key aspects of training such as the life history; in-depth description of behavior; dynamic formulations; introspection; the working alliance; and dealing with transference, countertransference, and resistance. The third category is verbal flow, emphasizing patient communication and the therapist's ability to recognize emerging themes. Technique, the fourth category, comprises knowledge about the theory of therapy and such technical skills as questioning, responding, and interpreting. The final category is analytic theory, emphasizing the basic theory essential and appropriate for each phase of learning.

Discussion.—This model presents an organized, integrated approach to training in psychodynamic psychotherapy. The proposed approach aids program directors in developing the curriculum, students in focusing their learning process, and supervisors in linking their individual teaching to the goals of the program. The model can help to make psychotherapy programs more consistent, clearer, and more efficient.

▶ The need for greater specificity in delineating training goals in psychotherapy education has long been recognized. Dr. Goldberg's approach, honed during years when we were colleagues in the department of Psychiatry at the University of Connecticut, provides a useful framework for psychodynamic psychotherapy education. Work like this helps us to focus on the need to be more clearly define what we wish to teach, to be more thoughtful about the appropriate sequence to teach the subject material, and to develop our ability to assess whether students have learned what it is that we are trying to teach. Such a process will undoubtedly produce better trained psychotherapists and better educators of psychotherapy.

A. Tasman, M.D.

Responsibilities of the Psychotherapy Supervisor
Whitman SM, Jacobs EG (Med College of Pennsylvania, Philadelphia)
Am J Psychother 52:166–175, 1998   2–43

Background.—The supervisor of psychotherapy is not merely an observer of the process; that person is a participant. The supervisor's responsibilities to the supervisee, to the patient, to the training program, and to the profession as well as to himself or herself were reviewed.

Responsibilities to the Supervisee.—The supervisor's goal is to help the supervisee develop professional values and knowledge. The supervisor must balance direct suggestions regarding what to do with encouraging the supervisee to explore new ideas and approaches. Personal psychotherapy with a person other than the supervisor can help the supervisee's development and should be encouraged. Supervisors must also help supervisees better understand their patients and recognize and deal with countertransference issues.

Responsibilities to the Patient.—The patient and the therapist enter into a therapy agreement in which the patient expects a satisfactory treatment. The supervisor must be ready to confront the supervisee if the treatment goals are not being met or if the therapeutic situation is unsatisfactory. However, the supervisor must be aware of the possible consequences of such a confrontation and should explore with the supervisee the issues leading to a confrontation. The supervisor must balance patient satisfaction with letting supervisees try out their own ideas and learn by trial and error when possible.

Responsibilities to the Training Program and to the Profession.—Supervisees need to know how they are doing, and regular evaluations by the supervisor provide necessary feedback. Evaluations may uncover issues relating to a lack of knowledge, cultural differences, one's own emotional responses, and countertransference. Furthermore, regular evaluations of the supervisors are beneficial because supervisors are role models. Supervisors should discuss educational techniques, supervisory techniques, and supervisory problems with other supervisors to share their experiences.

Responsibilities to the Supervisor.—The supervisor must keep up-to-date, not only regarding new knowledge, but also regarding one's own strengths and weaknesses as they relate to supervising. The supervisor's style and actions directly influence the supervisor-supervisee relationship and ultimately the therapy the patient receives. Furthermore, supervisors should keep current regarding relevant laws and their legal responsibilities and document important issues that arise during therapy.

▶ It is gratifying to see that a former resident of mine (Dr. Sarah Whitman) has focused her academic attention on the need to clarify the role and responsibility of the psychotherapy supervisor. Because the psychotherapy supervisor still plays the central role in transmitting the body of knowledge to be learned, in helping to integrate it in to the clinical setting, and in assessing the resident therapist's capacities, such a focus is clearly needed. As training curricula have become more hectic (mainly because of the change in mental health delivery systems) attention to the role of the supervisor has waned. Dr. Whitman and her colleague Dr. Jacobs are to be commended for raising our awareness of this important issue once again.

A. Tasman, M.D.

Supervision of Termination in Psychotherapy
Robb M, Cameron PM (Univ of Ottawa, Ont)
Can J Psychiatry 43:397–402, 1998   2–44

Background.—Most practitioners agree that a planned termination of psychotherapy is preferable to a more abrupt ending. These authors described a planned termination of psychoanalytic psychotherapy in which the final weeks took place in a group situation with psychiatric residents.

> *Case Report.*—Mrs. M was a 44-year-old divorced woman with 3 grown children who had been undergoing 2 years of weekly psychotherapy because she couldn't "have a normal relationship with a man." She had been taking low-dose antidepressants for years. When she was 18-years-old, she married a man she did not love, then divorced him 13 years later. Afterward she had 2 kinds of relationships with men, either calm, "safer" relationships with married men, or tumultuous relationships that inevitably ended with her rejecting the man. Her father had abused her physically and emotionally, and she felt that all her interpersonal problems existed because of her father's treatment of her. During the 2 years of therapy, Mrs. M and her therapist worked on her family relationships and her feelings about herself. The therapeutic alliance was good, and transference was mainly positive, with little interpretive emphasis on the transference. Mrs. M began feeling better

about herself, stopped taking antidepressants, and was maintaining a stable relationship with a man. When Mrs. M said she was ready to finish therapy, she and her therapist chose a closing date 12 weeks later.

The therapist was a fourth-year psychiatric resident. The therapist and her supervisor decided to perform the closing sessions in a group situation with 6 other residents interested in psychotherapy. During the closing weeks, Mrs. M reviewed the themes of her psychotherapy and for the first time talked freely about her frustrations with the therapist because of her feeling that she was not "100% cured." When she saw that her expressions of anger did not damage the relationship, but rather that their discussions could strengthen the therapist–patient relationship, she began expressing her pain and anger more freely to other important people in her life. Her relationships with these people improved also. By the end of therapy, she was also able to forgive her father and could admit to some of his positive attributes.

Benefits of the Group Termination Sessions.—All 6 residents reported that sitting in on the termination was a valuable learning experience. In particular, they were able to see therapy at its completion, see that the process worked, and note the patient's accomplishments. They also saw one of their peers successfully navigate a termination, which bolstered confidence in themselves. This modeling experience was a valuable, cost-effective way to teach the termination phase during psychotherapy training.

▶ No aspect of psychotherapy training is more complex than dealing with termination. This is in no small part due to the fact that most terminations of psychotherapy by residents are not carried out because the patient has improved sufficiently to warrant termination of treatment, but, rather, because of changes in the resident's rotations or the end of the resident's training experience. Robb and Cameron bring to our attention the importance of supervision of this key phase of psychotherapy and highlight a number of important issues regarding termination supervision.

A. Tasman, M.D.

Empirically Supported Treatments: Implications for Training
Calhoun KS, Moras K, Pilkonis PA, et al (Univ of Georgia, Athens; Univ of Pennsylvania; Univ of Pittsburgh, Pa; et al)
J Consult Clin Psychol 66:151–162, 1998   2–45

Background.—Empirically supported treatments (ESTs) can facilitate the training of clinical psychologists. ESTs can help a trainee understand the theory of psychopathology and its related therapy. They can help trainees know when and how to use specific intervention skills. ESTs can also help psychologists acquire general skills for enhancing the therapeutic process and specific skills for evaluating the effectiveness of a therapy. The authors reviewed the special challenges involved with ESTs and proposed a set of guidelines for their use.

Training at the Predoctoral, Internship, Postdoctoral, and Continuing Education Levels.—ESTs can provide a practical framework for the predoctoral student to formulate and implement intervention strategies. A primary goal of training at the predoctoral level is teaching the skills needed to develop the therapeutic alliance, and ESTs can play a role here. During the internship, training focuses on practical experience and an understanding of the relationship between basic and applied sciences. Training in specific EST skills is available at specialty or research clinics, or even (for more established ESTs) at clinics that offer parent training programs for children or psychoeducation programs. At the postdoctorate level, the goal is to train practitioners who can conduct ESTs with expertise and who can train others in their performance. One program of note is the postdoctoral training program for cognitive therapy at the University of Pennsylvania. Finally, ESTs can have a substantial impact on continuing education and keeping practitioners informed with the most up-to-date information in a field.

Guidelines for Training in ESTs.—Seven training guidelines are offered, based on experience with EST training but without data from systematic or controlled research. First, training programs should include videotapes that show the process of conducting the EST. Videotapes can communicate enormous amounts of information efficiently and should be implemented early in the training program. Second, supervisors should use audiotapes or videotapes to assess the therapy session; these tapes target more areas for critique than the trainee's self-report. Third, supervisors should determine the extent to which trainees adhere to how the EST should be implemented according to the EST manual. Fourth, trainees can learn from the mistakes of others, so programs should include videotapes of common errors. Fifth, several trainees can be taught at once by reviewing individual tapes within a group session. Sixth, developing skill with an EST requires experience with at least 3 prototypic cases and at least 4 nonprototypic cases. Seventh, trainees must be taught how to assess the patient's response to the EST on an ongoing basis; this ensures the efficacy of treatment.

▶ Too often academic psychiatrists practice and teach treatments with which they are most familiar by virtue of the fact that they have been trained in those treatments themselves. This article and the 1 by Davison (Abstract 2–46) challenge educators to raise the standard in how we teach what treatments should be prescribed for which patients.

A. Tasman, M.D.

Being Bolder With the Boulder Model: The Challenge of Education and Training in Empirically Supported Treatments

Davison GC (Univ of Southern California, Los Angeles)
J Consult Clin Psychol 66:163–167, 1998

2–46

Background.—In many "Boulder model" psychology training programs, much time and effort are devoted to approaches for which there is no empirical justification. Although controlled outcome and process studies of various interventions are now available, many different factors continue to serve as barriers to the scientist-practitioner model of training. Some key issues related to the incorporation of empirically supported treatments (ESTs) in training programs are discussed.

ESTs in Education and Training.—Academic faculty and internship supervisors alike may resist ESTs for a variety of reasons. Personally and politically, they may be invested in approaches that have been used for many years, but which lack empirical support. For students, the lack of experience with certain types of assessment and intervention may preclude placement in American Psychological Association (APA)-approved clinical programs. Still there are legitimate concerns about the use of ESTs and their reliance on treatment manuals as a mainstay of training. Most ESTs arise from studies using treatment manuals, which were originally designed to define independent variables in psychotherapy research. Manuals now play a key role in graduate training, where they place considerable limitations on clinician behavior and are associated with categorically defined treatment categories. Reliance on manuals can lead to neglect of the idiographic analysis of single cases, and limit functional analysis of complex individual cases. Using validated approaches only may also place limitations on innovation and the development of new approaches. Postdoctoral clinical training appears to be a highly appropriate setting in which to teach ESTs; in contrast, the issue of teaching ESTs in continuing education settings is far more complex.

Discussion.—The application of ESTs to the development of applied psychology faces difficult and ongoing challenges. The author believes it is time to be more assertive in bringing the teaching and practice of psychology more into line with empirical support.

▶ As a companion to the previous article (Abstract 2–45), Davison also challenges us to become more specific in teaching clinical decision-making regarding therapeutic interventions. We are, however, limited a great deal by the absence of adequate data. We anxiously await further work along the lines of that described by DeRubeis and Crits-Christoph.[1]

A. Tasman, M.D.

Reference

1. DeRubeis RJ, Crits-Christoph P: Empirically supported individual and group psychological treatments for adult mental disorders. *J Consult Clin Psychol* 66:37–52, 1998.

3 Alcohol and Substance-related Disorders

Introduction

The Director of the National Institute of Drug Abuse, Dr. Alan Leshner, has been vocal about the importance of disseminating new developments in the treatment of addiction and making sure that new psychosocial and pharmacological treatments are readily available to the general public. New findings, such as the utility of naltrexone in the treatment of alcoholism, and of methadone maintenance for opioid addiction, have not been as widely disseminated in practice as indicated by expert consensus. This is due in part to ideologic issues, such as Mayor Guiliani's opposition to methadone maintenance in New York, and in part to lack of adequate large-scale field trials which might convince more primary care doctors and psychiatrists to regularly prescribe naltrexone. The increase discussed last year in use by teenagers of marijuana, tobacco, and cocaine continues, and if our data are accurate and this trend continues by next year we will see the epidemic level of use in schools that occurred in the 1970's. Major public policy issues related to addiction include trying to achieve parity in insurance plans for mental health, including addictive disorders. At this writing several bills supporting parity are being discussed in Congress.

Some of the findings presented in this section are preliminary and some help further establish treatments that already have substantial credibility.

On the topic of diagnosis and comorbidity, Abstract 3–1 is an interesting collaboration between the fields of ophthalmology and addiction psychiatry and finds that color vision is impaired after cocaine withdrawal a finding that might prove useful in diagnostic studies. Abstracts 3–2 and 3–3 discuss issues in comorbidity related to schizophrenia and other psychiatric disorders. In the section on risk factors and complications, Abstract 3–4 finds an equal inheritability of alcohol dependence in both women and men, a new finding. Risk factors associated with cocaine use during pregnancy are studied in Abstract 3–5. Abstract 3–6 looks for risk factors for spread of HIV infection involving addiction. Risk factors for violent death in the home related to substance use are discussed in Abstract

3–7. Health risks in women living in a household with alcohol abuse are discussed in Abstract 3–8, and Abstract 3–9 discusses the high alcohol-related injury and death rates linked to alcohol availability in remote Alaska. Abstract 3–10 finds a very high instance of suicidal behavior in drug abusers admitted to psychiatric hospitals in Sweden.

Treatment outcome studies have become quite common in the substance abuse field and large field trials are needed to further disseminate results of these studies. Abstract 3–11 studies treatment matching, finding an increase of treatment effectiveness for targeting treatment. Compelling research findings indicate that adding psychotherapy, marriage counseling, employment counseling and skill training in medical care to substance abuse treatment results in better outcomes than drug and alcohol counseling alone. Abstracts 3–12 and 3–13 look at cognitive behavioral treatments and group treatments. Abstract 3–14 finds that a dual diagnosis model of treatment can be effective for those with a coexisting, severe mental illness and substance disorders. Abstract 3–15 finds a very helpful treatment for aftercare and demonstrates a good dovetailing between professionally led and self-help treatments. Abstract 3–16 discusses factors predictive of compliance in patients with schizophrenia and substance abuse. Abstracts, 3–17 and 3–18 further establish the value of naltrexone as a treatment for alcoholism and Abstract 3–17 emphasizes the use of naltrexone by primary care providers, a group that has been slow to implement this advance in treatment. One major problem with naltrexone has been patient compliance—Abstract 3–18 deals with this issue. Early studies indicated that buprenorphine might be superior to methadone with cocaine addicted patients. However, the study described in Abstract 3–19 did not find this to be the case. Abstract 3–20 looks at 3 good ways to detoxify opioid patients without finding any one clearly superior. However, it does help establish that buprenorphine may be more comfortable for some patients. Many of us await Food and Drug Administration approval for use of buprenorphine for detoxification, as it looks like it will be a positive addition to our treatment armamentarium for opioid detoxification. Abstract 3–21 provides pilot data on stimulant treatment for cocaine users with adult attention deficit disorder.

Findings from these articles can help us further refine treatment guidelines that are being developed in the field and form a basis for large field trials needed to test the most effective treatments. To help the general public, it is not enough for studies to be done in university settings. It is essential that treatments with proven effectiveness gain wide-spread acceptance. Unfortunately, not enough study is done on the complicated interactions between psychiatric disorders and substance abuse as it relates to treatment outcome. Clearly, a new generation of researchers has their work cut out for them.

Richard J. Frances, M.D.

Diagnosis and Comorbidity

Impaired Color Vision in Cocaine-withdrawn Patients

Desai P, Roy M, Roy A, et al (New Jersey Med School, Newark; Veterans Affairs Med Ctr, East Orange, NJ)
Arch Gen Psychiatry 54:696–699, 1997   3–1

Background.—The primary reinforcing effects of cocaine are caused by dopamine uptake inhibition in the nucleus accumbens and brain reward centers. Dopamine is also present in high concentrations in the retina, where is it is involved in color vision. Patients who had recently withdrawn from cocaine were evaluated for problems with color vision.

Study Design.—Thirty-one cocaine-withdrawn patients, including 1 woman, from the locked drug and alcohol rehabilitation unit for the Veterans Affairs Medical Center in East Orange, New Jersey were studied. All reported usage of at least 12 g of cocaine during the 3 months prior to admission and were drug-free at the time of testing. These patients were matched for sex and age with 31 healthy, drug-free controls. Participants received a complete eye examination, and then color vision was tested with the Lanthony desaturated D-15 and Farnsworth-Munsell 100-hue tests.

Findings.—The cocaine-withdrawn study participants had significantly higher error scores on both tests of color vision than did the matched controls. The most common change was blue-yellow color-vision loss.

Conclusions.—Color vision appears to be impaired several months after cocaine withdrawal, especially in the blue-yellow range. Color-vision testing may prove useful in studies of cocaine-dependent patients.

▶ This psychiatric and ophthalmologic team may have hit upon an interesting new finding indicating that cocaine causes color-vision loss, acting through the dopamine system. This could lead to development of another diagnostic tool for cocaine addiction.

R.J. Frances, M.D.

Reasons for Substance Use in Schizophrenia

Addington J, Duchak V (Univ of Calgary, Alberta, Canada)
Acta Psychiatr Scand 96:329–333, 1997   3–2

Background.—Substance abuse is common among schizophrenic patients. A better understanding of substance abuse in this population is necessary to design effective interventions. The reasons for abuse of alcohol and marijuana were examined in a group of relatively stable outpatients with schizophrenia.

Study Design.—The study group consisted of 41 schizophrenic outpatients, 34 males and 7 females, average age 35, who fulfilled the criteria for substance abuse or dependence. All participants were on antipsychotic medication. A questionnaire was used to assess reasons for drug use, subjective effects of drugs, and reasons for stopping drug use.

Findings.—The most common reasons for using either alcohol or marijuana were to relax, to increase pleasure, to reduce depression, and to be more sociable. Despite the desire to reduce depression, 65% of participants reported increased symptoms of depression with substance use. Those who used cannabis reported feeling happy and relaxed, but more than half also reported an increase in positive schizophrenic symptoms. The strongest motivating factors for stopping alcohol use were health reasons, cost, and disapproval of significant others. The strongest motivating factors for stopping cannabis use were cost, health reasons, disapproval of significant others, and paranoia.

Conclusions.—In this group of stable outpatients with schizophrenia, abused substances were chosen to relieve depression, to increase affect, or to decrease side effects of antipsychotic medication. This strategy was not successful, as the majority of patients reported an increase in both depression and positive psychotic symptoms with substance use. Pointing out that a patient's own subjective experience demonstrates that substance abuse is not helpful may provide motivation for stopping substance abuse in this population.

▶ These authors point to the importance of targeting reasons why particular schizophrenic patients abuse substances, if the planning of treatment interventions is to be appropriate. This article goes over the important ways in which patients self-medicate for both side effects and negative symptoms of schizophrenia. Though patients may rationalize their use of substances, this method can help us to better understand the patient's experience and to explore the self-medication hypothesis.

R.J. Frances, M.D.

Dual Diagnosis Subtypes in Urban Substance Abuse and Mental Health Clinics
Hein D, Zimberg S, Weisman S, et al (St Luke's Roosevelt Hosp Ctr, New York)
Psychiatric Serv 48:1058–1063, 1997   3–3

Background.—National psychiatric epidemiology studies of community samples have reported a high rate of lifetime comorbid psychiatric and substance abuse disorders. Studies that have compared individuals with single and dual disorders have consistently reported that those with dual disorders have a poorer outcome. The rate of dual psychiatric and substance abuse disorders in low-income, inner-city outpatients was determined, the rates in outpatient mental health and substance abuse treatment settings were compared, and the value of categorizing individuals with dual disorders into 3 subtypes was examined.

Methods.—There were 130 low-income, urban individuals who participated; 57 were receiving mental health treatment and 73 were receiving substance abuse treatment. In a semistructured interview, lifetime and concurrent DSM-III-R axis I disorders were determined. Patients with dual disorders were categorized into subtypes based on whether one disorder was caused by the other or both existed independently.

Results.—Of the 130 patients, 83 had a lifetime history of dual disorders; 34 of these were in mental health settings and 49 were in substance abuse treatment settings. Of the 83 patients with dual disorders, more than 50% had symptoms of both disorders in the last 12 months. For 24 patients receiving mental health treatment and 31 patients receiving substance abuse treatment, each of the disorders was considered primary.

Discussion.—In these mental health and substance abuse treatment settings, about two thirds of patients had a lifetime diagnosis of a dual disorder. These rates are consistent with data from similar studies. This high rate of comorbidity did not apparently result from one disorder causing the other. This high rate of comorbidity also indicates that there is a need for greater integration of mental health and substance abuse treatment in all settings.

▶ Few states have integration of their psychiatric and substance abuse services, and this article points to the necessity of having integrated services and cross-trained staff, especially in urban substance abuse and mental health clinics. The patients described in this article have complex biomedical and psychosocial problems that need to be addressed by sophisticated treatment teams.

R.J. Frances, M.D.

Risk Factors and Complications

Genetic and Environmental Contributions to Alcohol Dependence Risk in a National Twin Sample: Consistency of Findings in Women and Men
Heath AC, Bucholz KK, Madden PAF, et al (Washington Univ, St Louis; Queensland Univ, Brisbane; Royal Prince Alfred Hosp, Sydney, New South Wales, Australia)
Psychol Med 27:1381–1396, 1997   3–4

Background.—There is strong evidence for an important genetic component to alcoholism in men, but the evidence for a genetic contribution to alcoholism is weaker for women. Gender differences in the genetic influence on alcohol dependence (AD) were examined in a large study of both monozygotic and dizygotic twins.

Study Design.—The study group consisted of twins from a volunteer adult twin registry formed in 1978–1979 and maintained by the Australian National Health and Medical Research Council. There were 3,848 women and 2,041 men. For this study, telephone interviews were conducted with both members of 2,685 twin pairs and with 1 member of 519 pairs. Diagnostic assessments included lifetime history of *Diagnostic and*

Statistical Manual of Mental Disorders III-R alcohol dependence, as well as twin and family history. Sociodemographic variables were obtained from the 1981 baseline questionnaires.

Findings.—There were significantly higher twin pair concordances for alcoholism among monozygotic than among dizygotic same-sex twin pairs of either sex. AD risk was increased in younger birth cohorts, Catholic males, women without religious affiliation, those with a history of conduct disorder, and those with a history of Depression, high Neuroticism, Social Nonconformity, Toughmindedness, Novelty-seeking, or, only in women, high Extraversion scores. Alcohol dependence risk was decreased in "Other Protestants," weekly church attenders, and university-educated males. Even when these variables were controlled for, there was still a significant association with having an alcoholic monozygotic twin, suggesting a strong genetic component. There was no significant gender difference in the genetic variance in alcohol dependence.

Conclusions.—These findings indicate that the heritability of alcohol dependence is equally strong in both women and men. Approximately two thirds of the variance in risk of AD can be attributed to genetic factors in both sexes.

▶ This Australian group finds an equal genetic contribution to AD risk in women and men. Most studies have been done on men, and this study on a large N sample of 5,889 respondents is quite interesting. It has implications for theories of subtyping including that of Type 1 vs. Type 2 alcoholics, that have received prominent attention.

R.J. Frances, M.D.

Psychosocial Risk Factors Associated With Cocaine Use During Pregnancy: A Case-control Study
Hutchins E, Dipietro J (Maternal and Child Health Bureau, Rockville, Md; Johns Hopkins Univ, Baltimore, Md)
Obstet Gynecol 90:142–147, 1997   3–5

Background.—With the emergence of crack cocaine in the 1980s, the problem of drug abuse in America began to affect large numbers of pregnant women and their infants. It is currently estimated that 5.5% of all pregnant women use an illicit drug during pregnancy. Little is known about the characteristics of these women because most research has focused on the infant.

Methods.—A questionnaire measuring 7 psychosocial risk factors was administered to 229 pregnant women recruited from an urban prenatal clinic. Drug use was determined by urine toxicology and self-report. Multivariate analysis was used to determine the predictive relation between the risk factors and drug use.

Results.—Of the 229 women, 102 were classified as drug users and 127 as nonusers. After controlling for possible sociodemographic confounding factors, 6 of the 7 psychosocial risk factors were shown to be significant predictors of cocaine use during pregnancy in these individuals. These 6 factors were a family history of alcohol or drug problems, an introduction to drugs by a male partner, depression, less social support, current partners who use substances, and less stable living situations. There was a high rate of childhood sexual abuse in both groups of women, but this factor alone did not predict drug use. Cigarette smoking was also a strong predictor of drug use.

Discussion.—Information about psychosocial risk factors that help predict cocaine use during pregnancy is important for the identification and treatment of pregnant women who are substance abusers. In this study, drug users did not register for prenatal care later than nonusers. This does not support the public perception that pregnant women who abuse drugs do not seek prenatal care. There are opportunities to identify drug use in pregnant women relatively early in gestation.

▶ Crack cocaine has had devastating effects on urban areas, and these effects have been greatest in pregnant women. Severe potential teratogenic effects to the fetus, as well as social factors affecting parenting, are quite significant. Methods that aid in screening an urban population for those at high risk for crack abuse are important. Smoking status, family history of alcohol or drug problems, and current use by a male partner can be important tipoffs that should lead to a more vigorous diagnostic effort, which could include toxicology testing.

R.J. Frances, M.D.

Sociometric Risk Networks and Risk for HIV Infection

Friedman SR, Neaigus A, Jose B, et al (Natl Development and Research Insts Inc, New York; Emory Univ, Atlanta, Ga; Beth Israel Med Ctr, New York)
Am J Public Health 87:1289–1296, 1997   3–6

Background.—Network analysis is emerging as a means of helping researchers explain the spread of HIV infection and infection with other diseases, as well as HIV-related risk behaviors. Sociometric network structures, consisting of patterns of relationships involving risk behaviors among large numbers of individuals, were examined. Sociometric risk networks provide a structural model for studying the types of linkages used in contact tracing by describing direct and indirect linkages through which HIV and similar agents can be transmitted.

Methods.—A cross-sectional survey was conducted of 767 drug injectors in New York City. Chain-referral and linking procedures were used to measure large-scale or sociometric risk networks. Through graph–theoretical algebraic techniques, 92 connected components were identified (drug injectors linked to each other directly or through others). A 105-member 2-core within a large connected component of 230 members was also identified.

Results.—Drug injectors in the 2-core of the large connected component were more likely to have HIV infection. Members of the 2-core who were seronegative engaged in a variety of high-risk behaviors, some with infected drug injectors.

Discussion.—Among drug-injecting peer groups, sociometric risk networks appear to be pathways along which HIV travels. The cores of large connected components can become pockets of HIV infection. Analyzing sociometric networks may help researchers understand patterns of HIV infection within communities of drug users. Understanding these networks may help in the development of interventions to reduce transmission of HIV infection in areas with high prevalence, and prevent outbreaks in areas with low prevalence. This report also includes an illustration of terms used to describe network structures.

▶ The study of the spread of infectious diseases including AIDS through network analysis is an important, emerging field. The cultural practices, methods of using syringes, kinds of drugs used, and particular kinds of drug use behaviors are looked at. Studying factors that lead to high-risk behavior and prevention tell us a great deal about the probability that an individual will be infected with HIV, and whether a large-scale HIV epidemic will occur among drug injectors in a community. The differences in prevalence between HIV use in different cities and rapidity of spread has been a source of major interest. Why do sites like New York have high rates and sites like Los Angeles a lower incidence? Learning about patterns of changes in risk networks and risk behaviors that might spark rapid transmission is vital. Network-based interventions that supplement existing programs could be an important strategy to prevent new infections.

R.J. Frances, M.D.

Alcohol and Illicit Drug Abuse and the Risk of Violent Death in the Home
Rivara FP, Mueller BA, Somes G, et al (Harborview Injury Prevention and Research Ctr, Seattle; Univ of Washington, Seattle; Univ of Tennessee, Memphis; et al)
JAMA 278:569–575, 1997   3–7

Introduction.—Alcohol is a major contributing factor to violent deaths, including homicides and suicides. However, little is known about the role of chronic alcohol and drug use, as opposed to acute intoxication, in violent death. The risk of violent death in the home associated with alcohol and drug abuse was assessed.

Methods.—The analysis used medical examiners' data from 438 suicides and 388 homicides occurring in the victims' homes in 3 large American metropolitan areas. These cases were matched for age, sex, race, neighborhood, and county to the same number of controls. Proxy interviews were performed to gather information on the use of alcohol or illicit drugs by the deceased person, history of alcohol-related hospitalization, or any trouble at work because of drinking. Alcohol use by others living in the same household was assessed as well. The risk of violent death associated with alcohol and drug use was assessed, with adjustment for other potential risk factors.

Results.—Use of alcohol was associated with an approximate 2–fold increase in the risk of homicide or suicide (odds ratios [OR] 2.2 and 1.8, respectively). Use of other drugs also increased the risks of homicide or suicide (OR 5.2 and 7.1). Both risks were higher still for subjects who used both alcohol and other drugs (OR 12.0 for homicide and 16.6 for suicide). The risk of homicide was also increased for nondrinkers living with an alcohol user (OR 1.7) and for nondrug users living with a drug user (OR 11.3).

Conclusions.—Alcohol and illicit drug use are risk factors for violent death in the home. Homicide risk is increased not only for the substance users but also for nonusers living with drug or alcohol abusers. The homicide risk associated with substance abuse includes not only the abuser but also others at risk because of their exposure to a substance abuser.

▶ The role of chronic alcohol and drug abuse in victims of homicide and suicide is clearly important, and parameters that indicate problems with substance abuse, such as drinking and using drugs, trouble at work from drinking, or being hospitalized for drinking, lead to a vast overrepresentation in the population that is at risk of becoming a victim of homicide or suicide. With suicide, this is especially the case when additional psychiatric problems are also present. Even those who do not drink or use substances but who live with those who drink and use illicit drugs are at greatly increased risk of being a homicide victim. In this article, the issue of risk extends to being part of a network of drug- and alcohol-dependent people, and this increases risk.

R.J. Frances, M.D.

Health Outcomes of Women Exposed to Household Alcohol Abuse: A Family Practice Training Site Research Network (FPTSRN) Study
Ryan JG, Verardo LT, Kidd JM, et al (State Univ of New York, Stony Brook; North Shore Univ Hosp, Glen Cove, NY; Southside Hosp, Brentwood, NY; et al)
J Fam Pract 45:410–417, 1997   3–8

Background.—The effect of alcohol abuse by family members on non-alcohol abusers (such as the spouses of alcoholics) has not been well studied. Some research has suggested that members of alcoholics' families use more healthcare services. This suggests that screening for and treating these patients may be an important component of effective primary medical care. The health-related adverse effects of exposure to a family member who abused alcohol on nonalcohol-abusing women were examined in this study.

Study Design.—A historical prospective survey of female patients was performed at 5 sociodemographically diverse, hospital-based primary care practices on Long Island. All of these practices participate in the Family Practice Training Site Research Network (FPTSRN). Female patients, aged 18–45, were recruited from September 1995–September 1996, if there was a 2-year history in their medical records. Participants completed 4 CAGE questions, 5 items to screen for familial alcoholism, the Medical Outcomes Study 36–Item Short Form Health Survey (MOS SF-36), demographic questions, and 2 open-ended questions on experience of alcohol problems. Patient records were evaluated for specific diagnoses.

Findings.—The initial study group consisted of 267 women. Of these, 42 were potential alcohol abusers. These women were excluded, leaving 225 in the study group. Of these, 70 were potentially exposed to familial alcohol abuse. Although women exposed to alcohol in their homes were not at increased risk for specific diagnoses, their health-related quality of life was decreased, as measured by the MOS SF-36.

Conclusions.—Women exposed to alcohol abusers in their homes were more likely to experience decreased health-related quality of life. The needs of these women might be better served if primary care physicians screened for exposure to alcohol abuse in the home and for need for biopsychosocial medical care. These patients may benefit from referral to community-based support groups.

▶ The results of this study fit with much clinical experience in dealing with alcoholics' spouses, who frequently have problems with self-esteem and bottled-up feelings. This article helps to alert family practitioners to the importance of watching out for mental health needs of the spouses of alcoholics. If Lois Wilson, the founder of Al-Anon, were still alive, I know she would have been very interested in this study and would have agreed with its conclusions.

R.J. Frances, M.D.

Alcohol-related Injury Death and Alcohol Availability in Remote Alaska
Landen MG, Beller M, Funk E, et al (Ctrs for Disease Control and Prevention, Atlanta, Ga; Alaska Division of Public Health, Anchorage)
JAMA 278:1755–1758, 1997   3–9

Background.—Injury is a major health problem in remote Alaskan areas. Alcohol consumption has been shown to be associated with the injury death rate. The relationship between injury death and laws in remote Alaskan villages prohibiting the sale and importation of alcohol was investigated.

Study Design.—Information about injury deaths from 1990–1993, in remote Alaskan villages with fewer than 1,000 residents, was obtained from Alaska death certificate data. Dry villages were defined as those that prohibited both the sale and importation of alcohol. There were 78 wet and 72 dry villages at the end of the study period. Each injury was classified by blood alcohol concentration. Injury death rates were determined from U.S. census population estimates. Rate ratios were calculated to compare injury death rates for wet and dry remote Alaskan villages. Alaska Native is used to refer to Native Americans from Alaska.

Findings.—Blood alcohol concentrations were available for 200 of the 302 injury deaths during the study period. Of these 200 injury deaths, 130 involved a blood alcohol concentration of at least 17 mmol/L and were classified as alcohol-related. The total injury mortality rate and alcohol-related injury mortality rate were higher among Alaskan Natives from wet villages than among those from dry villages. This association was highest for deaths due to motor vehicle accident, homicide, or hypothermia.

Conclusions.—Small remote Native Alaskan villages that prohibit the sale and importation of alcohol have lower alcohol-related and total injury death rates. This suggests that in these remote locations, Alaskan villages can successfully use local alcohol laws to reduce the availability of alcohol to the benefit of their population.

▶ This article indicates that prohibition helps to reduce alcohol-related injury deaths. Injury death is a major problem in remote areas of Alaska with high Native populations and high alcoholism rates. These areas' very remoteness makes it difficult to obtain alcohol when there are prohibitions against it, and concomitant public health problems associated with alcohol are reduced with reduced availability. Though prohibition is not likely to occur on the mainland United States, this kind of study indicates the importance of maintaining prohibition on other currently illegal and very dangerous drugs. Legalization leads to greater availability, greater craving, and greater use.

R.J. Frances, M.D.

Suicide Attempts in a Cohort of Drug Abusers: A 5-year Follow-up Study

Johnsson E, Fridell M (Lund Univ, Sweden)
Acta Psychiatr Scand 96:362–366, 1997   3–10

Background.—Although drug abuse is a predictor of suicidal behavior, suicide attempts by drug abusers have not been well studied. To investigate suicidal behavior in this group, follow-up interviews were conducted with drug abusers who had been admitted to a psychiatric ward for detoxification and short-term rehabilitation.

Study Design.—The study group consisted of 125 drug abusers, 58% men and 32% women, consecutively admitted as inpatients to a detoxification ward during 1988. The average age of these patients was 30 and all had been hard-drug abusers for at least 3 years. Patients were contacted again 5 years later. At this time, 118 patients were still living and 92 were interviewed. None of the patients had died as a result of suicide.

TABLE 1.—Psychological/Psychiatric Symptoms in Drug Abusers With a History of Suicide Attempts and No History of Suicide Attempts: Interview Data

Last 12 Months Prior To Follow-up	SA (*n*=41)		NSA (*n*=51)	
	n	%	*n*	%
Suicidal thoughts (*n*=40)	33	83	20	39‡
Weariness of life	34	83	28	55†
Depressive mood	34	83	27	55†
Anxiety	37	90	36	72*
Irritability	33	81	34	67
Hopelessness	32	78	30	59*
Sleeping problems	21	51	26	51

*P less than 0.05.
†P less than 0.01.
‡P less than 0.001; Chi-square test.
Abbreviations: SA, history of suicide attempts; *NSA*, no history of suicide attempts.
(Courtesy of Johnsson E, Fridell M: Suicide attempts in a cohort of drug abusers: A 5-year follow-up study *Acta Psychiatr Scand* 96:362–366, 1997.)

Results.—Of the 92 patients interviewed, 45% had attempted suicide, with 17% making multiple attempts. Most suicide attempts occurred while the patients were in their 20s. Nearly half of suicide attempts involved prescribed psychotropic drugs. The most frequent reason for suicide attempts was loss and loneliness. Compared to the members of the study group who had not attempted suicide, patients who attempted suicide were more likely to have grown up in a home with a substance abuser, to have experienced the loss of a loved one in childhood, to have received childhood psychiatric treatment, and to have had significant levels of suicidal ideation and psychiatric problems (Table 1). There was no significant difference in drug abuse or treatment variables between these 2 groups.

Conclusions.—A sample of 125 drug abusers who were treated at a psychiatric detoxification center were interviewed 5 years later to examine suicidal behavior. Almost half of these patients had attempted suicide. Effective assessment and treatment strategies are necessary for this vulnerable patient group.

▶ This Swedish group found a particularly high (45%) rate of reported lifetime suicide attempts in drug abusers. This article points out the importance of both exploring issues of loss and loneliness, which may be major risk factors for suicide, in addicts, and suicide prevention in working with this population.

R.J. Frances, M.D.

Treatment and Outcome

Problem-Service 'Matching' in Addiction Treatment: A Prospective Study in 4 Programs

McLellan AT, Grissom GR, Zanis D, et al (Univ of Pennsylvania, Philadelphia; Compass Information Services, King of Prussia, Pa)
Arch Gen Psychiatry 54:730–735, 1997
3–11

Background.—In a previous study, the authors attempted to match individuals with substance abuse disorder to an optimal treatment setting, but were unsuccessful. No variables predicted better outcome by treatment setting or program. From a practical standpoint, patients could not be placed in the intended programs. This led to the current study, which was designed to identify specific patient problems and match them to treatment services within each of 4 treatment programs.

Methods.—There were 94 patients admitted to 4 substance abuse treatment programs. Patients were randomly assigned to standard treatment or "matched" services in which at least 3 sessions were directed at their major family, employment, or psychiatric problems.

Results.—Patients who received matched services stayed in treatment longer, were more likely to complete treatment, and had better outcomes than patients who received standard treatment in the same programs.

Discussion.—For various reasons, it is unlikely that patients will be matched to specific kinds of programs. Within any given treatment program, it is possible to match a patient's specific problems to specific treatment services. This treatment strategy resulted in a 20%-30% increase in treatment effectiveness for substance abuse disorders. This strategy may be applicable to other treatment programs for other addiction-related problems and may improve the results of treatment. More than 10 years of research have shown that adding psychotherapy, marriage counseling, employment counseling and skill training, and medical care results in better outcomes than drug and alcohol counseling alone.

▶ Although most studies show that addiction treatment is effective, it has been difficult to develop studies that show differential effectiveness. This group has been in the vanguard of studying treatment matching. The positive results found an improvement in matched patients compared with patients who had standard treatment. Strategies to address employment, family, or psychiatric problems with the addition of psychotherapy, employment counseling, and skill training produce clinically and significantly better outcomes from substance abuse treatment than do drug and alcohol counseling alone. This emphasizes the importance of having a sophisticated biopsychosocial approach and better trained personnel rather than having patients relying on treatment that is not professionally led.

R.J. Frances, M.D.

Cognitive-Behavioral Treatment for Depression in Alcoholism

Brown RA, Evans DM, Miller IW, et al (Brown Univ, Providence, RI)
J Consult Clin Psychol 65:715–726, 1997   3–12

Background.—Alcoholism and depression commonly occur together, and comorbid depression has a poor prognosis after alcoholism treatment. There is limited evidence to suggest that cognitive-behavioral therapy for depression (CBT-D) may be more effective than standard treatment for alcoholics with significant depressive symptoms. The efficacy of adding CBT-D to standard partial hospital alcohol treatment for alcoholics with depressive symptoms was assessed.

Methods.—The study included 35 alcoholic patients being treated in a daytime partial hospital program. All had depressive symptoms, scoring 10 or higher on the Beck Depression Inventory. All patients received standard partial hospital alcohol treatment, an abstinence-oriented, group treatment-based program. In addition, 19 patients received 8 individual sessions of CBT-D, modified for use in alcohol-dependent patients. For comparison, 16 patients received a relaxation training control program. Treatments were given to 5 sequential, nonoverlapping cohorts. Follow-up interviews were conducted to assess (1) dependent measures of depressive symptoms and depressed and anxious mood; (2) alcohol use; (3) diagnostic and descriptive participant data; and (4) cognitive-behavioral process measures.

Results.—The CBT-D group showed significantly greater reductions in somatic depressive symptoms and depressed and anxious mood during treatment. The percentage of days abstinent from alcohol was greater in the CBT-D group. However, there was no significant difference in overall abstinence or number of drinks per day during the first 3 months of follow-up. From 3–6 months' follow-up, patients receiving CBT-D had a greater total abstinence rate, 47% vs. 13%; a greater percentage of days of abstinence, 91% vs. 68%; and fewer drinks per day, 0.46 vs. 5.71. The change in depression symptoms was apparently a mediator of the relationship between assigned treatment and drinking outcomes.

Conclusions.—Adding CBT-D to standard alcohol treatment for alcoholics with depression leads to greater reductions in somatic depressive symptoms and in depressed and anxious moods. By 3 to 6 months' follow-up, patients receiving CBT-D show better outcomes on all measures of drinking behavior than those receiving a relaxation training intervention. The reduction in depressive symptoms is apparently an important mediator of the effect on drinking. Cognitive-behavioral therapy helped patients to better understand their depression and the factors affecting their moods. The depression coping skills gained are viewed as relevant to recovery from alcohol dependence.

▶ This study found a delayed positive outcome for CBT in depressed alcoholics compared with control patients who received relaxation training. The effect appeared between approximately 3 and 6 months into the follow-up with reduction of depressed symptoms and anxious mood. Perhaps an integrated CBT addiction and depression treatment needs to be designed that would be even more effective.

R.J. Frances, M.D.

Group Counseling Versus Individualized Relapse Prevention Aftercare Following Intensive Outpatient Treatment for Cocaine Dependence: Initial Results
McKay JR, Alterman AI, Cacciola JS, et al (Univ of Pennsylvania, Philadelphia)
J Consult Clin Psychol 65:778–788, 1997   3–13

Introduction.—Treatment for cocaine abusers is increasingly delivered in outpatient settings. However, even with intensive rehabilitation and aftercare, relapse continues to be a major problem for some patients. Few studies have compared the effectiveness of various approaches to aftercare for cocaine abusers, or the predictive factors of cocaine use during aftercare. Two approaches to aftercare for cocaine dependence, group counseling and individualized relapse prevention (RP), were compared.

Methods.—The study included 98 men patients who completed an intensive outpatient rehabilitation program for cocaine dependence at a VA medical center. On entering the aftercare phase of treatment, the patients were randomized to receive either standard group counseling (STND) or individualized RP aftercare. Based on standardized assessment tools, patients in the RP group received specific cognitive-behavioral interventions. The efficacy of the 2 approaches was compared, and predictors of cocaine use during aftercare were analyzed.

Results.—Predictors of cocaine use during treatment included higher levels of cocaine and alcohol use during the intensive outpatient program and low self-efficacy. Cocaine use was lower for patients with lifetime diagnoses of alcohol dependence, major depression, or any anxiety disorder. During the 6-month study period, patients in the STND group had higher rates of complete abstinence than those in the RP group. However, among patients who used cocaine during the first 3 months, those in the RP group were better able to limit the extent of their cocaine use. On matching analyses, RP produced better results in patients who did not stop using cocaine during their intensive outpatient program and in those who had a commitment to absolute abstinence. In contrast, patients with goals other than complete abstinence had better results in STND care. Analysis of episodes of cocaine use and "near-misses" during the first 3 months of aftercare suggested that relapse can be provoked by many different factors, including sensation seeking, protracted thoughts about using, situational cues, and failure to use social supports for abstinence.

Conclusions.—This study compares group counseling with individualized RP approaches to aftercare for patients with cocaine dependence. Although standard group counseling produced higher abstinence rates, RP may help to limit the extent of cocaine use. The results suggest that individualized RP aftercare may be helpful for patients who do not achieve abstinence during outpatient rehabilitation.

▶ This University of Pennsylvania group, which is prolific in producing fine outcome studies, looks at the important question of whether a group or individualized relapse prevention effort works better for cocaine addicts after intensive outpatient treatment. The results are very interesting and include a finding that individualized relapse prevention may be of additional value, especially to the cocaine abuser who continues to use during rehabilitation. Patients who are committed to absolute abstinence also did better in the individualized relapse prevention program. This is especially true of those patients who are committed to absolute abstinence but who get discouraged if they use cocaine during an intensive outpatient program and did not get an adequate opportunity in a group to work through these difficulties.

R.J. Frances, M.D.

Illness Severity and Treatment Services for Dually Diagnosed Severely Mentally Ill Outpatients

Ries RK, Comtois KA (Harborview Med Ctr, Seattle)
Schizophr Bull 23:239–246, 1997   3–14

Background.—A basic concept in managed care is that the intensity of treatment services delivered to an individual should relate to the severity of that individual's illness. This is particularly relevant in the treatment of individuals with severe mental illness and a substance abuse disorder because they reportedly use more acute treatment resources and have more symptoms than individuals with mental illness without substance abuse disorder. There is little information on the relationship between treatment service intensity and severity of illness in populations with dual diagnoses.

Methods.—A commonly endorsed but untested model of outpatient treatment for individuals with coexisting severe mental illness and substance abuse disorder was evaluated. The following topics were examined: the relationship between the amount of treatment services delivered and a subject's global severity of illness, how various modes of treatment relate to different aspects of illness, how noncompliance relates to severity of illness and amount of services delivered, and how schizophrenia/schizoaffective diagnoses affect these issues.

Results.—Patients with high total severity of illness scores received about twice as many appointments per month as those with low severity of illness scores. A relation was seen between higher total severity of illness scores and (1) DSM-IV diagnoses of schizophrenia/schizoaffective; (2) being in a lower phase of treatment; (3) representative payee benefit management; (4) homelessness; and (5) more hospitalizations. Patients with greater psychiatric symptom severity received substantially more case management and medication services, but not more group therapy or day treatment. There was a significant relation between severity of substance abuse disorder and case management only.

Discussion.—This model of outpatient treatment for individuals with coexisting severe mental illness and substance abuse disorder was successful in delivering higher levels of treatment services to the individuals that need them. More studies of the association between treatment services and patient condition, and how to measure this relation would be useful.

▶ This Washington State group is doing important clinical research on dually-diagnosed patients and is finding that severely mentally ill patients do better when they have "wrap-around" treatment availability with assertive case management and more intensive treatment services, including help with finances, help with finding living arrangements, and integration of treatment approaches. Substance-abusing mentally ill patients require a high intensity of treatment, and it is important to design ways to give more intensive treatment to those who need it when they need it.

R.J. Frances, M.D.

Affiliation With Alcoholics Anonymous After Treatment: A Study of Its Therapeutic Effects and Mechanisms of Action

Morgenstern J, Labouvie E, McCrady BS, et al (Mount Sinai School of Medicine, New York; Rutgers—The State Univ of New Jersey, New Brunswick)
J Consult Clin Psychol 65:768–777, 1997   3–15

Introduction.—Most formal treatment programs for substance use disorders in the United States are oriented toward the 12-step program of Alcoholics Anonymous (AA). The 12-step model is one of the most controversial, least understood, and least evaluated strategies for treating substance use disorders. The therapeutic effects of affiliation with AA were assessed in 100 individuals entering residential or intensive day treatment.

Methods.—Research subjects were followed for changes in 4 process factors: primary appraisal, self-efficacy, commitment to an abstinence goal, and cognitive and behavioral coping. A battery of measures was assessed at baseline and 1- and 6-month follow-up visits.

Results.—Increased affiliation with AA was predictive of better outcomes. Affiliation with AA after treatment was associated with maintenance of self-efficacy and motivation and increased active coping efforts. These process factors were significant predictors of patient outcome.

Conclusions.—Increased affiliation with AA after formal treatment for substance use disorders was associated with better patient outcomes. Findings differ from those of 12-step theorists, who suggest that AA works through its unique effects that share little with mechanisms that are mobilized by self-changers or other treatment approaches. The association of AA with outcome was mediated by its effects on sustaining beliefs in the cost-benefit of maintaining behavior change, commitment to a specific goal and ability to accomplish this goal, and through promoting active coping efforts.

▶ After all of these years, the issue of affiliation with AA after treatment has still not been adequately studied. This study shows that AA is useful, and It examines the mechanisms of its effectiveness, connecting them to various hypotheses such as self-efficacy, motivation, and coping efforts that are thought to be positive predictors of outcome.

R.J. Frances, M.D.

Prediction of Compliance With Outpatient Referral in Patients With Schizophrenia and Psychoactive Substance Use Disorders
Miner CR, Rosenthal RN, Hellerstein DJ, et al (Beth Israel Med Ctr, New York; Univ of Pennsylvania, Philadelphia)
Arch Gen Psychiatry 54:706–712, 1997   3–16

Background.—Outpatient treatment can be effective in individuals with concurrent schizophrenia and psychoactive substance use disorders, but many do not comply with outpatient referral and are at higher risk for rehospitalization. Studies have indicated that individuals with mental illness and psychoactive substance use disorder are less compliant with outpatient treatment than individuals with mental illness but no psychoactive substance use disorder. However, in many areas, mental health and substance abuse treatment programs are uncoordinated. The authors have previously shown that some patients with concurrent schizophrenia and psychoactive substance use disorders can be more effectively treated in settings that combine psychiatric and substance abuse services.

Methods.—A logistic regression model was developed to predict compliance with outpatient treatment in individuals with schizophrenia and psychoactive substance use disorders. Data from standardized interviews were collected during an index acute care hospitalization. The model was validated in a separate sample. Sensitivity and specificity were assessed in a cross-validation study of 1,000 random samples.

Results.—The model distinguished individuals who complied with treatment from those who did not comply in 37 of 49 cases in a reference sample, and in 11 of 14 cases in a confirmatory sample; sensitivity was 1.00 and specificity was 0.67. Women and individuals with negative syndrome schizophrenia complied with outpatient treatment. Individuals with mixed syndromes were most likely to be noncompliant. Cross-validation supported the stability of this model.

Discussion.—According to this logistic regression model, gender, presence of mixed syndrome, and lower scores on the Schedule for the Assessment of Negative Symptoms Affective Flattening and Blunting Scale predicted treatment compliance in 75% of this sample. Enhanced intervention in men with mixed syndrome schizophrenia regardless of substance abuse history may improve long-term outcome by addressing characteristics that contribute to noncompliance. These results would be strengthened by replication of the study in a larger population. It may be helpful to use knowledge of patient characteristics at the outset to design more effective treatment programs for those at high risk for noncompliance.

▶ Those patients who are candidates for an integrated treatment program do quite well. Resistance to outpatient treatment engagement at the outset leads to poor outcome. This article links positive outcome with both being female and with having a greater degree of negative symptoms of schizophrenia. There is a need for the development of new kinds of interventions for patients who have high dropout rates.

R.J. Frances, M.D.

Pharmacologic Treatment

A Preliminary Investigation of the Management of Alcohol Dependence With Naltrexone by Primary Care Providers
O'Connor PG, Farren CK, Rounsaville BJ, et al (Yale Univ, New Haven, Conn)
Am J Med 103:477–482, 1997   3–17

Introduction.—Patients identified in the primary care setting as having problem drinking or alcohol dependence are typically referred to specialized alcohol treatment programs. Those with problem drinking who continue to have primary care-based treatment often participate in minimal or brief interventions. Naltrexone, a new form of pharmacotherapy for alcohol dependence, was evaluated as an adjunct to a counseling strategy used by primary care providers.

Methods.—Twenty-nine alcohol-dependent patients were enrolled in the study. All were managed within a primary care model located at a university-affiliated substance research program. None had major comorbidity or was at high risk for complicated withdrawal. Participants were required to have current alcohol dependence by *Diagnostic and Statistical Manual III-R* criteria and abstinence for 5 days before study entry. On day 1, patients received 25 mg of naltrexone followed by 50 mg/day on subsequent days. An initial 45-minute counseling session was used to review substance-abuse history, develop a treatment plan, refer to Alcoholics Anonymous, and set goals for later follow-up sessions. Seven brief follow-up visits were scheduled for the 10-week study.

Results.—Most patients were employed Caucasian men. Twenty-one (72%) of those enrolled completed treatment. The percent of days abstinent increased significantly (from 36.6% to 88.8%), as did the percent days abstinent from heavy drinking (from 48.7% to 97.3%). The mean number of drinks per occasion significantly fell from 9.2 to 2.5. Mean serum gamma glutamyl transferase decreased compared with baseline, from 67.1 U/L to 45.3 U/L (Table 2). Providers reported that 33% of patients had improved "very much" and 24% "moderately." Participant ratings were "much better" for 29% and "somewhat better" for 19%.

TABLE 2.—Change in Measures of Alcohol Consumption:
Baseline vs. DuringTreatment (n = 29)

Measure	Baseline (Mean, SD)	Treatment (Mean, SD)	T	P
Days abstinent (%)	36.6 (±23.7)	88.8 (±16.7)	11.01	<0.0001
Days abstinent from heavy drinking (%)	48.7 (±24.9)	97.3 (±4.6)	10.46	<0.0001
Drinks per occasion (no.)	9.5 (±4.5)	2.5 (±3.7)	−6.93	<0.0001
Serum GGT (U/L)	67.1 (±47.3)	45.3 (±37.5)	−4.46	<0.0001

Abbreviations: GGT, gamma glutamyl transferase; *SD*, standard deviation.
(Reprinted from O'Connor PG, Farren CK, Rounsaville BJ, et al: A preliminary investigation of the management of alcohol dependence with Naltrexone by primary care providers. *Am J Med* 103:477–482, 1997 with permission from Excerpta Medica Inc.)

Seventeen of the 21 patients who completed the study continued treatment with their primary care provider and 4 were referred to other treatment.

Conclusion.—Counseling by primary care providers, combined with naltrexone treatment, proved to be both feasible and effective for alcohol-dependent patients. Overall, 45% of the 29 patients who enrolled remained abstinent and 35% relapsed to heavy drinking.

▶ This open-ended study found that primary care providers using a combination of naltrexone and counseling were successful in reducing drinking days and amount of drinking. The development of naltrexone provides the primary care physician with a new tool that is useful in the treatment of alcoholism. However, at this point the medication has not been heavily marketed and is not widely used by primary care physicians. There is a need for disseminating information to primary care physicians about both the effectiveness of this treatment approach and ways it can be integrated with a counseling model of advice and clinical management.

R.J. Frances, M.D.

Naltrexone and Alcohol Dependence: Role of Subject Compliance
Volpicelli JR, Rhines KC, Rhines JS, et al (Univ of Pennsylvania, Philadelphia; Rutgers Univ, Piscataway, NJ)
Arch Gen Psychiatry 54:737–742, 1997   3–18

Background.—In 2 randomized, double-blind, placebo-controlled studies, it was shown that naltrexone, 50 mg/day, reduced alcohol drinking in alcohol-dependent individuals. Treatment compliance was excellent in both studies, but analysis has shown a significant treatment effect size for naltrexone compared with placebo for compliant subjects, but not those who missed research visits. The effectiveness of naltrexone in individuals undergoing psychosocial treatment in a more naturalistic setting of treatment attendance and compliance was examined.

Methods.—Naltrexone or placebo was given to 87 alcohol-dependent individuals for 12 weeks. All subjects received individual counseling twice per week for a month, then once per week.

Results.—Overall, individuals given naltrexone showed only modest improvement in alcohol drinking for the 12-week study period. However, naltrexone was more effective across a variety of outcome measures in subjects who completed the 12-week treatment period and who were highly compliant.

Discussion.—The effectiveness of naltrexone in reducing alcohol drinking is dependent on compliance. Large treatment effect sizes are seen in individuals given naltrexone who comply with treatment compared with individuals given placebo. Naltrexone does not benefit individuals who are less compliant.

▶ It is not surprising that compliance with taking naltrexone is a crucial variable in determining whether it is clinically effective. Substance abuse patients have major problems with compliance, and strategies for improving compliance with taking medication need to be developed. I have had patients discover that they will not get a high when they drink on naltrexone, and this leads them to stop taking their naltrexone at times when they are about to relapse. A strategy that has often been used for Antabuse is having a family member or a loved one observe the patient taking the medication daily.

R.J. Frances, M.D.

Buprenorphine vs Methadone Maintenance Treatment for Concurrent Opioid Dependence and Cocaine Abuse
Schottenfeld RS, Pakes JR, Oliveto A, et al (Yale Univ, New Haven, Conn; APT Found, New Haven, Conn)
Arch Gen Psychiatry 54:713–720, 1997   3–19

Background.—Buprenorphine is a partial µ-agonist and κ-antagonist that may be an effective alternative to methadone for maintenance treatment of individuals with opioid dependence, especially those with concurrent cocaine dependence. However, buprenorphine has been associated with various problems, such as the need for daily dosing, potential diversion of take-home doses and overdoses, difficulty in withdrawing from methadone, and lack of availability. Treatment with methadone is not successful in all patients. Cocaine use during maintenance treatment with methadone is a special concern.

Methods.—In a double-blind, 24-week study, 132 patients were randomly assigned to 1 of 4 treatment groups. These groups used 12 mg or 4 mg of sublingual buprenorphine, or 65 mg or 20 mg of methadone. Outcome variables included treatment retention and opioid or cocaine use.

Results.—Final analysis was done in 116 patients. Illicit use of opioids or cocaine was determined by urine toxicology testing and self-report. Maintenance treatment had significant effects on the rate of opioid use, but no significant effects on treatment retention or rate of cocaine use. The rates of positive opioid toxicology tests were 45% for treatment with 65 mg of methadone, 58% for 12 mg of buprenorphine, 72% for 20 mg of methadone, and 77% for treatment with 4 mg of buprenorphine. The differences between these rates for 65 mg of methadone and both low-dose treatments, and for 12 mg of buprenorphine and both low-dose treatments were significant.

Discussion.—Higher doses of buprenorphine or methadone are superior to lower doses for reducing opioid use in individuals with opioid dependence and concurrent cocaine dependence. These findings do not demonstrate that buprenorphine is more effective than methadone for reducing cocaine use. These results are generally consistent with results of similar studies. Methadone and buprenorphine are well tolerated by patients. More research is needed to study the effectiveness of flexible and higher maintenance dosing regimens, and of combining maintenance treatment with buprenorphine or methadone with additional drug treatment or behavioral and psychosocial therapy.

▶ This article helps to establish that high-dose methadone works better than low-dose methadone or buprenorphine for both reducing the number of dirty urines with opioids and cocaine. Earlier reports from members of this group had hinted that buprenorphine might be superior to methadone in reducing cocaine abuse in this population. However, this article finds that this is not the case. Clinically, the problem of continued cocaine abuse in the opioid-addicted population remains a serious problem, even when methadone at high doses is used.

R.J. Frances, M.D.

Three Methods of Opioid Detoxification in a Primary Care Setting: A Randomized Trial
O'Conner PG, Carroll KM, Shi JM, et al (Yale Univ, New Haven, Conn)
Ann Intern Med 127:526–530, 1997   3–20

Background.—Treatment options for individuals who are opioid dependent, in addition to counseling, include maintenance with opioid agonists, or detoxification followed by maintenance with an opioid antagonist or followed by psychotherapy alone. Opioid maintenance is effective in decreasing drug use, but is highly restricted and may not be available to all individuals. An alternative may be detoxification and ongoing substance abuse treatment.

Methods.—In a randomized, double-blind trial, 3 pharmacologic protocols for opioid detoxification were compared in 162 heroin-dependent individuals. Patients were randomly assigned to 1 of 3 protocols: clonidine, clonidine and naltrexone combined, or buprenorphine. Outcome measures included successful detoxification, treatment retention, and withdrawal symptoms.

Results.—Successful detoxification was seen in 65% of patients given clonidine, 81% of patients given clonidine and naltrexone combined, and

81% of those given buprenorphine. Retention rates were similar in all groups: 65% of patients given clonidine, 54% of those given clonidine and naltrexone combined, and 60% of those given buprenorphine. Patients receiving buprenorphine had significantly lower withdrawal symptom scores than those given clonidine or clonidine and naltrexone combined.

Discussion.—Opioid detoxification in a primary care setting with 1 of these 3 pharmacologic treatment options may be effective in some patients with opioid dependency. There was no statistical difference between the percentage of patients assigned to clonidine or clonidine and naltrexone combined who completed detoxification. Detoxification with buprenorphine may be more comfortable for some patients.

▶ In spite of some of the benefits found for clonidine and naltrexone and buprenorphine, at this point clonidine therapy is likely to be the protocol of choice for primary care physicians, especially when methadone is unavailable or inappropriate, because clonidine therapy is less labor intensive and does not require as close observation as does treatment with clonidine and naltrexone (currently buprenorphine is an experimental drug). Buprenorphine did show promise in this study in that it provides a more comfortable detoxification for patients.

R.J. Frances, M.D.

Methylphenidate Treatment for Cocaine Abusers With Adult Attention-Deficit/Hyperactivity Disorder: A Pilot Study
Levin FR, Evans SM, McDowell DM, et al (Columbia Univ, New York; New York State Psychiatric Inst)
J Clin Psychiatry 59:300–305, 1998   3–21

Introduction.—Lack of treatment for comorbid disorders may play a role in the poor results of treatment for cocaine dependence. Cocaine abusers with adult attention-deficit/hyperactivity disorder (ADHD) may be at particularly high risk of treatment dropout or early treatment failure. Methylphenidate is an efficacious treatment for childhood ADHD. The use of this psychostimulant was evaluated in cocaine abusers with adult ADHD.

Methods.—The open trial included 12 cocaine abusers who also met DSM-IV criteria for cocaine dependence. All patients received 12 weeks of treatment with sustained-release methylphenidate, 40–80 mg in divided daily doses. In addition, all received standardized behavioral therapy for relapse prevention. The effects of treatment on ADHD symptoms were assessed. Regular assessment of vital signs and urine toxicologic studies were performed as well.

Results.—Eight patients completed the entire study, and 10 completed at least 8 weeks of treatment. Methylphenidate treatment was associated with reductions in attention difficulties, hyperactivity, and impulsivity. The patients also reported significant decrease in cocaine use and craving. Reductions in cocaine use were confirmed by urine tests.

Conclusions.—In cocaine abusers with ADHD, treatment with methylphenidate can reduce ADHD symptoms as well as cocaine craving and cocaine use. By reducing impulsivity and improving concentration, methylphenidate may heighten the effectiveness of relapse prevention and other treatments for cocaine abuse. A double-blind trial of methylphenidate for this difficult-to-treat population is recommended. There is some controversy regarding the use of methylphenidate in substance abusers.

▶ Although it may seem counterintuitive, sustained-release methylphenidate and relapse prevention therapy may help those with both adult ADHD and cocaine dependence who are self-medicating with cocaine for their underlying ADHD symptoms. This research group has been doing important studies to establish the safety and efficacy of stimulant treatment in selected patients with cocaine addiction. Other treatments that do not involve addicting substances for ADHD patients with addiction are also available and should be considered.

R.J. Frances, M.D.

4 Psychiatry & The Law

Introduction

The issue of physician-assisted suicide has heated up this year with the passage of a statute in Oregon permitting this practice. The federal government has warned physicians that the use of controlled substances for this means is against federal regulations. This issue parallels the controversy about medical uses of marijuana; the federal government has warned physicians in California and Arizona not to prescribe marijuana because state law may conflict with federal law. Both of these situations place physicians in an untenable situation in that state law may run counter to federal law. When state legislatures write laws that are counter to federal policies, it is unfair to place the burden of resolving these conflicts on physicians.

This year's psychiatry and law chapter is divided into four sections, covering the topics of end-of-life decisions (Abstracts 4–1 to 4–4); criminality (Abstracts 4–5 to 4–9); forensic and ethical issues (Abstracts 4–10 to 4–13); and informed consent and treatment issues (Abstracts 4–14 to 4–18).

This has been an important year for comment on physician-assisted suicide and end-of-life decisions. The Supreme Court handed down a decision refusing to define physician-assisted suicide as a right; however, the decision gives states leeway to develop their own approaches (Abstract 4–1). New reports from Holland about end-of-life decisions are covered in Abstracts 4–2 and 4–3. The accuracy of substituted judgments in patients with terminal diagnoses is discussed in Abstract 4–4. The section on criminality includes articles on sexual offenders (Abstracts 4–5, 4–6, and 4–7) and focuses on violence in Abstracts 4–7 and 4–8. Abstract 4–9 discusses an interesting longitudinal study from Finland. In the section on forensic and ethical issues, Abstract 4–10 discusses ideas for setting guidelines for conducting forensic examinations. Abstract 4–11 offers a theory of ethics for forensic psychiatry by a leading forensic psychiatrist. Abstract 4–12 discusses the effects of laws on mandatory parental involvement in minors' abortions, and Abstract 4–13 discusses discrimination against physicians on the basis of their sexual preferences. The last section in this chapter covers the topic of informed consent and treatment issues. Abstract 4–14 is an American Psychiatric Association document on principles of informed consent in psychiatry and provides an expert consensus from the American Psychiatric Association Counsel on psychiatry and the law.

Abstract 4–15 predicts physician judgments of capacity to consent, based on cognitive models. Abstract 4–16 describes issues related to public conservatorship related to age. Abstract 4–17 discusses the undertreatment of older persons with cognitive impairment, depression and incontinence, and Abstract 4–18 gives a broad international perspective on the evolution of laws of involuntary commitment.

With the development of a growing number of fellowships in forensic psychiatry and added qualifications, we are seeing an increasing number of peer review data-based articles related to forensic psychiatry. In my work as the Chief Executive Officer and Medical Director of Silver Hill Hospital, I find that a strong knowledge of forensic psychiatry can be very useful in reducing risk and claim issues, and plays an important part in the knowledge base required of psychiatric administrators.

Richard J. Frances, M.D.

End-of-Life Decisions

Physician-assisted Suicide and the Supreme Court: The *Washington* and *Vacco* Verdicts
Candilis PJ, Appelbaum KL (Univ of Massachusetts, Worcester; Worcester State Hosp, Mass)
J Am Acad Psychiatry Law 25:595-606, 1997   4–1

Objective.—The U.S. Supreme Court recently ruled in 2 cases concerning physician-assisted suicide. Both cases were related to state statutes that prohibited giving assistance to individuals wishing to end their lives. Analysis and commentary of these 2 decisions are presented.

Washington v. Glucksberg.—This case reached the Supreme Court after the Ninth Circuit Court ruled that Washington State's ban on assisted suicide was unconstitutional. Although the Supreme Court vote on this case was 9-0 in support of the state law, it still provided significant leeway for states to determine their own approaches to the issue. The opinion differentiated between the physician's obligation to respect a patient's right to refuse treatment and the physician's involvement in assisted suicide. The Court expressed concern that physician-assisted suicide could blur the distinction between healing and harming, and thus undermine trust between the physician and patient. The Court also expressed concern about vulnerable populations who might be at risk of coercion regarding end-of-life decisions, and about whether assistance in committing suicide might not be limited to physicians. Concurring opinions reinforced the notion that there is no generalized right to commit suicide.

Quill v. Vacco.—In this case, the Second Circuit Court refused to define physician-assisted suicide as a new fundamental right. At the same time, the circuit court agreed that the New York statute regarding physician-assisted suicide as second-degree manslaughter violated equal protection, in that it did not treat all competent individuals equally. The Supreme Court agreed that the New York statutes did not infringe on any fundamental rights. It also ruled that the law does not necessarily treat certain groups differently, even if groups are affected unevenly. As in the *Washington* decision, the court affirmed the distinction between withdrawal of life-sustaining treatment and assisted suicide. The intent in removing treatment is compliance with the patient's autonomy, whereas the intent in assisted suicide is to cause the patient's death. This distinction was a sound one, even though the line may be blurred in individual circumstances.

Discussion.—In these 2 decisions, the Supreme Court has ruled that state laws prohibiting physicians from providing lethal medications to competent, terminally ill patients do not violate the Due Process or Equal Protection Clauses of the Constitution. The Court returns the issue of physician-assisted suicide to the states, while not ruling out review of statutes that might place too many restrictions on end-of-life care. Key issues in future discussions of this controversial issue include the conceptual distinctions among assisted suicide, refusal of life-sustaining treatment, and administration of pain medication to terminally ill patients.

▶ These 2 important Supreme Court cases regarding physician-assisted suicide give the states leeway to establish their own approaches. The Supreme Court clearly did not want to follow the slippery slope toward involuntary euthanasia, looking to avoid using Holland as a model. While not accepting a right to assisted suicide, the Court does not equate this with a right to refuse unwanted treatment. The *Vacco* case supported the conceptual difference between withdrawing life-sustaining treatment and assisted suicide.

R.J. Frances, M.D.

Active Voluntary Euthanasia or Physician-assisted Suicide?
Onwuteaka-Philipsen BD, Muller MT, van der Wal G, et al (Vrije Universiteit Amsterdam; Naarderheem Ctr for Rehabilitation and Long-Term Care, Naarden, The Netherlands)
J Am Geriatr Soc 45:1208-1213, 1997   4–2

Background.—In The Netherlands, euthanasia is defined as the intentional termination of life by someone other than the patient, at the patient's request. Physician-assisted suicide is defined as a physician intentionally helping a patient to terminate the patient's own life. In 1990, 2 investigations were conducted into these practices in The Netherlands.

Study Design.—The studies were retrospective, covering the period from 1986 through 1990, and descriptive. Two random samples were obtained from all independently established general practitioners (GPs) registered with The Netherlands Institute of Primary Health Care. All 713 nursing home physicians (NHPs) who were members of the Association of Nursing Home Physicians were contacted for the second study. All studies were conducted by questionnaire. All nonresponders were contacted by telephone.

Findings.—Among those who used euthanasia, 48% of the GPs, 78% of the NHPs, and about 50% of the patients chose this option because of the patient's physical condition. The most common reason for GPs, NHPs, and patients to choose the physician-assisted suicide option was to give the patient ultimate responsibility.

Conclusions.—In general, active voluntary euthanasia was chosen by patients, GPs, and NHPs for medical or technical reasons, whereas physician-assisted suicide was chosen for moral reasons. GPs performed euthanasia more often than NHPs. Euthanasia is the only option possible for many patients because of their physical condition.

▶ With attention focused on physician-assisted suicide, it is fascinating to study the Dutch experience. It appears that in Holland, GPs would prefer to perform active, voluntary euthanasia, whereas most NHPs preferred assisted suicide. With euthanasia, the patient's life is terminated by someone other than the patient at the patient's request. With physician-assisted suicide, the physician is intentionally helping a patient to terminate his or her own life at his or her request. It is not clear to me whether this fine distinction, which may or may not make some doctors feel more comfortable with physician-assisted suicide, is important. However, the experience of those who have been involved in this controversy is interesting, especially as physician-assisted suicide becomes more common in the United States. The debate about whether, when, how, and by whom physician-assisted suicide should be allowed needs to be aired.

R.J. Frances, M.D.

Retrospective Study of Doctors' "End of Life Decisions" in Caring for Mentally Handicapped People in Institutions in the Netherlands
van Thiel GJMW, van Delden JJM, de Haan K, et al (Utrecht Univ, The Netherlands)
BMJ 315:88-91, 1997   4–3

Background.—Most mentally handicapped patients are dependent on others to make decisions for them, including decisions that might hasten death or end-of-life decisions. A nationwide retrospective study of end-of-life decisions for institutionalized mentally handicapped patients was performed in The Netherlands.

Study Design.—The study consisted of a survey of a random sample of 89 doctors who care for mentally handicapped patients, who reported all patient deaths from 1991 to 1996. The doctors completed a questionnaire and 68 mentioned at least 1 case in which they had taken an end-of-life decision. During 1996, 67 of these doctors were interviewed.

Findings.—These doctors reported 222 deaths in 1995. An end-of-life decision was made in 97 cases. In 75 of these cases, the decision was to withdraw or withhold treatment, and in 22, it was to relieve pain with dosages of opiates that may shorten life. In the 67 most recent cases, the patients were generally incompetent and younger than 65 years. Only 2 patients asked to die, but 23 communicated with their doctors in some fashion. In 60 cases, the doctor discussed the decision with the nursing staff, and in 46 cases, the doctor discussed the decision with a colleague.

Conclusions.—End-of-life decisions are an important aspect of the care of mentally handicapped people, but little is known about these decisions. An open discussion about these decisions could contribute to the quality of care for mentally handicapped patients.

▶ As end-of-life decisions become a more important topic for discussion because of state laws that are being passed to permit physician-assisted suicide in the United States, it is important to look at the Dutch experience. Many physicians in the United States might be especially worried about mentally handicapped patients who are not competent to participate in this decision and who, in this study, for the most part had not explicitly asked to die. In only 2 of the 222 cases reported in 1995 had patients actually requested to die. Therefore, developing a careful way of making sure that abuses do not occur and that attention be paid to developing a well thought-out approach to these important end-of-life decisions is essential.

R.J. Frances, M.D.

The Accuracy of Substituted Judgments in Patients With Terminal Diagnoses
Sulmasy DP, Terry PB, Weisman CS, et al (Georgetown Univ, Washington, DC; Johns Hopkins Med Institutions, Baltimore, Md)
Ann Intern Med 128:621-629, 1998   4–4

Introduction.—Loved ones are often called upon to make end-of-life decisions for patients who cannot speak for themselves. Although this is regarded as an important means of preserving the dying patient's autonomy, the accuracy of such substituted judgments has been questioned. A better understanding is needed of the accuracy of substituted judgments and the factors associated with accurate judgments. These issues were examined in an interview study of patients with terminal diagnoses and their surrogates.

Methods.—A total of 250 patients with various terminal diagnoses, such as congestive heart failure, AIDS, amyotrophic lateral sclerosis, lung cancer, and chronic obstructive pulmonary disease, were studied. Fifty pairs of patients and surrogates from each diagnostic group participated in the study, along with 50 general medical patients and their surrogates. The patients and surrogates were presented with hypothetical clinical scenarios and potential treatments. The accuracy of surrogate judgments was assessed, as were the beliefs, practices, and clinical and demographic factors associated with accurate judgments. Patient preferences regarding life-sustaining treatment were assessed, and the various diagnostic groups were compared for accuracy of surrogate decisions.

Results.—The surrogates' predictions agreed with the patients' preferences in two thirds of cases. A clinical scenario involving permanent coma was associated with higher accuracy scores than scenarios involving severe dementia or coma with a small chance of recovery. Factors associated with a greater chance of accurate surrogate decisions included having spoken with the surrogate about such decisions, odds ratio (OR) 1.9; having private insurance, OR 1.4; surrogate's educational level, OR 1.5; and patient's level of education, OR 1.7. Factors decreasing the likelihood of accurate predictions were patients' belief that they would live more than 10 years, OR 0.6; surrogate experience with life-sustaining treatment, OR 0.4; surrogate participation in religious services; and patient diagnosis of heart failure. Accuracy was unaffected by age, ethnicity, marital status, religion, or the presence of advance directives.

Conclusions.—Many different patient and surrogate factors influence the accuracy of substituted judgments regarding end-of-life decisions. These variables can be used to assess the likelihood that a given judgment is accurate or inaccurate, and to target educational interventions to increase the accuracy of surrogate judgments. Several testable strategies of this type are suggested.

▶ This article points to the importance of increasing public education about end-of-life decisions, the limitations of surrogates' judgment, and the importance of having frank discussions with loved ones about one's wishes in a terminal situation. Some of the factors that promote more accurate judgments, such as a greater level of education and a greater degree of communication between the patient and the surrogate, are what might be expected. However, it was surprising that those involved with religious services are more likely to have inaccurate judgments. Clinicians clearly need to use their judgment and to look closely at whether the surrogate is likely to be representing a patient's true preferences.

R.J. Frances, M.D.

Criminality

Predicting Relapse: A Meta-analysis of Sexual Offender Recidivism Studies

Hanson RK, Bussière MT (Solicitor Gen of Canada)
J Consult Clin Psychol 66:348-362, 1998   4–5

Introduction.—The prediction that sexual offenders will relapse can have a considerable impact, because those likely to repeat such behavior may receive a permanent label as a sexual offender. Although there is extensive research on prediction of recidivism among nonsexual criminals, sexual offending may be different from other types of crime. A meta-analysis of data from 61 studies sought to identify factors most strongly related to recidivism among sexual offenders.

Methods.—Data were obtained from computer searches of PsycLIT and the National Criminal Justice Reference System, from reference lists, and

TABLE 4.—Correlations With Recidivism for Each Category of Predictor

Predictor	Sexual	Type of Recidivism Nonsexual Violence	Any
Criminal lifestyle	.12 ± .02	.16 ± .03	.21 ± .02
Sexual deviance	.19 ± .01	.01 ± .03	.12 ± .02
Psychological maladjustment	.01 ± .03	.02 ± .08	.02 ± .03
Negative clinical presentation	.00 ± .07		.15 ± .07
Failure to complete treatment	.17 ± .07	.08 ± .09	.20 ± .07

Values represent average correlations ± 95% confidence interval.

(Reprinted with permission from Hanson RK, Bussière MT: Predicting relapse: A meta-analysis of sexual offender recidivism studies. *J Consult Clin Psychol* 66:348-362, 1998, copyright by the American Psychological Association.)

from communication with 32 established sexual offender researchers. All eligible studies examined a sample of sex offenders, reported recidivism and nonsexual violent offenses, and contained sufficient statistical information for analysis. Quality of the study was also a consideration.

Results.—Each of the eligible studies had small sample sizes, but information was provided for a total of 28,972 sexual offenders. With an average follow-up period of 4 to 5 years, the overall sex offense recidivism rate was 13.4%: 18.9% for rapists and 12.7% for child molesters. Recidivism rates were considerably higher if all reoffenses by the sexual offenders were included. Sexual offense recidivism was best predicted by measures of sexual deviancy, such as deviant sexual preferences and previous sexual offenses. Also at increased risk of relapse (Table 4) were offenders who failed to complete treatment. Predictors of nonsexual violent recidivism were similar for sexual and nonsexual offenders.

Discussion.—Predictors of nonsexual recidivism among sexual offenders were similar to those found in general offender populations (young, unmarried individuals with a history of antisocial behavior), whereas the strongest predictors of sexual recidivism were factors related to sexual deviance. With sexual offenses, many years of follow-up may be required to determine whether the offender has responded to treatment.

▶ I found it surprising that only 13.4% of the sample of sexual offenders committed a new offense within an average of 4 to 5 years. I was also surprised that treatment programs can make a greater contribution to community safety than I might have expected, and are more effective than most people think. This article identifies risk factors that might predict higher rates of recidivism, such as attitudes tolerant of sexual crimes. More research needs to be done to develop new and better treatment approaches for this population, who often spend long periods in prison.

R.J. Frances, M.D.

Stalking Part II: Victims' Problems With the Legal System and Therapeutic Considerations

Abrams KM, Robinson GE (Univ of Toronto)
Can J Psychiatry 43:477-481, 1998

4–6

Background.—The victims of stalking or criminal harassment are usually women who have had a relationship with the offender. This article is the second of a 2-part review of the crime of stalking. Part I summarizes stalking behavior, types of offenders, the relationships between victims and offenders, and mental health consequences for the victims. Part II summarizes the problems that victims have with the legal system, and the psychotherapeutic tasks for victims and therapists.

Methods.—Relevant articles from psychiatric and legal journals were identified by a computerized search. Publications from victims' and women's organizations were also reviewed.

Results.—Victims suffer emotional consequences of being stalked, and stress from the lack of understanding that they encounter in the legal system, and from laws that are either inadequate or unenforced. Treatment for the victim should include education, psychotherapy, and discussion of practical and safety measures. Therapists may overidentify with the patient's sense of powerlessness, or may be unwilling to take the case of a stalking victim because of fear of the stalker. Female therapists may blame the victim as a way of avoiding the realization of their own vulnerability. Male therapists may feel defensive or guilty and project their own anger onto the patient, or may feel overprotective, thereby reinforcing the message that the victim is helpless and vulnerable.

Discussion.—Stalking is a crime that is not well understood by society and that causes major mental health consequences. Therapists need to be aware of the victim's emotional reactions, available legal and practical support, and the biases of society. Therapists should encourage education and research in this area by working with the police, as well as the medical and legal fields, to increase understanding of and effective interventions for this crime.

▶ Victims of crimes, especially stalking, are often doubly victimized by the process of dealing with the legal system. This article discusses the powerful countertransference reactions to these vulnerable people, and the need to have a practical approach to the patient. This issue would benefit from collaborative study between police and mental health professionals.

R.J. Frances, M.D.

Natural Born Killers?: The Development of the Sexually Sadistic Serial Killer
Johnson BR, Becker JV (Univ of Arizona, Tucson)
J Am Acad Psychiatry Law 25:335-348, 1997   4–7

Objective.—Case studies of so-called serial killers have provided little clinically useful information, including how to identify children and adolescents at risk of becoming serial killers. Many adolescents fantasize about committing violent crimes at a young age. Nine clinical cases of adolescents who fantasize about becoming serial killers were described.

Patients.—Most of the patients were referred for forensic evaluation after having committed a legal offense. Some were referred by mental health workers concerned about unusual behavior. The age range was 14 to 18 years; only 1 was female. Many of the patients had histories of killing animals. All fantasized about killing and/or mutilating individuals. Many became sexually excited when killing animals or fantasizing about killing individuals. Histories of sexual abuse were common. Some specifically mentioned being excited by the movie "Silence of the Lambs," or wishing to emulate the serial killer character in that movie. Two had already committed murders.

Discussion.—These case reports of adolescents who fantasize about becoming serial killers are similar in many ways to retrospective studies and case reports of real serial killers. Young patients who have sexually sadistic fantasies and talk about killing must be followed up over time. This information may aid in understanding whether there is any way to distinguish between those who will and will not go on to kill. More study is needed to evaluate potentially helpful treatments for this population.

▶ The violent crimes of children and adolescents have received a great deal of media attention. Clearly, there is a need to determine the factors that might lead to high-risk situations and look for ways to prevent these crimes from being committed. Tip-offs that indicate who will become a psychopathic sexual sadist, a crime spree killer, a member of organized crime, or a violently psychotic individual may be difficult to recognize. The value of obtaining a detailed sexual history in adolescents prone to crime, especially a history of sexual sadism and paraphilia, appears to be important. I would find it hard to predict whether any of the patients described in this article will actually become a serial killer. Clearly, there is a need for longitudinal study. Currently, I think our ability to predict who will become a murderer is limited. It is also very hard to determine the immediate risk vs. the long-term risk for developing homicidal behavior. It is also not clear how many individuals share characteristics with serial killers but do not become murderers. Narcissism, paranoia, antisocial features, and sexual paraphilias are far more common than actual murders. It is still hard to know the best ways to treat an individual with these characteristics and prevent him from becoming a murderer.

R.J. Frances, M.D.

Violence and Severe Mental Illness: The Effects of Substance Abuse and Nonadherence to Medication

Swartz MS, Swanson JW, Hiday VA, et al (Duke Univ, Durham, NC; North Carolina State Univ, Raleigh)
Am J Psychiatry 155:226-231, 1998   4–8

Introduction.—Some patients with severe mental illness who live in the community are at risk for committing violent behavior. To identify such individuals and design more effective ways to prevent their violent and threatening behavior, investigators examined the effects of selected predictors of recent community violence in a study of 331 hospitalized patients.

Methods.—The longitudinal outcome study enrolled involuntarily admitted inpatients with severe mental illness; all were awaiting a period of outpatient commitment at the time of participating in an extensive face-to-face interview. A family member or other individual who knew the patient well completed a telephone interview. Data from patients, family members, and hospital records were combined to determine the patient's illness history, clinical status, medication noncompliance, substance abuse, insight into illness, and violent behavior during the 4 months before hospitalization. Multivariable logistic regression was used to analyze associations between serious violent acts and individual characteristics and problems.

Results.—Serious violent acts were more likely to be committed by those who were male, African-American, had been victims of crimes in the past 4 months, or had co-occurring substance abuse problems. Variables not associated with serious violent acts were urban residence, medication noncompliance, or low insight into illness. After controlling for sociodemographic and clinical characteristics, however, there was a significant association between the combination of medical noncompliance and alcohol or substance abuse problems and serious violent acts in the community.

Conclusion.—To prevent violent behavior and institutional recidivism in severely mentally ill patients after hospital discharge, careful attention must be paid to medication adherence and to the availability of integrated substance abuse and mental health treatment. Neuroleptic medications are often difficult to take regularly because of adverse side effects and complicated dosing regimens.

▶ In the summer of 1998, a severely mentally ill schizophrenic attempted to "shoot up" Congress. Newspaper accounts said that he had not taken medication for schizophrenia and that he had a history of drug abuse, both of which, according to this article, may signal a higher risk of violent behavior among persons with severe mental illness. Factors such as integrating mental health and substance abuse treatment, outpatient commitment, and broadening commitment laws for those who have severe mental illness and do not take their medication would be useful. Unfortunately, patients with severe mental illness and substance abuse often have low levels of insight and low motivation for treatment. We need to find better ways to get these patients the help they need. An additional problem is lack of adequate funding for treating mental illness in the United States, a problem that leads to greater numbers of these mentally ill patients ending up in prison. Congress should now be more aware that the costs of mental illness go beyond the financial costs and that it is important to sensitize the public to the need for adequate funding to treat the mentally ill or chemically dependent.

R.J. Frances, M.D.

Juvenile Mortality, Mental Disturbances and Criminality: A Prospective Study of the Northern Finland 1966 Birth Cohort

Räsänen P, Tiihonen J, Isohanni M, et al (Univ of Oulu, Finland; Univ of Kuopio, Finland)
Acta Psychiatr Scand 97:5-9, 1998

4–9

Background.—Various types of samples can be used to study relationships among mortality, criminality, and mental disorders. Total population studies suggest a high frequency of mental disorders in individuals dying of unnatural causes. The associations among mortality, criminality, and mental illness were examined in juveniles in an unselected birth cohort.

Methods.—Data were used from a prospective longitudinal cohort of 12,058 children born in northern Finland during 1966. Data on cohort members' mental health, criminality, and mortality were prospectively collected up to the age of 27 years.

Results.—Of the 117 deaths observed, 79.5% were of unnatural causes—i.e., suicide or other violent death. Eighty-two percent of the violent

TABLE 3.—Causes of Death for Each Diagnostic and Criminality Group, Including Male and Female Subjects

	Unnatural deaths (*n*)			Natural Deaths (*n*)	Total (*n*)
	Suicide	Accident Or Trauma	Homicide		
Diagnosis (*DSM-III-R*)					
Schizophrenia	4	1	0	0	5
Schizophrenia spectrum	0	0	0	0	0
Other psychoses	2	1	0	0	3
All psychoses	6	2	0	0	8
Personality disorder	3	0	0	0	3
Alcohol abuse	0	1	0	0	1
Other mental disorder	1	4	0	0	5
No diagnosis	21	53	2	24	100
Registered crimes	7	8	0	0	15
Mental disorder and criminality	4	1	0	0	5

(Courtesy of Räsänen P, Tiihonen J, Isohanni M, et al: Juvenile mortality, mental disturbances and criminality: A prospective study of the Northern Finland 1966 Birth Cohort. *Acta Psychiatr Scand* 97:5-9. Copyright 1998, Munksgaard International Publishers Ltd., Copenhagen.)

deaths occurred in males. Mortality was significantly increased for men with schizophrenia, odds ratio (OR) 9.31; other psychoses, OR 10.28; and personality disorders, OR 4.28. By comparison, mortality was lower for criminality alone (OR 2.60) or criminality combined with mental disorders (OR 3.27). Mental disturbance did not significantly increase mortality among females. Among individuals with major mental disorders, three fourths of the deaths resulted from suicide (Table 3).

Conclusions.—In young males, mortality is significantly increased in association with psychotic and personality disorders and with criminality. Males are more than 3 times as likely to die as females, and much more likely to die of unnatural causes. This is the first study to examine associations among juvenile mortality, mental disorders, and criminality using a large birth cohort and structured validation of psychiatric diagnoses.

▶ The high mortality rates for young men, and especially for those with mental illness, are a striking finding in this study. That 75% of the deaths of those with major mental disorders are suicides is even more striking in this cohort who were followed up to age 27. Apparently, violence and suicide are major risk causes of death in this young population, and most of the suicides occur in the severely mentally ill and those with substance abuse.

R.J. Frances, M.D.

Forensic and Ethical Issues

Toward the Development of Guidelines for the Conduct of Forensic Psychiatric Examinations

Simon RI, Wettstein RM (Georgetown Univ, Washington, DC; Univ of Pittsburgh, Pa)
J Am Acad Psychiatry Law 25:17-29, 1997　　　　　　　　　　4–10

Purpose.—There are no clear guidelines for conducting independent forensic psychiatric consultations and evaluations. Although statements by the American Academy of Psychiatry and the Law and the American Psychiatric Association provide some relevant information, they do not include specific guidelines. Guidelines designed to maintain the integrity of the forensic psychiatric consultation were proposed and discussed.

Guidelines for Forensic Psychiatric Examinations.—The guidelines are based on clinical practice, on the ethical principles of general and forensic psychiatry, and on relevant case and statutory law. Their premise is that the forensic psychiatrist is offering clinical knowledge and expertise for use in litigation, with the goal of objectivity and without any alliance to the patient. The first guideline is to maintain objectivity and neutrality. This guideline includes correcting for personal biases, not attempting to influence or coerce the examinee, or creating the illusion of a treatment relationship. The forensic psychiatrist should make every effort to personally examine the individual; if this is not required or feasible, the psychiatrist should note that the opinion is a limited one. The examination should respect examinee autonomy, including allowing the examinee to contact counsel or to terminate the interview. The evaluation should protect confidentiality to the maximum possible extent, within the context of the legal situation. The forensic examiner should obtain informed consent, providing the examinee with information on the nature and purpose of the examination at the start. This includes the information that there is no treatment relationship. The primary mode of evaluation should be verbal; if any type of physical examination or special procedure is to be performed, specific permission should be obtained.

To ensure a credible, objective examination, there should be no previous, current, or future personal relationship between the examiner and examinee. There should be no romantic or sexual contact between the examiner and examinee, any member of the examinee's family, or any other party involved in the legal case. Anonymity between the examiner and examinee should be preserved to the greatest extent possible. The fee policy for the examination should be clearly established in advance, in writing. There should be no contingency fee. The examination should take place in a suitable setting that is reasonably private and comfortable, especially if outside the examiner's office. The evaluation should be scheduled in advance, allowing sufficient time for a thorough review of all relevant issues.

Discussion.—These guidelines for forensic psychiatric examinations are intended to enhance the performance of competent, honest, and objective forensic examinations. The authors hope that their proposed guidelines will promote further discussion and additions.

▶ These authors propose guidelines for forensic psychiatric examinations based on clinical practice as well as ethical principles in general psychiatry, and provide a practical starting point for discussion. I'm glad that the guidelines take into account the ethical principles in general psychiatry, because I feel that psychiatrists should, even in subspecialty roles, be responsible for maintaining the general principles and standards of being a psychiatrist as well as being a physician. Elaborating particular issues that psychiatrists face when they testify or take on forensic work can also be useful. Guidelines such as these need to be tested against both the empirical literature and the consensus of experts and practitioners in the field.

R.J. Frances, M.D.

A Theory of Ethics for Forensic Psychiatry

Appelbaum PS (Univ of Massachusetts, Worcester)
J Am Acad Psychiatry Law 25:233-247, 1997   4-11

Purpose.—At least 1 commentator has not only pointed out the lack of ethical principles in forensic psychiatry, but also suggested that it was futile to try to develop such principles. Although certain principles have been discussed, no comprehensive schema of ethics in forensic psychiatry has been put forth. An outline of a theory of ethics for forensic psychiatry was presented.

Ethics in Forensic Psychiatry.—The proposed principles are based on the specific societal functions performed by forensic psychiatrists, consistent with the theory of professional ethics in general. The goal of these principles is to intensify the efforts by forensic psychiatrists to promote certain key moral values. The main value of forensic psychiatry is to promote the interests of justice. Two principles were identified that are relevant to this effort: truth-telling and respect for individuals. General medical ethics do not necessarily apply to physicians operating outside the usual clinical setting, such as in clinical research. That is because medical ethics is centered on the physician-patient relationship, which is not a factor in forensic psychiatry. Any effort to preserve aspects of the physician-patient relationship and its associated ethical principles is likely to lead to confusion for both the forensic psychiatrist and their evaluees. This approach could also lead to increased problems with double agency. In contrast, basing the ethics of forensic psychiatry on the pursuit of justice, rather than the pursuit of health, draws a clear distinction between the roles of the forensic and therapeutic psychiatrist.

Discussion.—It is suggested that a separate theory of ethics is needed for forensic psychiatry, based on the principle of advancing the interests of justice. Such a code of ethics is essential to deal with the problem of double agency. The author hopes that his efforts will stimulate discussion of the ethical foundation of forensic psychiatry.

▶ A thoughtful and thorough examination of the ethical foundations of forensic psychiatry is presented in this important article. Although exigencies related to the court situation lead to a need to elaborate ethical principles specific to the forensic psychiatrist, I find myself uncomfortable when arguments are made for not using traditional medical and psychiatric ethics as the basis for developing principles of ethics that need to be followed by forensic psychiatrists. Paul Appelbaum feels that there are enough differences to warrant the development of whole additional ethical principles for forensic psychiatrists and gives a rationale for doing so. Even when testifying in court, however, I feel that psychiatrists need to act on the principles of being a psychiatrist first and a forensic psychiatrist second. As long as Dr. Appelbaum's principles do not conflict with core medical and psychiatric principles, I think they are useful.

R.J. Frances, M.D.

Mandatory Parental Involvement in Minors' Abortions: Effects of the Laws in Minnesota, Missouri, and Indiana
Ellertson C (Population Council, New York)
Am J Public Health 87:1367-1374, 1997   4–12

Objective.—Several states have parental involvement laws that require notification or consent of parents before a minor can have an abortion. There is heated debate over the claimed beneficial vs. harmful effects of these laws. Empirical data on the impact of these laws could be useful to advocates, policy makers, and legislators. Vital records data were analyzed to assess the effects of parental involvement laws.

Methods.—Data were used from 3 states with parental involvement laws: Minnesota, Missouri, and Indiana. Records from before and after parental involvement legislation was implemented were analyzed by Poisson and logistic regression models. The analysis sought to determine the laws' effects on birth rate, in-state abortion rate, likelihood of interstate travel, and likelihood of late abortions among minors.

Results.—Compared with older women, the in-state abortion rate for minors decreased in each state after parental involvement laws were implemented. Neither was there any increase in the minors' abortion rate when Minnesota's parental involvement laws were lifted. The data did not support the hypothesis that births to minors would increase. Minors appeared more likely to travel out of state to obtain abortions. Although data on this subject were incomplete, they suggested that—at least in Missouri—minors traveling out of state might have accounted entirely for the reduction in in-state abortions. Parental involvement appeared to be associated with a delay of abortions past the eighth week of gestation, but probably not into the second trimester (Table 5).

Conclusions.—Laws requiring parental notification or consent for abortions in minors do not appear to increase the rate of births to minors. Although there is evidence that these laws reduce the in-state abortion rate for minors, this may be counterbalanced by minors traveling to other states to get abortions. The available empirical data do not support many of the arguments used either in favor of or against parental involvement legislation.

▶ When parental involvement laws went into effect, birth rates for minors did not rise in the states affected, nor did they fall when the states' laws were lifted. One effect of the law was to increase interstate travel for minors looking for an abortion, which may have led to a slight delay in abortions for these minors. Certainly forcing minors to travel out of state for their abortions didn't improve family unity, help resolve family problems, protect the rights of the parents to raise their children, or reduce sexual behavior among minors in those states. If policy makers are indeed looking to enact such laws, perhaps they should think about imposing them on a regional or

TABLE 5.—Estimated Change in Outcome Measures for Women of 3 Age Groups (Minors and 2 Control Groups) During Period of Parental Involvement Law Relative to Period Immediately Prior to the Law*

Outcome Measure	Minnesota		Missouri†		Indiana	
	% Change	z Ratio‡	% Change	z Ratio‡	% Change	z Ratio‡
Birth rate						
<18	+0.9		+4.4		−9.2	
18–19	−0.4	0.750	+7.4‖	2.900	−3.4§	4.692
20–24	+1.7	10.000	+2.7	1.625	−3.3§	6.300
In-state abortion rate						
<18	−26.0		−20.1		−16.9	
18–19	−7.8§	11.000	−8.2§	7.875	+9.2§	12.909
20–24	+4.4§	18.556	+2.8§	16.800	15.3§	18.000
In-state pregnancy rate						
<18	−9.1		−2.3		−10.6	
18–19	−1.6§	6.583	+3.3§	6.000	+0.1§	10.363
20–24	+1.7§	10.182	+2.1§	6.143	−0.6§	11.778
Odds of ending preg- nancy by in-state abortion						
<18	−28.3		−23.6		−7.7	
18–19	−9.3§	9.400	−14.2§	5.421	+8.2§	8.231
20–24	+1.5§	15.818	+0.0§	15.882	+15.2§	12.318
Odds of traveling out of state for abortion						
<18	NA		+52.9		NA	
18–19	NA		+12.9§	8.758	NA	
20–24	NA		+18.2§	7.355	NA	
Odds of delaying abor- tion > 12 weeks						
<18	NA		+10.1		NA	
18–19	NA		+12.7	0.719	NA	
20–24	NA		+17.5¶	2.167	NA	
Odds of delay, in state, > 12 weeks						
<18	−0.7		16.6		−28.4	
18–19	−6.5	1.200	3.9‖	3.026	−50.0	1.671
20–24	−8.4¶	1.761	21.7	1.229	−46.6	1.547
Odds of delay, out of state, > 12 weeks						
<18	NA		−9.4		NA	
18–19	NA		34.6§	7.014	NA	
20–24	NA		−3.1§	0.353	NA	
Odds of delay, in state, > 8 weeks						
<18	+9.5		NA		−5.4	
18–19	−3.2§	2.860	NA		−9.9	1.600
20–24	−2.2§	3.289	NA		−7.4	0.600

*Estimates are percentage change in fitted values derived from legal period by age interaction coefficients from models that also include terms for time (linear and quadratic), age group, legal period, and legal period by time interactions.

†Out-of-state abortions refer to abortions performed on Missouri residents in the states of Arkansas, Kansas, Nebraska, Oklahoma, and Tennessee. A small number of abortions performed in other states (not including Illinois) are included.

‡Absolute z ratios of the original test statistics.

§Significantly different from change for minors at $P < 0.001$.

‖Significantly different from change for minors at $P < 0.01$.

¶Significantly different from change from minors at $P < 0.05$.

Abbreviation: NA, not available.

(Courtesy of Ellertson C: Mandatory parental involvement in minors' abortions: Effects of the laws in Minnesota, Missouri, and Indiana. *Am J Public Health* 87:1367-1374. Copyright 1997, American Public Health Association.)

national basis to have a bigger impact on behavior without increasing the risk and expense created by having minors travel out of state for an abortion.

R.J. Frances, M.D.

Discrimination Against Gay, Lesbian and Bisexual Family Physicians by Patients

Druzin P, Shrier I, Yacowar M, et al (McGill Univ, Montreal)
Can Med Assoc J 158:593-597, 1998   4–13

Introduction.—Individuals who are gay, lesbian, or bisexual (GLB) face discrimination within the medical community as well as in other areas. It may be more difficult for GLBs to enter medical school, be selected for a residency program, and have patients referred to them. A study based upon telephone interviews sought to determine the attitudes of patients toward GLB physicians.

Methods.—Questions posed in the interviews were drawn from suggestions by 10 GLBs and 10 heterosexuals. Each of the 6 potential reasons why a patient might refuse to see a GLB physician had been proposed by more than 10 of the 20 individuals questioned. The 500 respondents were randomly selected from Montreal residential telephone listings.

Results.—The survey had a refusal rate of 30%. Of those who were reached and agreed to participate, 249 (72%) were aged 50 years or younger and 194 (56%) were women. Forty-one (11.8%) respondents stated that they would refuse to see a GLB family physician. The 2 most common reasons cited were incompetence on the GLB physician's part and an "uncomfortable" feeling on the patient's part. Men were more likely than women to discriminate against a GLB physician, and most men and women expressed more discrimination with increasing age.

Conclusion.—The rate of discrimination by patients against GLB physicians was lower than that found in some previous reports, and younger individuals were less likely to discriminate. Responses indicate that discrimination against GLB physicians is caused by misinformation and a general negative view of homosexuality.

▶ Clearly, the public needs to be better educated about the lack of any relation between clinical competence, education, and credentials and sexual preference. Although there are professional and societal prohibitions against physicians' discrimination against patients, discrimination by patients is not sanctionable in any way, and demands efforts to destigmatize homosexuality in general.

R.J. Frances, M.D.

Informed Consent and Treatment Issues

American Psychiatric Association Resource Document on Principles of Informed Consent in Psychiatry

The American Psychiatric Association Council on Psychiatry and Law
J Am Acad Psychiatry Law 25:121-125, 1997   4–14

Introduction.—The principle of informed consent involves legal, ethical, and clinical dimensions. This resource document discusses the legal principles and clinical aspects of informed consent in psychiatry.

Legal Principles.—Before initiation of psychiatric treatment, informed consent should be obtained from all adult patients and from the parents or legal guardians of minors who cannot provide consent. Patients are to be advised about the nature of their condition and of the proposed therapy, the benefits and risks of the treatment, and available alternatives. Exceptions to these guidelines include emergency situations, incompetence on the part of the patient, patients who have waived their right to receive information, therapeutic privilege (information withheld because of possible harm to the patient), and involuntary treatment (patient's refusal of treatment overridden).

Clinical Aspects.—Patients should be encouraged to ask for additional information relevant to their condition. Disclosure can continue during treatment as the patient's condition changes or as alternative treatments become available. Minors who cannot provide informed consent should still be given as much information as possible. Consent should be documented, using either printed forms or chart notes. Discussion with families or institutional review can be helpful if the patient's capacity to give informed consent is questionable. Informed consent should be sought for psychotherapy as well as for invasive procedures and medications.

▶ In this fast-paced world where sessions with psychiatrists are often reduced to between 15 and 30 minutes, there can be inadequate explanation of the risks and benefits of treatment. The value of patient and family education clearly exists and these guidelines are useful in describing the clinical aspects of informed consent. Patients may be able to give more informed consent as their condition improves, and therefore obtaining consent is an ongoing process.

R.J. Frances, M.D.

Cognitive Models That Predict Physician Judgments of Capacity to Consent in Mild Alzheimer's Disease

Marson DC, Hawkins L, McInturff B, et al (Univ of Alabama, Birmingham)
J Am Geriatr Soc 45:458-464, 1997   4–15

Purpose.—There has been surprisingly little research in the area of competency loss in dementia, including the natural history of loss of competency, factors affecting physicians' decisions regarding competency, and interventions to assist decision-making capacity in patients. Physician judgments are widely accepted as the standard for determining capacity to consent in patients with dementia; yet, there have been no studies of how specific cognitive changes in Alzheimer's disease (AD) are related to loss of competency judgments by physicians. Cognitive factors predicting consent capacity, as judged by experienced physicians, were researched.

Methods.—Five experienced physicians made competency decisions regarding 45 patients: 29 with mild AD, as reflected by a Mini-Mental State Examination score of 20 or greater, and 16 normal older controls. These judgments were based on videotaped interviews of the subjects responding to a standardized consent capacity interview. The same patients were also assessed on various neuropsychological measures linked or potentially linked to competency. The physicians' judgments of competency or non-competency to consent to treatment were made without knowledge of the subjects' diagnoses or neuropsychological test results. Data on the overall sample were used in stepwise discriminant function analyses (DFAs) to identify neuropsychological variables affecting each physician's competency judgments. These models were then tested for accuracy in classifying competency outcomes by classification DFAs.

Results.—The individual physicians varied in their cognitive models, and the variation was unrelated to the stringency of judgments for patients with AD. Judgments were predicted by delayed verbal recall in 1 physician, by short-term verbal recall in another, by phonemic word fluency in another, and by visuomotor tracking–sequencing in another. The percentages of patients with AD judged incompetent by these physicians were 90%, 52%, 24%, and 14%, respectively. The rates of correct classification by these single-predictor solutions were 93%, 87%, 87%, and 96%, respectively. (The fifth physician judged all research subjects with AD to be competent; therefore, he had no predictor model for incompetence.) When 2 predictor solutions were used, rates of successful classification improved from 98% to 100%.

Conclusions.—Physicians' judgments of consent capacity can be described by 2 cognitive models: verbal recall and simple executive function. Under the verbal recall model, physicians are likely to judge patients with mild AD to be incompetent. Under the executive function model, the judgment is more likely to be for competency. Physicians evaluating capacity to consent to treatment in patients with dementia may find it useful to assess the patients' verbal recall and simple executive functions.

▶ The use of specific tests such as verbal recall and simple executive function can help physicians in making judgment calls that are difficult to make with regard to capacity consent in mild AD.

R.J. Frances, M.D.

Criteria for Placing Older Adults in Public Conservatorship: Age as Proxy for Need

Reynolds SL (Univ of South Florida, Tampa)
Gerontologist 37:518-526, 1997

4–16

Background.—Public conservatorship or guardianship provides the services of a surrogate decision maker for impaired adults. Older adults have been thought to be inappropriately subject to conservatorship. California's conservatorship practice was evaluated to determine whether it is age blind as specified by law.

Study Design.—The Los Angeles County Office of Public Guardian (LACOPG) provides public guardianship services of 2 types. Lanterman-Petris-Short (LPS) conservatorship provides decision-making services to mentally ill adults who enter the system through civil commitment. Probate conservatorship provides decision-making services for those who enter through the process of a judicial petition. A needs-based definition is used to determine service requirements. A cross-sectional study was performed of California public conservatees in Los Angeles County in July 1993. The data were obtained from the LACOPG's management information system. The total study population consisted of 2,151 adults ranging in age from 18 to 103 years. The study group was 55% male and 59% single. Latinos and Asians were underrepresented. Median income was $7,236 and median estate value was $11, 630. Approximately 34% of conservatees had problems with at least 3 activities of daily living, whereas 36% had no problems with activities of daily living. Most conservatees had diagnoses of psychoses. This study investigated the time LACOPG staff spent on investigating proposed conservatees and their assignment into the 2 conservatorship programs.

Findings.—Age was not a factor in the amount of time LACOPG staff spent on investigations of proposed conservatees. Being older and having more income increased the probability of probate conservatorship by 1 percentage point for each year or each $1,000.

Conclusions.—The findings of this study of public conservatorship in California suggest that the process by which adults are assigned to public conservatorship is not age blind, as specified by California law. Further studies should be conducted to determine the reasons behind this finding.

▶ I have seen clinical cases where elderly who are in need of conservatorship do not get it and where this leads to their being taken advantage of or being mistreated, and I have seen other situations in which the very old feel deprived of their rights unjustly because of their age. This article poses the problems and discusses criteria and discrimination related to ageism. There needs to be more precise criteria for probate conservatorship based on need.

R.J. Frances, M.D.

To Treat or Not to Treat: Issues in Decisions Not to Treat Older Persons With Cognitive Impairment, Depression, and Incontinence
Silverman M, McDowell BJ, Musa D, et al (Univ of Pittsburgh, Pa)
J Am Geriatr Soc 45:1094-1101, 1997   4–17

Background.—Successful identification of problems of cognitive impairment, depression, and urinary incontinence by geriatric assessment units (GAUs) at 4 geriatric centers was previously described. However, despite the identification of these problems, not all were addressed by treatment recommendations. The decisions not to treat problems identified by GAUs were investigated in a descriptive study.

Study Design.—A multicenter, randomized, controlled trial of geriatric assessment and short-term follow-up was conducted between 1988 and 1992. The 442 adult participants lived in the community or in personal care homes, were at least 65 years of age, and had health problems. Of the 442 participants, 239 were randomly allocated to receive geriatric assessment. The complete medical charts were available for review in 192 cases. Recommendations of the GAU were communicated to the patient directly and to the referring physician by telephone or letter. These patients were studied for 1 year by monthly telephone calls and quarterly in-home interviews.

Findings.—Although treatment was recommended for most of the cognitive impairment, depression, and incontinence problems of this older patient group, approximately one third of cognitive impairment and depression and one half of incontinence problems did not receive treatment recommendations. Decisions not to treat were categorized as treatment refusal, incomplete assessment, intervention already in place, concurrent problems interfered with treatment, no documented diagnosis, problem was ruled out, or no documented reason for the decision not to treat. There was no documented reason for lack of treatment in 24% of incontinence, 13% of depression, and 4% of cognitive impairment cases.

Conclusions.—Chart records were reviewed for patients undergoing geriatric assessment who were identified as having problems in cognitive impairment, depression, or incontinence. Treatment recommendations were documented in the majority of cases, but in a number of cases, there was no evidence of treatment recommendation. With the increasing number of older adults with multiple problems in our community, guidelines for how to make treatment decisions, especially in cases of comorbidities, need to be established.

▶ This article documents the problem of inadequate assessment, intervention, and treatment planning in situations in which a decision is made not to treat elderly individuals with cognitive impairment, depression, and incontinence. It will be helpful to develop better guidelines in the treatment of this population. Increasing skills of staff in dealing with cognitive impairment, depression, and incontinence are important parts of improving treatment efficacy in this area.

R.J. Frances, M.D.

Almost a Revolution: An International Perspective on the Law of Involuntary Commitment
Appelbaum PS (Univ of Massachusetts, Worcester)
J Am Acad Psychiatry Law 25:135-147, 1997   4–18

Introduction.—One of the most significant and controversial areas of mental health law is the law governing involuntary commitment of mentally ill individuals. This article considers to what extent developments in commitment law around the world have paralleled trends in the United States in the last 3 decades.

Reform of Civil Commitment Law in the United States.—The focus of civil commitment law in the United States remained unchanged and unchallenged from the early 19th century to approximately the mid-1960s. Judicial oversight was inconsistent, and members of the medical profession were usually in charge of the procedures by which commitment was effected. At the time of the civil rights revolution, many voices were raised against involuntary hospitalization and the conditions of state hospitals. Costs to taxpayers also made hospitalization less desirable. The law allowing hospitalization solely because an individual was "in need of treatment" was abandoned and a set of procedural rights imported from criminal law was adopted.

Reform of Civil Commitment Law Elsewhere in the World.—Reforms similar to those in the United States began to be seen in other countries within a decade. Costs were an important consideration, but individual rights were also cited. The American model, however, has not become the dominant approach around the world; most countries have not turned to strict danger-based standards and criminal-style procedures. In England and Wales, review occurs automatically after 6 months of commitment, and again every 3 years. Overall, the British approach, which focuses on the "health and safety" of the patient as well as on the protection of others, is more typical of international trends than is the more rigorous American model.

Consequences of Reform.—Reforms are generally resisted when they are seen as shifting the focus away from patients' treatment needs. Changes resulting from the new laws have been quite difficult to document, but it appears that the decrease in public-sector psychiatric beds, rather than changes in the law, accounts for obstacles to hospitalizing patients in need of care. Decision makers, including judges, apply intuitive criteria, rather than a narrow reading of the law, for involuntary commitment. Similar responses have been seen in Europe and elsewhere when commitment law appears to restrictive. In the future, an expanded menu of options may be adopted.

▶ This noted expert on psychiatry and the law gives us a nice glimpse of involuntary commitment practices in other parts of the world and opens up our thinking about the recent narrowing of commitment laws in the United States. The commonsense intuition that the majority of severely mentally ill people should receive treatment when they need it, even if it must be provided against their will, is basically sound and likely to lead to an expansion of interpretation of what have become too restricting laws in the United States.

R.J. Frances, M.D.

5 Community Psychiatry

Community Psychiatry

Continuity of Care for Patients With Schizophrenia and Related Disorders: A Comparative South-Verona and Groningen Case-Register Study

Sytema S, Micciolo R, Tansella M (Rijksuniversiteit Groningen, The Netherlands; Università de Verona, Italy; Università di Trento, Italy)
Psychol Med 27:1355–1362, 1997   5–1

Background.—Continuity of care is generally thought to be essential to ensure better outcomes and prevent long-term hospitalization among the severely mentally ill. However, little progress has been made in the operationalization and measurement of this concept. Continuity of care was compared in a community mental health system without mental hospital back-up and in an institution-based system in which mental hospitals still predominate.

Methods.—Two indicators of continuity of care were used to compare these 2 systems: readiness of aftercare (the time from hospital discharge to the first day- or out-patient contact) and flexibility of care (combinations of in-, day-, and out-patient care during 2 years of follow-up). Survival analysis was used to correct for censored observations.

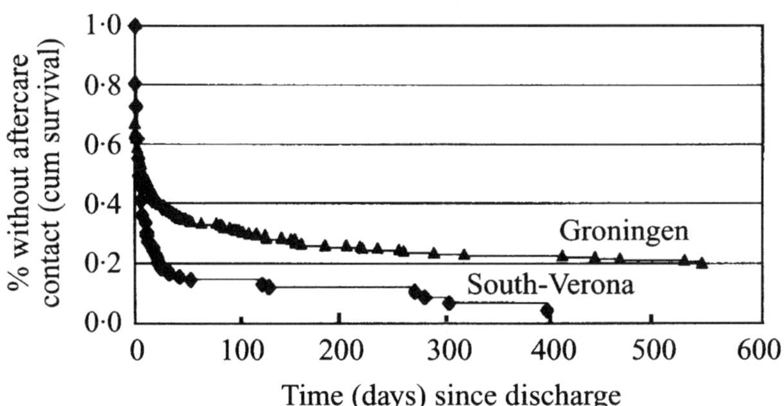

FIGURE 1.—Time from discharge to next out- or day-patient contact. (Courtesy of Sytema S, Micciolo R, Tansella M: Continuity of care for patients with schizophrenia and related disorders: A comparative South-Verona and Groningen case-register study. *Psychol Med* 27:1355–1362, 1997. Reprinted with the permission of Cambridge University Press.)

Findings.—Within 2 weeks after discharge, 71.5% of the patients in the community mental health system and 54.6% in the institution-based system received community care. Survival functions were significantly different. Significant predictors for aftercare in both systems, according to Cox regression analysis, were contact before admission, time between this contact and admission, and duration of admission. Sixty-two percent of the patients in the community mental health system had multiple service use, compared with 45% in the institution-based system (Fig 1).

Conclusions.—Both indicators used in the current study showed a greater continuity of care in the community mental health system than in the institution-based system. However, statistical analyses suggest that comparable processes are at work in the 2 systems.

▶ I am convinced from my review of the literature[1] that the 2 things that prevent or forestall exacerbations of illnesses, rehospitalization, or both among patients suffering from chronic schizophrenia are continued medication and continuance in a program (what used to be called "aftercare"), both of which cannot be delivered without continuity of care. Therefore, it is very encouraging to see the report of its operationalization and the proof of its superiority.

J.A. Talbott, M.D.

Reference

1. Ancill R, ed: Lessons Learned About the Chronic Mentally Ill Since 1955, *Schizophrenia: Exploring the Spectrum of Psychosis*, NY: John Wiley, 1955.

A Randomized Trial of Assertive Community Treatment for Homeless Persons With Severe Mental Illness

Lehman AF, Dixon LB, Kernan E, et al (Univ of Maryland, Baltimore)
Arch Gen Psychiatry 54:1038–1043, 1997   5–2

Background.—One fifth to one third of homeless persons reportedly experience severe and persistent mental illness (SPMI). There is a great need for more effective community-based services for such people. The efficacy of an innovative program of assertive community treatment (ACT) for homeless persons with SPMI was assessed.

Methods.—By random assignment, 152 homeless persons with SPMI received ACT or usual community services. Assessments, performed at baseline and at 2, 6, and 12 months, included the Structured Clinical Interview for *Diagnostic and Statistical Manual of Mental Disorders, Third Edition, Revised,* Quality-of-Life Interview, Colorado Symptom Index, and the Medical Outcomes Study 36-Item Short Form Health Survey.

Findings.—Persons receiving ACT had significantly fewer psychiatric inpatient days, fewer emergency department visits, and more psychiatric outpatient visits than those receiving the usual community services. Also, the former group spent significantly more days in stable community housing and had significantly greater improvements in symptoms, life satisfaction, and perceived health status.

Conclusions.—The ACT program for homeless persons with SPMI shifts the treatment focus from crisis-oriented services to ongoing outpatient care. This program resulted in better housing, clinical, and life satisfaction outcomes than usual community care.

▶ As the authors point out, this is the first study (without methodological problems) demonstrating the superiority of ACT teams to "usual community treatment" in the homeless mentally ill. I have a huge conflict of interest in selecting this article, but given its peer-reviewed publication and its stunning results, it needs wide dissemination.

J.A. Talbott, M.D.

Fact: Integrating Family Psychoeducation and Assertive Community Treatment
McFarlane WR (Maine Med Ctr, Portland)
Adm Policy Ment Health 25:191–198, 1997   5–3

Introduction.—Unusual effectiveness in randomized clinical trials has been demonstrated by family psychoeducation and assertive community treatment, both state-of-the-art service systems with rich empirical foundations. When the 2 approaches are integrated, there may be a possible additive effect. The role of family support and intervention in the care of persons with serious mental illness and the benefits of merging the multiple-family versions of this approach with community treatment programs are reviewed.

Family Therapy.—To create a home environment that minimizes relapse-inducing stress and to create a convalescent environment that can facilitate recuperation from illness episodes, families are informed of the scientific understanding of mental illnesses. This approach is known as family psychoeducation. Rates of relapse have been shown to be reduced with this approach. In medical and psychiatric illness, lack of social support appears to increase vulnerability to ordinary stressors. Family isolation and stigma are countered when family psychoeducation is provided to several families at a time, and the family has an opportunity to rebuild a network. For avoidaning future relapse, improving medication compliance, and improving quality of life for both patients and families, multiple family format psychoeducation is a powerful tool.

Community Treatment.—Unequivocal evidence of efficacy in schizophrenia occurred with family intervention and assertive community treatment. Integrating the 2 techniques combines the unique efficacies of each approach. The family is encouraged to expand its network by cross-family problem solving and out-of-group socializing. Desired outcomes have been further enhanced by combining assertive community treatment with multiple family psychoeducation. Nearly double the employment rates of assertive community treatment were achieved by the combined approach.

Conclusion.—A major shift in resource allocation can be achieved by reducing rehospitalization rates by 75%. The combination approach increases the size and complexity of a patient's social network; provides a forum for mutual aid and encouragement; exposes families to others; and creates a holistic service context for reinforcing information about treatments, coping strategies, and management approaches.

▶ Over the years, several key individuals have demonstrated or espoused the utilization of combined modalities of treatment because of their ability to improve outcome or decrease relapse. Here, McFarlane demonstrates and advocates the increased efficacy of 2 novel community approaches—assertive community treatment and family psychoeducation—much as Keith and Klerman did for combined psychopharmacologic and psychosocial interventions and Hogarty did for combined psychopharmacologic, social skill, and family interventions. I have always believed it made intuitive sense, and I think this report strengthens our data base as we advocate what we believe, and now know, is better.

J.A. Talbott, M.D.

Individual and Community-level Variation in Intensity and Diversity of Service Utilization by Homeless Persons With Serious Mental Illness
Rosenheck R, Lam JA (Veterans Affairs Northeast Program Evaluation Center, West Haven, Conn; Yale Univ, West Haven, Conn)
J Nerv Ment Dis 185:633–638, 1997   5–4

Background.—The need for an integrated, multimodal approach to service delivery for homeless persons with major mental illnesses has been emphasized. Individual client- and community-level sources of variation in service use among clients entering 18 community treatment programs as part of a national project were assessed.

Methods and Findings.—Data on 1,828 clients were analyzed to determine the relationship of individual client characteristics and site of entry to the intensity and diversity of service use. The relative importance of client characteristics and site of entry were identified in a hierarchical multiple regression analysis. Only 2%–3% of the variance in service use was explained by client characteristics. Two to three times more of the variance was explained by intersite variation.

Conclusions.—Intersite differences account for much more of the variance in service use than the individual characteristics of homeless persons with mental illness. Additional research is needed to identify specific community-level factors accounting for intersite variations.

▶ If I read this study correctly, the site of entry is a more important factor in predicting service utilization in the homeless mentally ill than patient and client factors. Site of entry is a proxy for "diverse service system characteristics," and therefore, the results support the belief that we can improve care and treatment through "availability of services and the degree of integration." I agree more needs to be done, but this is a welcome finding.

J.A. Talbott, M.D.

Trends in Siting Strategies
Zippay A (Rutgers Univ, New Brunswick, NJ)
Community Ment Health J 33:301–310, 1997   5–5

Introduction.—The value and ethics of notifying neighbors in advance of the development of group residential housing sites for the chronically mentally ill have been debated for decades. Some say the strategy promotes neighborhood acceptance, but others say it stirs community opposition. Mental health administrators were given the legal authority to forego such notification with the federal 1988 Fair Housing Amendments and the 1990 American Disabilities Act. Seventy-two mental health agencies described the strategy used in their most recent group housing development.

Methods.—Mental health administrators from 72 agencies that provide housing for the chronically mentally ill participated in a telephone interview. They responded to a 30-minute questionnaire and described the siting strategy used in their most recent housing development. They were asked the degree of opposition to a site. Ninety percent were private nonprofit representatives and 10% were representatives of for profit organizations with budgets ranging from $255,000–$40 million. Together, they provided housing to 4,500 consumers through 750 residences. There were 49 group homes, 11 apartments, 4 halfway houses, and 1 residential school.

Results.—Neighbors were notified by 61% of the agencies before the site opened, whereas 39% did not notify neighbors. Agencies have been influenced to do less outreach and education than in previous years because of the Federal Housing Amendments and the American Disabilities Act. Eight respondents said that legislation stopped them from notifying neighbors before establishing the site. Of those who notified neighbors, 36% notified the neighbors 6–12 months in advance, 21% notified neighbors 3–5 months in advance, and 36% notified them 2 months before the opening. Of those who gave notification, 73% had some level of neighborhood opposition, and of those sites in which no advance notice was given, 25% had some level of neighborhood opposition. Where opposition was the strongest, educational and outreach activities helped diffuse the opposition. Of those who notified neighbors, 79% held an open house after the site was opened, whereas 35% of those who did not notify neighbors held an open house.

Conclusion.—Most respondents still were loyal to the practice of notifying neighbors before opening a site because they believe it yields long-term gains in building positive community connections. To determine long-term associations between neighborhood integration and siting strategies, a follow-up study is planned.

▶ As the authors note, this is an old question: do you move into community sites under the stealth of darkness and then tell the community or do you conduct elaborate community education and preparation in advance of the move? I've seen both methods work and both fail; the problem is that it is not always clear why. This article is valuable in giving us the picture of such efforts in 1 state but lacks the in-depth analysis of when 1 approach should be used and when the other. Such an analysis should be undertaken.

J.A. Talbott, M.D.

Randomised Controlled Trial of Two Models of Care for Discharged Psychiatric Patients

Tyrer P, Evans K, Gandhi N, et al (Imperial College School of Medicine, London; Central Middlesex Hosp, London)
BMJ 316:106–109, 1998
5–6

Introduction.—Assertive community care of patients with severe mental illness is reported to reduce hospital admissions without any loss of efficacy in treatment. Recent studies, however, also suggest that the community care program approach has increased the demand for inpatient care. The hypothesis that there would be better outcomes when care of discharged patients was organized by community multidisciplinary teams instead of a hospital-based team was tested.

Methods.—The setting of the randomized controlled trial was inner and outer London psychiatric services. Participants were 155 patients with severe mental illness and an admission within the past 2 years. The primary outcome measure was improvement in clinical symptoms; cost was the main secondary outcome. Patients were allocated to community or hospital care programs and assessed before discharge. The community teams were closely integrated with a common base, common case records, frequent information sharing, and team supervision. In contrast, hospital services had more formal liaison with several agencies, mainly at review meetings.

Results.—After 1 year of follow-up, clinical outcomes were available for 133 patients and cost data for 144. The 2 models of care had essentially similar outcomes, but there were more admissions in the hospital-based care group. Costs of health care were nevertheless 14% greater per patient in the community group. There was a rapid reduction in hospital beds at the time of the study, leading to considerable pressure on psychiatric beds and twofold higher costs in the outer London services (Fig 2).

Conclusion.—Clinical outcomes were similar for discharged patients with severe mental illness who entered community or hospital-based care, but more patients in the hospital-based group were admitted to hospital. When psychiatric bed requirements are insufficient and greater use of beds

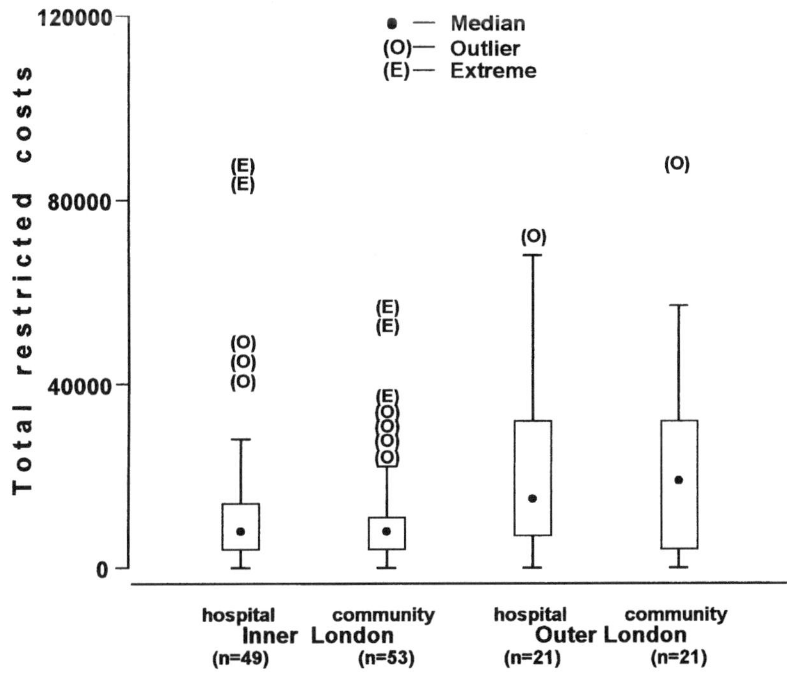

FIGURE 2.—Box plot of (restricted) total costs per patient in community and hospital teams separated by services in inner London (North Kensington and Paddington) and outer London (Brent), with outliers (O) and extreme (E) cases identified and median shown as *dot*. (Courtesy of Tyrer P, Evans K, Gandhi N, et al: Randomised controlled trial of two models of care for discharged psychiatric patients. *BMJ* 316:106–109, 1998. This article was first published in the *BMJ* and is reproduced by permission of the BMJ.)

outside the catchment is required, there is no advantage in providing better community care.

▶ The take-home lesson here is that community care works only when you have a sufficient number of beds. This flies in the face of statements of zealots who believe we don't need any beds, ever. Their finding of the cost-effectiveness of community care comes through loud and clear.

J.A. Talbott, M.D.

Scheduled Intermittent Hospitalization for Psychiatric Patients

Dilonardo JD, Connelly CE, Gurel L, et al (Ctr for Substance Treatment, Rockville, Md; Marymount Univ, Arlington, Va; Arlington, Md; et al)
Psychiatric Serv 49:504–509, 1998
5–7

Introduction.—Since the deinstitutionalization of psychiatric care, several comprehensive community treatment programs have been designed and evaluated. Earlier work has shown that short hospitalizations are beneficial for patients with serious and persistent mental illness. The effects of scheduled intermittent hospitalization on hospital use, community adjustment, and self-esteem in patients with serious and persistent mental illness were assessed.

Methods.—Fifty-seven male veterans with a primary axis 1 psychiatric diagnosis were randomized to either an experimental group or a control group. Patients were aged 65 or younger and were frequent users of inpatient care during the previous 2 years. Patients randomized to the experimental group were prescheduled for 4 yearly hospitalizations for 2 years. Each hospitalization ranged from 9 to 11 days. The control group had traditional access to hospital care. Both groups were assessed for number of psychiatric bed days, community adjustment, and self-esteem during and after the intervention.

Results.—There were no between-group differences in demographic or clinical variables at baseline. At 1-year follow-up, patients in the experimental group had improvement of measures in self-esteem, less negative emotions, and fewer complaints of physical symptoms. Both groups were similar in hospital use, financial management, substance abuse, and psychological well-being at 1 year.

Conclusion.—Scheduled intermittent hospitalization has potential as a promising alternative to traditional, crisis-oriented psychiatric hospitalization for patients who are frequent users of psychiatric hospital care.

▶ It is unusual to see a true innovation in mental health services; this program represents such an innovation and an intriguing 1 at that. Imagine scheduling admissions without a "medical necessity!" I would want to see true costs rather than the proxies they used, and I'd want to see if this holds up in areas where there are strong community programs, but as I said, it is unusual to see a truly innovative program introduced.

J.A. Talbott, M.D.

Case Management

Models of Community Care for Severe Mental Illness: A Review of Research on Case Management
Mueser KT, Bond GR, Drake RE, et al (Dartmouth Med School, Hanover, NH; Indiana Univ, Indianapolis)
Schizophr Bull 24:37–74, 1998

5–8

Introduction.—The removal of patients with severe psychiatric disorders from hospital to the community led to the growth of community mental health centers near the patients' homes. These centers began to provide more psychiatric services, a development with both positive and negative consequences. In particular, the needs of many severely mentally ill (SMI) patients were not being met because of their inability to seek out services. Different models (Table 1) of community care provided for the SMI population were identified and the literature on case management was reviewed.

TABLE 1.—Features of Different Community Care Models

Community Care Model

Program Feature	Broker Case Management	Clinical Case Management	Strengths	Rehabilitation	Assertive Community Treatment	Intensive Case Management
Staff to patient ratio	1:50(?)	1:30+	1:20–30	1:20–30	1:10	1:10
Outreach to patients	Low	Low	Moderate	Moderate	High	High
Shared caseload	No	No	No	No	Yes	No
24-hour coverage	No	No	No	No	Often	Often
Consumer input	No	Low	High	High	Low	Low
Emphasis on skills training	No	Low	Moderate	High	Moderate(?)	Moderate(?)
Frequency of patient contacts	Low	Moderate	Moderate	Moderate	High	High
Locus of contacts	Clinic	Clinic	Community	Clinic/Community	Community	Community
Integration of treatment	Low	Moderate	Low(?)	Low(?)	High	High(?)
Direct service provision	Low	Moderate	Moderate	Moderate	High	High
Target population	SMI	SMI	SMI	SMI	SMI high service users	SMI high service users

Note.—(?), area of model that is unclear; SMI, severely mentally ill.
(Courtesy of Mueser KT, Bond GR, Drake RE, et al: Models of community care for severe mental illness: A review of research on case management. *Schizophr Bull* 24:37–74, 1998.)

Community Care Models.—The models that have generated the most discussion and research are the broker service model, the clinical case management model, the assertive community treatment (ACT) model, the intensive case management (ICM) model, the rehabilitation model, and the strengths model. A review of research studies sought to find those that evaluated the effectiveness of one or more models of case management. To be included, studies had to conduct assessments at a follow-up point for 2 groups of patients receiving different models of community care and to conduct assessments at baseline and follow-up for patients receiving 1 model of case management. Most of the 75 studies meeting inclusion criteria dealt with ACT (44) or ICM (16) models.

Results.—Controlled research on ICM and ACT indicates that hospital time is reduced and housing stability improved in these models, especially for patients who are high service users. The 2 models appear to have a moderate effect on symptom reduction and quality of life, but little effect on social functioning, vocational functioning, and arrests or time spent in jail. There was a trend for ACT or ICM programs to result in higher patient satisfaction and, to a lesser extent, higher satisfaction among patients' relatives. Few studies were conducted on other models of community care, and findings were described as inconclusive.

Conclusion.—Although ACT and ICM services have areas of strength, there is a need for these models to address problems such as social and vocational functioning and substance abuse. Suggested topics of future research include evaluating implementation fidelity, exploring patient predictors of improvement, and assessing the role of the helping alliance in mediating outcome.

▶ It is unusual for me to select a review of the literature for abstraction, because a reading of the full article is really required to grasp their review's richness fully. But I think this 1 is nicely done and important. Two points: first, the authors advice to ascertain which model works for which patients is very well taken, and, second, the fact that different models differ in their long-term or short-term economic impact means that policymakers should resist the impulse to go for the short-term saving. Finally, the authors' historical recapitulation of how the case management system evolved— going from institutionalization to brokered case management to a combination of brokered and clinical case management to ACT and ICM—is most insightful.

J.A. Talbott, M.D.

Styles of Case Management: The Philosophy and Practice of Case Managers
Hromco JG, Lyons JS, Nikkel RE (Northwestern Univ, Chicago; Oregon Mental Health and Developmental Disability Division, Salem)
Community Ment Health J 33:415–428, 1997   5–9

Background.—Much discussion and research have gone into clarifying the role of case manager (CM) for severely mentally ill persons. Case management as it is currently practiced was described, using data from a cross-section of CMs in 3 states.

Methods and Findings.—The CMs were asked to rank 5 case management functions in terms of their importance to positive outcomes. These rankings were then used to classify CMs according to their case management philosophy. Cluster analysis suggested 4 styles of case management: supportive social worker, individual therapist, therapist broker, and community advocate. Overall, the CMs ranked supportive interventions as the most important and formal psychotherapy as relatively unimportant. The style of the CM was associated with CM activity.

Conclusions.—The styles of case management as practiced in 3 states were defined in the current study. These styles have implications for research on outcomes in case management and for CM training.

▶ A lot has been written about styles and types of case management, but clear direction from this literature has not been forthcoming. While this study demonstrates clear results as to what case managers *think* is important and how this translates into what they *do*, the next step is to test their beliefs against *outcomes* in various subpopulations of the chronically mentally ill.

J.A. Talbott, M.D.

Improving Publicly Funded Substance Abuse Treatment: The Value of Case Management
Shwartz M, Baker G, Mulvey KP, et al (Boston Univ; Boston Dept of Health and Hosps)
Am J Public Health 87:1659–1664, 1997   5–10

Introduction.—A retrospective cohort study was conducted to evaluate the impact of adding case managers to publicly funded substance abuse treatment programs. Although such a strategy would appear to be effective in keeping clients in treatment and reducing short-term relapse, there has been little hard research in support of case management in this setting.

Methods.—The study was conducted in Boston and used data from the Massachusetts Bureau of Substance Abuse Services management information system. Clients included in the analysis had been discharged in 1993 and 1994 from 4 treatment settings: short-term residential (3,112 clients), long-term residential (2,888 clients), outpatient (7,431 clients), and residential detoxification (7,776 clients). Discharge forms were available for more than 97% of short-term residential and detoxification program admissions, more than 88% of long-term residential admissions, and 65% of outpatient program admissions. Logistic regression models were used to examine the association of case management with outcome variables, after adjustment for differences in baseline characteristics.

Results.—Overall, more than half of the clients were minorities, many were unemployed, and more than 40% were not high school graduates. Case management was used for a higher percentage of clients in short-term (45%) and long-term (68%) residential facilities than in outpatient (10%) and detoxification (16%) programs. Across all treatment modalities, the percentage of clients reaching the long-stay category was at least 30% higher among case-managed than non–case-managed clients. Case-managed clients were also less likely to be admitted to detoxification within 90 days of discharge (with the exception of those discharged from outpatient treatment), and, in the detoxification group, more likely to experience transition to postdetoxification treatment within 30 days of discharge. When case management was statistically significant with univariate analyses (all-client analyses), it remained so with multivariate analyses.

Conclusion.—The evidence gathered for this study suggests that the case management model offered to these clients of a publicly funded substance abuse treatment system had a favorable impact on short-term outcomes. Case management provides a low-cost enhancement for such programs.

▶ Maybe I am straying over the border into the area covered by Richard Frances' chapter on alcohol and drug addiction in this volume, but it seemed to me that the subject of the occurrence and treatment of substance abuse as well as dual diagnosis in community psychiatry programs merited the inclusion of this study. Although the results are impressive, one wonders whether the authors' belief that this is a "low-cost enhancement" is shared by the managed care industry and their purchasers of care.

J.A. Talbott, M.D.

Case Managed Residential Care for Homeless Addicted Veterans: Results of a True Experiment
Conrad KJ, Hultman CI, Pope AR, et al (Edward Hines Jr VA Hosp, Hines, Ill; Northwestern Univ, Chicago; Loyola Univ, Maywood, Ill)
Med Care 36:40–53, 1998   5–11

Introduction.—Up to 51% of homeless men are veterans and up to one half of the homeless have psychiatric or substance abuse disorders. The case-managed residential care program provides transitional residential care for up to 6 months with ongoing and follow-up case management for 1 year. The effectiveness of transitional residential treatment, however, is still not known. Homeless veterans who received case-managed residential care were followed during a 2-year period and were compared with a

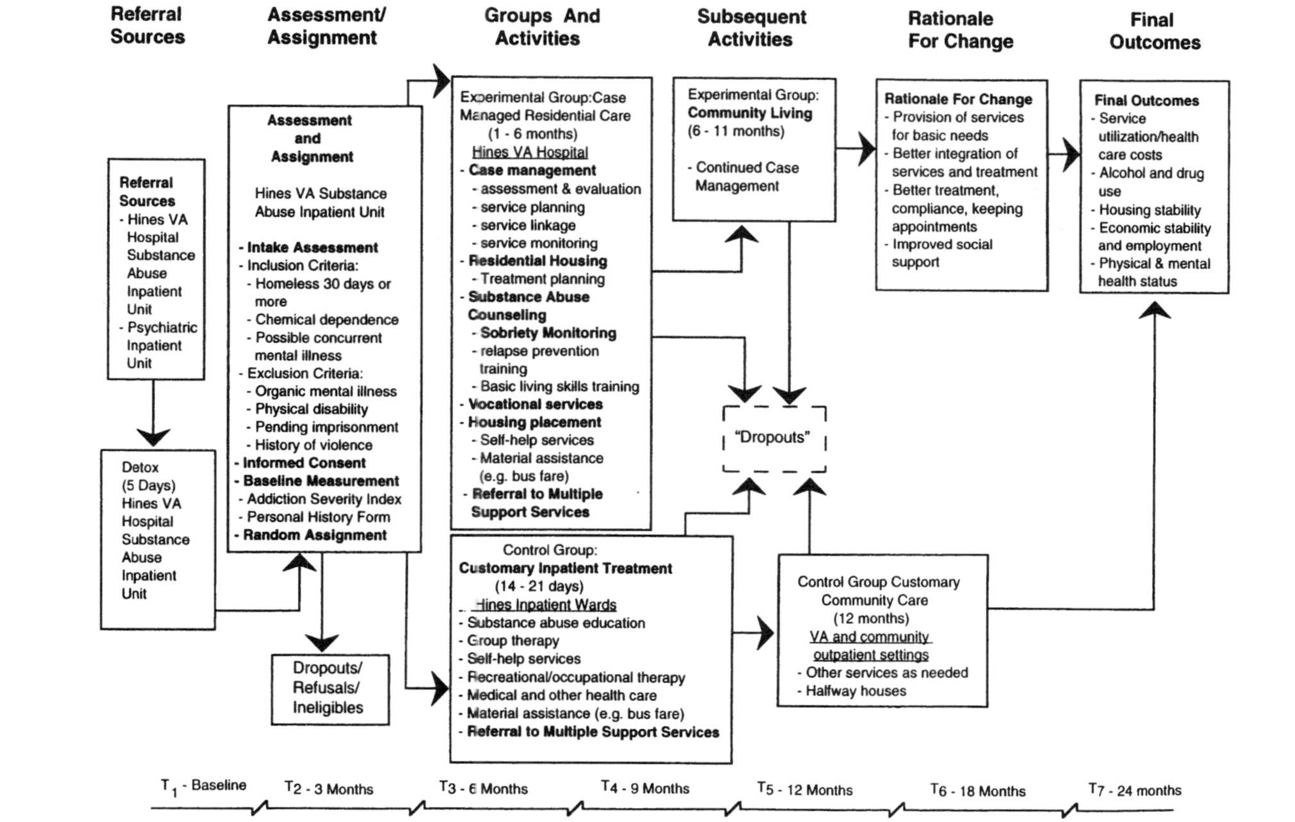

FIGURE 1.—Logic model. (Courtesy of Conrad KJ, Hultman CI, Pope AR, et al: Case managed residential care for homeless addicted veterans: Results of a true experiment. *Med Care* 36:40–53, 1998.)

control group receiving Veterans Administration customary care to test the effectiveness of case-managed residential care in reducing substance abuse, decreasing homelessness, increasing employment, and improving health.

Methods.—There were 358 homeless addicted male veterans included in the 5-year prospective experiment. They were followed up at 3, 6, and 9 months during their enrollment and at 12, 18, and 24 months after they completed the case-managed residential care program. The program had a 30-bed facility. The expected length of stay was 3–6 months. The program followed a model that focused on here-and-now issues (Fig 1). Essential components of treatment were relapse prevention skills training, assertive drink and drug refusal, coping with relapse, social networking, and anger management. The veterans participated in a 21-day hospital program and then were referred to community services.

Results.—With ongoing and follow-up case management for a total of up to 1 year of treatment, the experiment group averaged 3.4 months in transitional residential care. During the 2-year period, the experimental group showed significant improvement compared with the control group on medical, alcohol, employment, and housing measures. During the treatment year, these group differences tended to occur, but they tended to diminish during the follow-up year.

Conclusion.—On the 4 major outcomes, significant improvements were observed with time from baseline to all posttests. Even without the special case-managed residential care program, veterans had access to, and used, significant amounts of services. Similar services for the control group may account for improvements in that group and may have muted the differences between groups.

▶ Aside from the major findings in this study, which are of interest, I was struck by 2 other things: first, the finding that the impact of interventions with the chronically mentally ill is stronger at first than later; second, that employment, usually so unbudgeable a goal with this population, was improved in this study. As for first, the unremitting power of the illness often breaks through over time, despite good treatment, but regarding the second, at least this intervention cracks what I have always thought to be the most difficult outcome to achieve—employment.

J.A. Talbott, M.D.

Does Outreach Case Management Improve Patients' Quality of Life?
Curtis JL, Millman EJ, Struening EL, et al (Harlem Hosp, New York; Columbia Univ, New York; New York Univ)
Psychiatric Serv 49:351–354, 1998   5–12

Introduction.—An effective means of providing support services to deinstitutionalized psychiatric patients has been outreach case management. It was assumed that outreach case management would reduce psychiatric rehospitalization rates, improve social functioning and health care, and reduce mortality. A previous study, however, showed that patients who received outreach case management did not fare better than patients who received routine aftercare services with regard to rehospitalization rates or mortality outcomes. For patients who received outreach case management, whether certain aspects of quality of life were improved was examined.

Methods.—Follow-up research interviews were conducted with 147 patients to determine their reported sense of improvement in physical well-being and competence in performing activities of daily living; in emotional well-being as shown in emotional expressiveness, sadness, suicidal thoughts, and substance abuse; and in interpersonal relationships, living arrangements, friendships, income maintenance, and employment. These patients were compared with a control group of 145 patients who did not receive outreach case management. In all, 39 measures of quality of life were reviewed. All of the patients were followed up for 15–52 months.

Results.—In any of the quality-of-life variables, no differences were found between the groups. There were no differences between the groups in ethnicity, gender, age, education, entitlements, residential status, or clinical characteristics.

Conclusion.—Improved quality of life was not associated with outreach case management. Patients in the intervention group did not demonstrably improve their quality of life in comparison to the controls. However, the patients were not eligible for community support services because their illness was not regarded as chronic, and these findings cannot be generalized to patients in case management programs serving those eligible for community support services or to those whose biopsychosocial characteristics differ from these patients.

▶ One always has the impulse to ignore or underreport negative findings. But this finding prompts me to ask why? It seems like a good idea to augment aftercare with outreach case management; why didn't their quality of life improve? Maybe because of what the authors' imply, that is, because the patients did not have "chronic" illness and thus were not eligible for community support services, but maybe it was attributable to our overly optimistic view of the power of case management.

J.A. Talbott, M.D.

Mental Health Systems

The Use of Outpatient Mental Health Services in the United States and Ontario: The Impact of Mental Morbidity and Perceived Need for Care
Katz SJ, Kessler RC, Frank RG, et al (Univ of Michigan, Ann Arbor; Harvard Univ, Boston; Johns Hopkins Univ, Baltimore, Md; et al)
Am J Public Health 87:1136–1143, 1997   5–13

Introduction.—There is widespread concern that service use is poorly matched to need when it comes to the organization and financing of

TABLE 1.—Prevalence (%) of Mental Morbidity, Impairment, and
Perceived Need for Mental Health Care: United States vs. Ontario, 1990

	United States (n = 5393)	Ontario (n = 6261)
Disorder		
Any affective†	10.5	4.9
Any anxiety†	16.8	12.3
Two or more mental health diagnoses†	9.1	4.6
Any substance dependence*	6.8	4.5
Any substance abuse	3.3	2.4
Self-rated mental health†		
Excellent	31.4	40.0
Very good	38.6	40.9
Good	22.2	15.8
Fair	6.9	2.8
Poor	0.9	0.6
Disability†	7.4	4.0
Perceived need†	19.4	11.7

*U.S.:Ontario differences significant, $P < 0.01$.
†U.S.:Ontario differences significant, $P < 0.05$.
(Courtesy of Katz SJ, Kessler RC, Frank RG, et al: The use of outpatient mental health services in the United States and Ontario: The impact of mental morbidity and perceived need for care. *Am J Public Health* 87:1136–1143, 1997. Copyright American Public Health Association.)

mental health care in the United States. Professional help may not be given to some of those with serious mental health problems, while those with little need are using services of uncertain value. Because of concerns that an overuse of services would increase, some payers are reluctant to expand coverage. Those in favor of expanded coverage say there is little evidence of overuse in countries with more generous insurance coverage, such as in the province of Ontario, Canada, where there is no limit on inpatient stays or outpatient visits for psychiatric care. The associations of individual disorders, disability, and self-rated mental health were compared between countries with the use of mental health services.

Methods.—Reviewers used a cross-sectional study design and compared data from the 1990 Mental Health Supplement to the Ontario Health Survey with the 1990 U.S. National Comorbidity Survey. In the United States, the sample size was 5,393 and in Ontario, it was 6,261. Both surveys used identical structured psychiatric interviews and questions about the use of services for psychiatric disorders.

Results.—For persons with any affective disorder, the odds of receiving any medical or psychiatric specialty services were 3.1 in the United States vs. 11 in Ontario. For those with fair or poor self-rated mental health, the odds were 2.7 in the United States vs. 5 in Ontario. For persons with mental health-related disability, the odds were 3 in the United States and 1.5 in Ontario. Most of the between-country differences in use disappeared when perceived need was controlled for. In the United States, the prevalence of mental morbidity, impairment, and perceived need was consistently higher than in Ontario (Table 1).

Conclusion.—A combination of a higher prevalence of mental morbidity and a higher prevalence of perceived need for care among those with low mental morbidity in the United States accounts for the higher use of mental health services in the United States than in Ontario. There are noninsurance related barriers to receiving care, because this study shows that even under a more generous insurance plan, most with recent mental health disorders do not receive treatment from any source.

▶ Comparisons between the United States and Canada are always useful because, despite some financing, cultural, and political differences, there are abundant similarities in our populations and degree of scientific advancement. One wonders, therefore, why Americans perceive the need for care as so much higher than Canadians, especially in those with no morbidity or impairment. In addition to the authors' speculations on an explanation, I would add that perhaps we have educated our population better, perhaps "over-psychologized" situations, or perhaps Canadians retain more vestiges of the Anglo-Saxon stiff upper lip or are more sensitive to the inefficiencies of overuse of services in a national heath system.

J.A. Talbott, M.D.

Mental Illness and Nursing Home Reform: OBRA-87 Ten Years Later

Snowden M, Roy-Byrne P (Univ of Washington, Seattle)
Psychiatric Serv 49:229–233, 1998   5–14

Introduction.—For mental health care of nursing home residents, passing of the nursing home reform provisions of the Omnibus Budget Reconciliation Act was the major policy event. The new law prohibited the use of physical restraints and required preadmission screening and annual resident review to ensure that mentally ill persons were not inappropriately admitted to nursing homes. The law also intended to decrease the inappropriate use of antipsychotic medications as chemical restraints. The use of antipsychotic medications, physical restraints, and preadmission screening was reviewed to determine the effects of nursing home reform initiated by the Omnibus Budget Reconciliation Act of 1987.

Methods.—A MEDLINE search of peer-reviewed articles in a 12-year period and a PsycINFO search of articles in a 20-year period were conducted.

Results.—The intended impact, particularly in reducing the use of antipsychotic medications and physical restraints in nursing homes, has resulted, according to survey and observational data. The most widely criticized component of the reform is preadmission screening of nursing home residents with mental illness. This has also been the component that has been the subject of the fewest data-based studies. The survey data revealed that 20% of residents noted an improvement in the quality of care and only 31% of nursing home industry workers feel no improvement from the reform.

Conclusion.—To link the reform to improvements in nursing home residents' quality of life and to describe the economic costs of the reform, more data are needed. To further standardize assessment of mental illness in nursing homes, more needs to be done to ensure that the methods used are reliable and valid.

▶ Many experts have been distressed for years over the conditions of the chronic mentally ill in settings designed for patients recovering from severe medical and surgical illnesses or the frail elderly (e.g., nursing homes). There have been horrible problems in such facilities, e.g., overprescription of psychotropic medication, underutilization of psychosocial interventions, and problems in staff training and quality. The Omnibus Reconciliation Act promised to address some of these and it has partly fulfilled its promise. I still think, however, that many staffing issues (e.g., insufficient numbers of nurses and activities therapists) could be addressed.

J.A. Talbott, M.D.

Consumers/Patients/Families

Psychiatrists and Their Patients: Views on Forms of Dress and Address
Gledhill JA, Warner JP, King M (Royal Free Hosp, London)
Br J Psychiatry 171:228–232, 1997   5–15

Introduction.—An important element of psychiatric practice is the ability to form a trusting, confiding relationship between patient and doctor. This relationship can be influenced by the way a psychiatrist dresses or is addressed by the patient. White coats have been discarded by psychiatrists and most dress in a casual manner. Preferences for dress styles and forms of address were examined among patients and psychiatrists.

Methods.—There were 49 inpatients who participated in a semi-structured interview. There were 69 junior and consultant psychiatrists who filled out a questionnaire about how they prefer to dress and how they preferred to be addressed. The preferences of psychiatric inpatients about the attire of their doctor were examined. They were asked to look at photographs of female and male doctors dressed casually or more formally (Fig 2). The views of junior and senior psychiatrists were obtained on what they consider to be appropriate dress for work. Whether psychiatric inpatients preferred that their doctor call them by their first name or title and surname was also determined. They were also asked how they like to address their psychiatrist. Finally, the psychiatrists were asked how they like to be addressed and how they like to address their patients.

Results.—Smart attire and a white coat was the preference among the patients. The majority of doctors also supported smart dress as the most appropriate attire. Patients preferred to address doctors by their title and surname, but preferred that doctors call them by their first name. First names were preferred by junior doctors when talking to patients, whereas the title and surname was used by almost all consultants. Doctors of all grades preferred to be addressed by their title and surname.

Conclusion.—The therapeutic alliance may be better facilitated by paying more attention to the way psychiatrists present themselves. In this

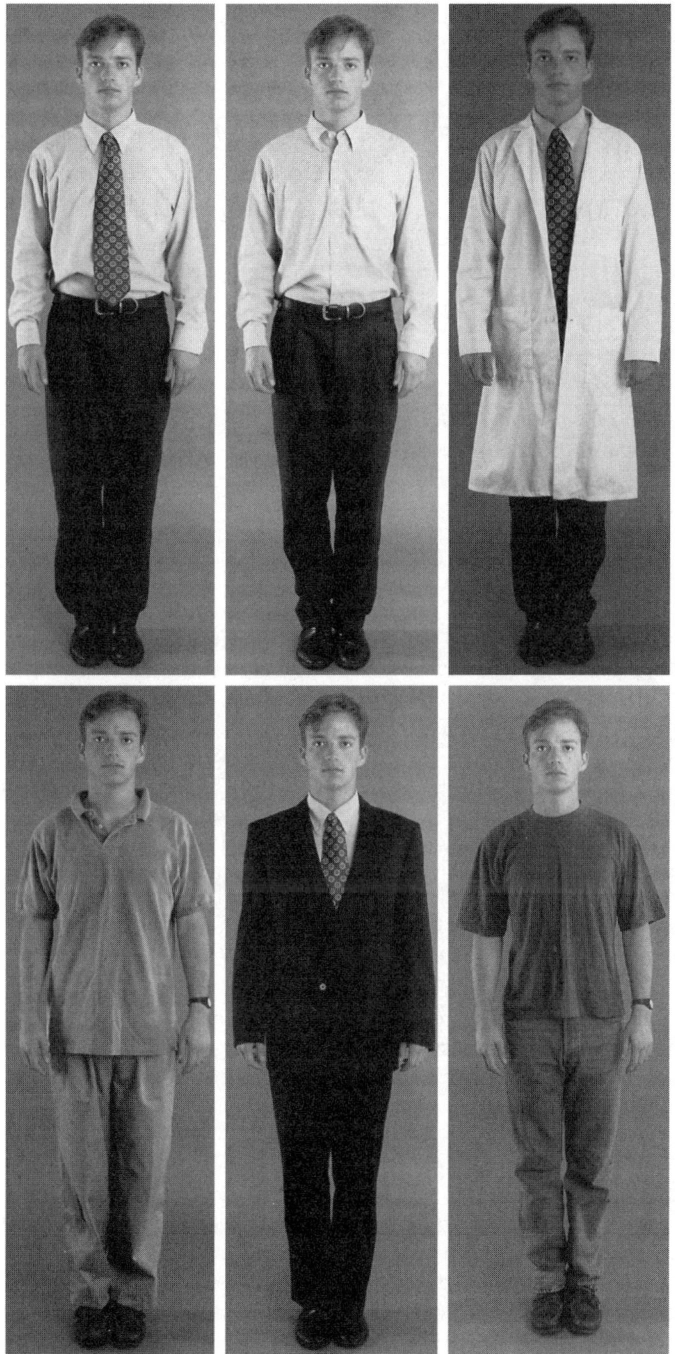

FIGURE 2.—Dress styles of male doctors. (Courtesy of Gledhill JA, Warner JP, King M: Psychiatrists and their patients: Views on forms of dress and address. *Br J Psychiatry* 171:228–232, 1997.)

especially vulnerable inpatient group, careful consideration of attire and forms of address may facilitate the therapeutic relationship.

▶ In the excesses of the 1960s, psychiatrists threw away their white laboratory coats and suits and nurses their uniforms in the spirit of breaking down hierarchical barriers. How revealing, then, to learn from this modest but fascinating study that patients see laboratory coats as implying understanding and suits as portraying competence. I remember the uncomfortable feeling I had when meeting the physician of a friend I had visited in a California hospital who was clad like a beach-bum. Certainly, in the competitive 1990s, dress can be important.

J.A. Talbott, M.D.

A Consumer-constructed Scale to Measure Empowerment Among Users of Mental Health Services

Rogers ES, Chamberlin J, Ellison ML, et al (Boston Univ)
Psychiatric Serv 48:1042–1047, 1997   5–16

Introduction.—Few researchers have attempted to define, measure or put into practice the word "empowerment," despite its widespread use in the lexicon of mental health programs. In the mental health arena, it seems to be associated with self-help programs. Few studies, however, have been conducted on empowerment as a process, a construct, or an outcome. The construct of personal empowerment was further defined and operationalized from the perspective of consumers, survivors, and former patients. A scale was constructed and validated that could be used in a variety of settings.

Methods.—There were 271 members of 6 self-help programs in 6 states who participated in the testing of a 28-item scale to measure empowerment. This scale has 15 attributes, including having decision-making power and having access to information and resources (Table). To identify the underlying dimension of empowerment, factor analyses were used. Responses were factor analyzed to establish the scale's reliability and validity. There were other analyses conducted as well, such as a checklist of 22 traditional mental health services, a 5-item scale to assess the effect of self-help on social supports, and an 11-item scale to assess the effect of self-help on quality of life.

Results.—There were 5 factors according to the analyses: optimism—control over the future, righteous anger, community activism, power-powerlessness, and self-efficacy—self-esteem. Quality of life and income were related to empowerment, but not the demographic variables of employment status, education level, marital status, ethnicity, gender, and age. The use of traditional mental health services was inversely related to empowerment. Community activism was positively related to empowerment.

Attributes of Empowerment Developed by an Advisory Board of
Leaders of the Self-help Movement

Having decision-making power
Having access to information and resources
Having a range of options from which to make choices (not just yes-no and
    either-or)
Assertiveness
A feeling that one can make a difference (being hopeful)
Learning to think critically; unlearning the conditioning; seeing things dif-
    ferently. For example, learning to redefine who one is (speaking in one's
    own voice), learning to redefine what one can do, and learning to redefine
    one's relationships to institutionalized power
Learning about and expressing anger
Not feeling alone; feeling part of a group
Understanding that a person has rights
Effecting change in one's life and one's community
Learning skills (for example, communication) that one defines as important
Changing other's perceptions of one's competency and capacity to act
Coming out of the closet
Growth and change that is never-ending and self-initiated
Increasing one's positive self-image and overcoming stigma

(Reprinted by permission, from Rogers ES, Chamberlin J, Ellison ML, et al: A consumer-
constructed scale to measure empowerment among users of mental health services. *Psychiatric
Serv* 48:1042–1047, 1997. Copyright 1997, the American Psychiatric Association.)

Conclusion.—A clearer understanding of the overused and imprecise concept of empowerment was established within a framework. Some evidence of validity and adequate internal consistency was demonstrated with the scale. To establish whether it is sensitive to change and whether it has discriminant validity, further testing must be done. Programs of empowerment should focus on increasing self-esteem and self-efficacy, increasing financial resources, decreasing feelings of powerlessness, and heightening sociopolitical consciousness and community activism.

▶ I always cringe or am confused when hearing the overused word "empowerment." But, surprisingly, the authors put some interesting substance to their examination of the issue. When you dissect out what is important to consumers, it demonstrates that the elements *are* understandable and are not vague. Maybe we should junk the term and go to the specifics desired by patients.

J.A. Talbott, M.D.

Care-related Decision-making Satisfaction and Caregiver Well-being in Families Caring for Older Members

Smerglia VL, Deimling GT (Univ of Akron, Ohio; Case Western Reserve Univ, Cleveland, Ohio)
Gerontologist 37:658–665, 1997   5–17

Introduction.—The degree of stress experienced by caregivers of older relatives is known to be related to impairment levels and care requirements of the elderly individual, but care-related decision making can also lead to caregiver strain. Data from 244 adult child and spouse caregivers were analyzed to determine the impact of decision-making satisfaction on caregiver well-being.

Methods.—Research data were drawn from 2 larger studies of caregivers in the Cleveland, Ohio, Standard Metropolitan Statistical Area. These studies were conducted between 1982 and 1986, and the analysis reported here is based on the fourth data collection wave (1984). This group of respondents included 169 adult children and 75 spouses. Caregivers were interviewed for information related to the impact of structural variables and family environment on satisfaction with care-related decision making and caregiver well-being.

Results.—The first regression analysis, which examined the impact that the caregiving context and network structure had on caregiver decision-making satisfaction, showed that only the cognitive impairment of the care recipient had a modest significant net effect. Neither caregiver type nor elder physical functioning significantly predicted satisfaction with the decision-making process. Regression analysis indicated that the best predictors of decision-making satisfaction were aspects of family environment, such as adaptability and conflict within the family. Spouse caregivers had higher levels of depression than adult child caregivers, independent of the care recipient's cognitive impairment. Less likely to be depressed were caregivers who perceived greater adaptability in the broader family environment.

Conclusion.—Caregiver satisfaction with decision making appears to be largely a function of the adaptability and lack of conflict in the larger family environment. Variables not related to decision-making satisfaction were the care recipient's level of dependence or cognitive impairment, the caregiving context, and the sizes of helping and decision-making networks. Service providers and families may be unable to reduce the effects of impairment on caregivers, but they can frequently offer helpful strategies to increase flexibility and adaptability.

▶ The topic of families and their burden in caring for their chronically mentally ill relatives is one of critical importance, given their predominant role in supporting and caring for their ill relatives. Obviously, all of us want to reduce as much as possible their burden and its resultant symptoms, e.g., depression, poor physical health, and negative affect. Therefore, this study helps us define and design strategies for reducing such burdens and, as such, it is most welcome.

J.A. Talbott, M.D.

Diagnosis, Epidemiology, Genetics, Followup

Use of Health Care Services by Persons With Panic Symptoms

Katerndahl DA, Realini JP (Univ of Texas, San Antonio)
Psychiatric Serv 48:1027–1032, 1997   5–18

Introduction.—In the community, panic disorder and infrequent panic are prevalent. Episodes of intense fear or panic attacks characterize the disorder. Symptoms include sweating, chest pain, nausea, dizziness, hot flushes or chills, and a sensation of choking. The person fears losing control, going crazy, or dying during a panic attack. Higher rates of physician visits and ambulatory health care visits are seen among this population. The health care utilization of persons with panic attacks was documented

Methods.—There were 97 patients with panic symptoms, mostly Mexican American and female, and matched controls. Data were collected on 2-month use of services of health care within and outside the mainstream health care system, levels of medical insurance coverage, and barriers to access of care. Rates of ambulatory and medical health visits and hospitalization were determined. The study also determined whether those with panic attacks specifically sought a remedy for their panic disorder.

Results.—There were higher rates of use for the services of psychiatrists and psychologists and for ambulance services among those with panic symptoms than among the controls. The differences between the group with panic symptoms and the control group were accounted for by those who met criteria for panic disorder and who sought care specifically for panic symptoms. Barriers to access were similar among both groups; however, the controls said that their medical insurance covered more types of services.

Conclusion.—Despite having less insurance coverage and having similar barriers to access, those with panic symptoms had higher rates of health care use than the controls. Increased use of health care by those who met criteria for panic disorder and seeking help specifically for alleviating symptoms of panic accounted for the higher rate.

▶ I am always surprised by the degree of chronicity, disability, and distress exhibited by persons suffering from panic symptoms. Perhaps my surprise is because we do not include them in our drumbeat definition of "severe and persistent mental illnesses." But here again, we see another manifestation of their crippling effect—in their high utilization of services despite their relative lack of insurance. The implications of this are that if we can design and disseminate more effective treatment of symptoms, we as a society, and the patients, will reap great rewards.

J.A. Talbott, M.D.

The Genetic Epidemiology of Schizophrenia in a Finnish Twin Cohort: A Population-based Modeling Study
Cannon TD, Kaprio J, Lönnqvist J, et al (Univ of Pennsylvania, Philadelphia; Univ of Helsinki; Natl Public Health Inst, Helsinki; et al)
Arch Gen Psychiatry 55:67–74, 1998

5–19

Introduction.—It is no longer controversial that genetic factors play an important role in schizophrenia, but the nature and extent of the genetic contribution is still uncertain. It is also unknown whether environmental and genetic contributions to schizophrenia differ by sex. Structural equation modelling was used in a total population of twins born in a 17-year period to determine the significance and magnitude of genetic and environmental contributions to schizophrenia and to determine whether these contributions differ by sex.

Methods.—A screening for nonorganic psychotic disorder diagnoses was conducted on all monozygotic twins (1,180 male and 1,315 female pairs) and same-sex dizygotic twins (2,765 male and 2,613 female pairs) born between 1940 and 1957 in Finland. The diagnoses were recorded from an eligibility review for a disability pension or on an inpatient or outpatient basis.

Results.—There was a 2% lifetime prevalence of schizophrenia with a marginally lower prevalence in women (1.8%) than in men (2.2%). Additive genetic factors accounted for 83% of the variance in liability, with the remaining 17% caused by unique environmental factors. Sex-limitation modeling revealed no evidence of sex-specific genetic effects and no sex difference in the magnitude of heritability. A multiple threshold model was rejected that incorporated affective and other psychoses as a phenotype intermediate between schizophrenia and no diagnosis.

Conclusion.—There was an estimated 83% heritability in a population-based twin study of schizophrenia, with the remaining variance in liability attributed to environmental factors not shared in common among cotwins. The heritability estimate in this study is almost identical to those reported in recent studies of index pairs using standardized applications, despite the notable limitation of using diagnoses ascertained through treatment contacts. Future studies should determine whether similar estimates are obtained with kinships other than twins. Studies in other countries should be conducted to establish the generalizability of these findings.

▶ Eighty-three percent heritability lies within the range of findings of prior studies, so why did I include this article? Because, although heritability remains the strongest single component in a person's liability in the development of schizophrenia, 17% comes from other factors. The authors point to obstetric complications as a cause, and this is well worth following up on, because until we have the genetics pinned down, reducing obstetric complications could have a payoff.

J.A. Talbott, M.D.

Long-term Follow-up of Patients Hospitalized for Schizophrenia, 1913–1940
Stephens JH, Richard P, McHugh PR (Johns Hopkins Univ, Baltimore, Md; Centre Hospitalier Spécialisé Esquirol, Paris)
J Nerv Ment Dis 185:715–721, 1997   5–20

Introduction.—Data on schizophrenics were collected from 1 clinic in the early 1900s and provide an invaluable picture of the characteristics of various clinical entities before the introduction of the somatic therapies. The ability provided for comparing outcomes during drug and nondrug treatment eras is the chief value of follow-up data on patients of an earlier era. One expert even declared that recovery rates for patients admitted since the introduction of the antipsychotic drugs are no better than for those admitted after the Second World War or during the first 2 decades of this century.

Methods.—Of 1,357 schizophrenic patients hospitalized between 1913 and 1940, 484 who were followed up for 5 or more years were studied. Ten percent from the sample of 1,357 patients committed suicide; none of these suicides were included in the sample of 484. This sample also did not include any patients with previous psychiatric admissions or episodes of mental illness.

Results.—There was a rating of recovery for 13% of the 484 patients. Fifty-eight percent were rated unimproved. Discharge status was highly correlated with long-term global follow-up. Long-term follow-up in the sample of 484 patients was significantly related to retrospective diagnosis by Diagnostic and Statistical Manual of Mental Diseases, edition IV criteria, with a continuum of poor outcomes ranging from the diagnoses of schizophrenia through schizophreniform to schizoaffective. Poor follow-up was significantly correlated with poor premorbid history, gradual onset, lack of depressive symptoms and heredity, seclusive personality, lack of precipitating events, lack of confusion, single status, onset before age 21, delusions of control, onset 6 months or more before admission, and emotional blunting.

Conclusion.—A validated prognostic scale was constructed from these variables. Schizophrenics who were hospitalized more than 50 years ago had poor outcomes. Better long-term outcomes have been linked with more recent treatment results, especially those with a long-term follow-up when contrasted with findings of an earlier era.

▶ What a wonderful data set! Most striking are the improved outcomes since the introduction of modern treatments. But the authors' ability to design a valid prognostic scale is also most helpful.

J.A. Talbott, M.D.

A Computer-administered Telephone Interview to Identify Mental Disorders

Kobak KA, Taylor LvH, Dottl SL, et al (Univ of Wisconsin, Madison)
JAMA 278:905–910, 1997   5–21

Introduction.—Primary Care Evaluation of Mental Disorders (PRIME-MD) is a diagnostic instrument designed for use by primary care physicians to detect the most commonly found mental disorders in primary care settings. It includes a 26-item patient questionnaire and a structured clinical interview. Computer interviews have been found to be a valid method for identifying and measuring psychopathology for disorders such as generalized anxiety, social phobia, depression, and obsessive-compulsive disorder. With an interactive voice response system, patients can answer the questions over the telephone and respond by pressing a number on their touch-tone telephone. Recently, a computer-assisted telephone-administered version of PRIME-MD has been developed. The validity of this method was tested.

Methods.—There were 200 outpatients with eating disorders, alcohol treatment, and psychiatric problems. Controls were also used in this study. Diagnoses obtained by computer over the telephone using this new technology were compared to diagnoses obtained by a trained clinician over the telephone using the structured clinical interview for *Diagnostic and Statistical Manual of Mental Disorders*, ed. 4 (DSM-IV). The clinician-administered version of PRIME-MD in a face-to-face interview was also used for comparison.

Results.—There were similar prevalence rates for any psychiatric disorder between diagnoses made by the computer and those made by a mental health professional using the structured clinical interview for the DSM-III. The versions showed similar prevalence rates for individual diagnoses. Twice as much alcohol abuse was reported on the computer among primary care patients as on either the clinician-administered PRIME-MD or the structured clinical interview. High and roughly equivalent levels of sensitivity and specificity were found among the computer- and clinician-administered version of PRIME-MD, using the structured clinical interview as the criterion.

Conclusion.—For assessing psychopathologic disorders in primary care patients, the computer-administered PRIME-MD appears to be a valid instrument. Increased availability is allowed with interactive voice response technology. An increase in quality of patient care is the result for primary care physicians who have access to more information without needing more time and money.

► We are told that telemedicine is 1 of the looming technologic trends that will revolutionize our field in the near future. Certainly, the Internet has provided patients and providers alike with a massive body of easy-to-access information, advice, and expertise. Not only are computers about as good as trained interviewers in diagnosing most mental illnesses, they are better in eliciting alcohol abuse. One wonders also if it's not easier to tell the computer about domestic violence, drug abuse, etc., than another human being.

J.A. Talbott, M.D.

Telephone Surveys as an Alternative for Estimating Prevalence of Mental Disorders and Service Utilization: A Montreal Catchment Area Study
Fournier L, Lesage AD, Toupin J, et al (Centre de recherche Philippe Pinel, Montreal; Centre de recherche Fernand Séguin, Montreal; Université de Sherbrooke, Quebec; et al)
Can J Psychiatry 42:737–743, 1997   5–22

Introduction.—Large-scale epidemiologic surveys have provided useful information about mental health issues. The high cost of these surveys prevents many countries from gathering data that could be helpful in service planning. The Diagnostic Interview Schedule created in the 1980s is a highly standardized instrument that can be administered by lay interviewers educated in its application. A telephone mental health survey may be a feasible, low-cost alternative for collecting information to determine the needs of a local area. A telephone survey with a sample of 893 residents from a Montreal catchment area was used to validate a new procedure for evaluating needs for mental health care and services in the community.

Methods.—The Composite International Diagnostic Interview Simplified is an instrument designed for mail or telephone surveys. It was used by lay interviewers to conduct telephone surveys in the Montreal catchment area. Service utilization was assessed by an instrument similar to those used for recent large Canadian and American surveys.

Results.—The prevalence rate for any mental disorder was lower in this investigation, compared to some earlier large-scale epidemiologic surveys (13.0% vs. 17.1% to 29.5%). This may be explained by methodological differences, such as number of disorders surveyed and period of reference. For specific mental disorders, results seemed very similar to those of other reports. Utilization rates tended to be higher than in other investigations. This could reflect real differences between Quebec and other Canadian provinces or the United States.

Conclusion.—Telephone surveys are lower in cost and produce results comparable to those provided by large-scale epidemiologic surveys conducted by face-to-face interviews. These findings will be helpful in service planning and policy making.

▶ There's not much to say about this result, except that it makes sense and is good to know. I agree with the authors that it is/was necessary to do big costly studies *but* that some stuff can be done more easily and inexpensively.

J.A. Talbott, M.D.

Primary Care

Integration Between Primary and Secondary Services in the Care of the Severely Mentally Ill: Patients' and General Practitioners' Views
Bindman J, Johnson S, Wright S, et al (Inst of Psychiatry, London)
Br J Psychiatry 171:169–174, 1997   5–23

Introduction.—General practitioners have played an increasing role in the care of patients with severe mental illness as community care has developed. The importance of the involvement of general practitioners in the care of their patients with severe mental illness has been emphasized. General practitioners should be receiving copies of care plans from specialists and the names of the patients' keyworkers should be known by the general practitioners. Professional bodies have been advocating shared care for patients with severe mental illness between primary and secondary services. Communication and joint working between general practitioners and psychiatric teams were measured.

Methods.—Interviews were conducted with 100 patients with severe mental illness and their general practitioners. The patients had one of the following disorders: schizophrenia, bipolar affective disorder, schizoaffective disorder, or recurrent depressive disorder. Questions to the general practitioners were about information from the psychiatric team about the patient, their knowledge of the patient's care by mental health services, and the types of contacts with the team in the preceding 6 months. Patients were asked about their contact with the general practitioners.

Results.—There was limited knowledge by general practitioners on the care that their patients received. Providing physical care and prescribing medications were perceived to be the principal goals of general practitioners. General practitioners were rarely consulted by their patients for mental health care. When it came to the care of Black Caribbean or Black African patients, general practitioners perceived themselves to be less involved.

Conclusion.—Much discontinuity was found between secondary and primary care. There is limited involvement by general practitioners for severely mentally ill patients. If care is to be shared, better communication is necessary.

▶ These are rather startling and disappointing findings. We have long known of the difficulty primary care practitioner's have in recognizing and adequately treating mental illnesses. However, when so much of American health care is hurtling off toward primary care treatment and gate-keeping, this should give us great cause for concern. The treatment of persons suffering from schizophrenia is not easy or simple or uncomplicated. The authors conclude that better communication is necessary. Sure, but we've been saying that for at least 40 years.

J.A. Talbott, M.D.

Can Case-finding Instruments Be Used to Improve Physician Detection of Depression in Primary Care?
Klinkman MS, Coyne JC, Gallo S, et al (Univ of Michigan, Ann Arbor)
Arch Fam Med 6:567–573, 1997   5–24

Introduction.—Studies of depression in the primary care setting indicate that depressive disorders are common but often go undetected. A study of patients seen in the practices of family physicians in southeastern Michigan sought to determine the relative accuracy of 3 methods for detecting major depression in primary care: a case-finding instrument alone, unaided physician identification, and "augmented" physician detection by use of a case-finding instrument.

Methods.—Patients were recruited from the practices of 50 board-certified family physicians. In the first stage of sampling, 1,928 consecutive adult patients were asked to complete screening forms while waiting for a scheduled visit. The forms included the Center for Epidemiologic Studies–Depression scale (CES-D), demographic questions, and self-rating items. Although unaware of these responses, physicians evaluated each of the patients for clinical depression. In the second stage, a weighted random subsample (425 of the 1,580 patients who completed the initial screening) completed the Structured Clinical Interview (SCID) for the Diagnostic and Statistical Manual of Mental Disorders, Third Edition, Revised (DSM-III-R).

Results.—Those completing the SCID were predominantly white (92.9%), female (76.7%), and currently married (59.8%). The mean age of the group was 39.6 years. In the final weighted sample, 57 patients (13.4%) had major depression. Both the CES-D and unaided physician detection methods had a low rate of success in identifying major depression. For each detected case, physicians missed almost 2 cases. The CES-D had high sensitivity but low specificity at standard and high cut points. Detection of depression was not improved by raising the CES-D threshold for a positive test. Only minimal improvement was seen when physicians used CES-D scores in an attempt to identify patients meeting DSM-III-R criteria for major depressive disorder.

Conclusion.—The findings of this study do not support the routine use of CES-D scores as a primary care screening instrument. Neither high scores on the CES-D nor unaided physician detection successfully identified patients with major depression, and physician access to CES-D scores had little effect on the accuracy of detection.

▶ Regarding the point about recognition I mentioned in my comments about (Abstract 5–23), here is an attempt to improve the recognition of depression in primary care that demonstrates how difficult it is. Neither standardized instruments nor personal observation were helpful. This is 1 of the few articles that make me wish the authors had speculated on how we might be more effective; what we have done so far certainly has not worked.

J.A. Talbott, M.D.

Integrating Mental Health Services Within Primary Care: A Canadian Program

Kates N, Craven M, Crustolo AM, et al (Hamilton-Wentworth HSO Mental Health Program, Hamilton, Ont, Canada)
Gen Hosp Psychiatry 19:324–332, 1997

5–25

Introduction.—Family physicians may fail to identify patients with mental health problems, and only a small percentage of individuals with an identified psychiatric illness are referred to a mental health service or psychiatrist. The Canadian program described in this study was designed to enhance the role of the family physician in delivering mental health care.

Methods.—Since 1994, the Hamilton-Wentworth Mental Health Program has linked mental health counselors and psychiatrists with primary care practices in the southern Ontario community. A central management team works with each health service organization to improve its mental health services and increase the skills of family physicians when managing mental health problems. Mental health counselors are attached permanently to each practice, and psychiatric consultants visit every 1–3 weeks. Even after a referral, family physicians remain integrally involved in patient care and are available by phone if a crisis arises. A comprehensive evaluation procedure is in place to ensure continuing quality improvement.

Results.—The program received 3,085 referrals during its first year of operation. Most of those referred (70%) were women, and the most common causes for referral were depression (38%) and marital/relationship problems (22%). The average hours of service provided by a counselor for each client per episode of care was 5.5. Overall, 61% of referrals to the consulting psychiatrist were made by the family physician and 39% by the counselor. Most of these 439 referred patients had a diagnosis of mood disorder (59%) or anxiety disorder (23%). On a 5-point Likert Scale, satisfaction with the program was rated at 4.6 by family physicians, counselors, and psychiatrists. All psychiatrists and 95% of counselors would recommend this style of practice to a colleague.

Conclusion.—The mental health program brought counselors, psychiatrists, and a management team to primary care practices to make mental health care more available in the primary care setting. Continuity of care was increased, communication improved, and opportunities for physician and patient education expanded. This type of program appears to be an efficient way of providing mental health care for large numbers of patients, many of whom would not otherwise be treated.

▶ On the other hand, in contrast to the Bindman study (Abstract 5–23), here is a program in which the linkage to primary care really pays off in continuity of care, reduction in referrals to tertiary care, and patient satisfaction. Having heard Dr. Kates present the program orally, however, I am convinced that it takes a lot of hard work, targeted helpful intervention, and someone like Dr.

Kates to make such a program work. But the results are well worth the effort!

J.A. Talbott, M.D.

Providing Psychiatric Backup to Family Physicians by Telephone
Kates N, Crustolo A-M, Nikolaou L, et al (McMaster Univ, Hamilton, Ont, Canada; Hamilton-Wentworth HSO Mental Health Program, Canada)
Can J Psychiatry 42:955–959, 1997   5–26

Introduction.—A problem identified by family physicians is lack of communication between psychiatrists or mental health services staff and family physicians. Family physicians rarely have the opportunity to discuss difficulties encountered with a patient with a psychiatrist. Psychiatry and family care need to find ways to improve communication and provide mutual support if they are to work together more productively. One effective strategy would be for a psychiatrist to be available to respond to telephone calls from family physicians. The experience of a psychiatrist who established such an arrangement was reviewed.

Methods.—Telephone backup concerning mental health problems the family physicians encountered was provided by 1 psychiatrist who visited 18 family physicians in 5 practices on a regular basis to provide clinical consultations. The psychiatrist visited each of the practices for half a day every 2 weeks. At the end of a 12-month period, all calls received by the psychiatrist were documented and analyzed.

Results.—Five practices made 128 calls in the course of 1 year. There were 78 that involved routine management or medication issues and 50 that were considered urgent. Family physicians were able to handle these patients more effectively with telephone advice, and this often provided support that was not otherwise available and reduced utilization of other mental health services. Eight minutes was the average time spent per call, which meant the psychiatrist spent 20 minutes per week on the phone in response to family physicians' requests.

Conclusion.—A time-efficient and effective method of supporting family physicians and reducing utilization of mental health services is providing telephone backup to family physicians. This practice can be applied by psychiatrists working any clinical setting.

▶ This is another article by the Kates group and I included it because it shows how simple things can be both meaningful and cost effective. I recall my reservations, long ago, of giving my home telephone number to visiting nurses and community care social workers, but it was unfounded; once they knew I was there, they used it sparingly and well, and I agree that its "bang for the buck" is enormous.

J.A. Talbott, M.D.

Psychiatric Morbidity and Physician Visits: Lessons from Ontario
Tweed DL, Goering P, Lin E, et al (Clarke Inst of Psychiatry, Toronto; Inst for Clinical Evaluative Sciences in Toronto)
Med Care 36:573–585, 1998
5–27

Introduction.—It is well known that persons with psychiatric disorders use more health services than the general population. The association between psychiatric morbidity and use of general and family practitioners by persons with psychiatric disorders in Ontario, Canada were assessed.

Methods.—Data was obtained from the 1990 Ontario Health Survey (OHS) and the companion Mental Health Supplement. The OHS surveyed 35,479 sample households, including 61,239 individuals. The Mental Health Supplement assessed mental health, related disability, and a range of factors known to place individuals at risk for mental health problems. This comprehensive survey of physical and mental health included the UM-CIDI standardized diagnostic interview.

Results.—It was estimated that 19.6% (14.8% single diagnosis and 4.8% multiple diagnosis) of the Ontario population, aged 15 to 64 years, had 1 or more diagnosable psychiatric disorders in the year before the interview. There was a disproportionately higher use of medical services in individuals with a psychiatric disorder, compared with the general population. This trend was strongest in persons with multiple psychiatric disorders. Contributing factors included comorbid physical conditions, subjective distress, psychiatric disability, and deliberate use of the general medical sector for mental health problems.

Discussion/Conclusion.—Psychiatric morbidity is correlated with higher rates of health service use, particularly in persons with multiple psychiatric disorders. Economic pressures within the system necessitate that many patients with psychiatric illness will continue to be seen by family physicians. Interventions need to be tailored to the level of morbidity and complexity of each patient.

▶ There's something wrong with this picture. Somehow, regardless of insurance or system of care, mentally ill and especially comorbidly mentally ill persons go to nonpsychiatric physicians more often than their medical status warrants. Don't we need some research and some recommendations as to specific remedies to this "dually-diagnosed" population just as we have done with those suffering from mental illness and mental retardation and mental illness and addictive disorders?

J.A. Talbott, M.D.

The Care of Patients With Chronic Schizophrenia: A Comparison Between Two Services
Gater R, Goldberg D, Jackson G, et al (Univ of Manchester, England; Inst of Psychiatry, London)
Psychol Med 27:1325–1336, 1997   5–28

Background.—The use of community multidisciplinary teams to deliver coordinated comprehensive mental health care is widespread. However, few published data on the quality of care and cost-effectiveness of such care are available.

Methods and Findings.—Quality of care for patients with chronic schizophrenia treated by a multidisciplinary community team with close links to primary care and a traditional psychiatric service in a district general hospital psychiatric unit was studied in a clustered, randomized, controlled comparison. Two years after the community team was established, patients with access to it had more of their needs met and were more satisfied with their care. These patients also had more service contacts and received more interventions. Though the community team resulted in a cost savings associated with the use of some hospital resources, these savings did not offset the cost of the new service. Four years after the establishment of the community team, it met a higher proportion of needs for underactivity, daily living skills, use of public amenities, and managing finances (Table 3).

TABLE 3.—Extent to Which Different Areas of Need Were Met by Study Group (The Denominator of the Number in Parentheses Represents the Number of Times a Meetable Need Was Identified in That Area and the Numerator the Number of Times That Need Was Met)

	Met Needs as a Percentage of Meetable Needs	
	Index	Control
Symptoms and behavioural problems		
Psychotic symptoms	92 (35/38)	76 (32/42)
Underactivity	80 (16/20)	22 (6/27)†
Side effects of medication	88 (15/17)	65 (11/17)
Neurotic symptoms	70 (14/20)	20 (3/15)†
Physical disorder	70 (12/17)	66 (12/18)
Behaviour difficulties†	100 (9/9)	45 (5/11)*
Distress	80 (8/10)	36 (7/19)
Skills and abilities		
Daily living skills‡	83 (40/48)	61 (36/59)†
Use of public amenities and transport	83 (5/6)	44 (4/9)
Vocational skills	26 (4/15)	25 (4/16)
Communication skills	45 (5/11)	16 (2/12)
Managing finances and affairs	68 (22/32)	47 (24/51)

Note: Educational difficulties and dementia have been omitted from the Table as there were only 2 patients with problems in these areas.

Chi-squared test: *significance of difference between groups, 0.05 greater than *P* greater than 0.01; †significance of difference between groups, *P* less than 0.01.

†Embarrassing or dangerous behavior.

‡Personal care, shopping, getting meals, managing the household chores.

(Courtesy of Gater R, Goldberg D, Jackson G, et al: The care of patients with chronic schizophrenia: A comparison between two services. *Psychol Med* 27:1325–1336, 1997. Reprinted with the permission of Cambridge University Press.)

Conclusions.—The multidisciplinary community service provided better quality of care at 2 and 4 years than did the traditional hospital-based service. The community services also targeted resources more efficiently.

▶ The 2 elements here that stand out as contributing to the success of the community team are the increased coordination of the team members and the linkage to primary caregivers. It is too bad that the cost offset was not powerful; I'm afraid that in the United States the increase in quality of care and patient satisfaction won't carry the day with managed care.

J.A. Talbott, M.D.

Financing, Cost, Managed Care

How Expensive Is Unlimited Mental Health Care Coverage Under Managed Care?
Sturm R (RAND, Santa Monica, Calif)
JAMA 278:1533–1537, 1997

5–29

Purpose.—Under the Mental Health Parity Act of 1996, employers are required to increase the limits for mental health coverage to equal those for medical care, but are not required to offer either type of coverage. Little is known about the impact of such policies; it will depend on how employers perceive the cost consequences. Older data on the costs of mental health coverage do not consider trends in the health care market or in treatment patterns—including the trend toward outpatient care—and, thus, may overestimate the costs of the new legislation. The cost consequences of unlimited mental health coverage in the managed care setting were studied.

Methods.—The study analyzed 1995 and 1996 claims data on 24 new managed care plans, all of which provided unlimited mental health coverage with minimal copayments. The costs of removing various coverage limits for mental health care were analyzed, including limits not affected by the Mental Health Parity Act but possibly affected by newer state laws. The probability of care, intensity of care, and total costs were analyzed in terms of service type and type of enrollee. The findings were compared with the assumptions made in recent policy debates.

Results.—The debate over the Mental Health Parity Act overestimated the actual costs of managed care by fourfold to eightfold. Factors leading to lower costs in the plans analyzed included reduced hospitalization rates, the shift toward outpatient care, and reduced payments per service. At the same time, 7% of enrollees had access to mental health specialty care, compared with 6.5% in previous fee-for-service plans and 5% with free care in the RAND Health Insurance Experiment. Eliminating a $25,000 annual limit on mental health care would raise insurance rates by only about $1 per year per enrollee. The greatest beneficiaries of mental health parity would be families with seriously mentally ill children.

Conclusion.—The debate over the Mental Health Parity Act was limited by incorrect assumptions and old data, which overestimated the impact of removing limits on mental health coverage. This study shows that the cost impact under managed care will actually be quite small. Children will be the greatest beneficiaries of the new legislation, a fact that has not received adequate attention.

▶ The estimated increase of $1 per managed care enrollee per year to remove restrictions on the mental health benefit is certainly a far cry from what the insurance industry, and even the Congressional Research Service, estimate, e.g., $100.00. How do we get this communicated without stirring up opposition?

J.A. Talbott, M.D.

Outpatient Utilization Patterns of Integrated and Split Psychotherapy and Pharmacotherapy for Depression
Goldman W, McCulloch J, Cuffel B, et al (United Behavioral Health, San Francisco; Duke Univ, Durham, NC)
Psychiatric Serv 49:477–482, 1998   5–30

Introduction.—The role of the psychiatrist has become limited to writing prescriptions for state and county institutions, community health centers, and other organized service settings in the public and nonprofit sectors. Psychotherapy services are primarily provided by nonphysician mental health specialists. Outpatient use and costs among depressed patients in 2 treatment models (integrated vs. split psychotherapy and pharmacology) were assessed in a quasi-experimental retrospective trial.

Methods.—Psychotherapy and pharmacotherapy were provided by a psychiatrist in the integrated group. Pharmacology was provided by a psychiatrist and psychotherapy was provided by a nonphysician psychotherapist in the split-treatment group. Claim data from a nationally managed mental health care organization was retrospectively collected from 191 patients in integrated treatment and 1,326 patients in split treatment.

Results.—Over an 18-month period, patients receiving integrated treatment used significantly less outpatient sessions and had significantly lower treatment costs, compared with patients in the split-treatment group. Integrated treatment was apparently associated with a pattern of use that was characterized by frequent treatment episodes. Split treatment was characterized by more sessions with fewer breaks of 90 days or more.

Conclusion.—These preliminary findings indicate that integrated treatment is more costly than split treatment in a managed care network. It apparently is more efficient for patients to see a single therapist for consolidated treatment.

▶ Here is another study whose findings fly in the face of all the widespread belief that integrated treatment costs more than splitting psychotherapy and psychopharmacology. We know from the extensive literature over the past 45 years since deinstitutionalization began, which I referred to in the first abstract in this section,[1] that the evidence is overwhelmingly favorable in clinical terms for integrated-combined care; this article demonstrates its economic power as well.

J.A. Talbott, M.D.

Reference

1. Talbott JA: Lessons learned about the chronic mentally ill since 1955, in Ancill R (ed): *Schizophrenia: Exploring the Spectrum of Psychosis*, New York, John Wiley & Sons, Ltd, 1994, pp 1–20.

Tennessee's Failed Managed Care Program for Mental Health and Substance Abuse Services
Chang CF, Kiser LJ, Bailey JE, et al (Univ of Memphis, Tenn)
JAMA 279:864–869, 1998   5–31

Introduction.—On January 1, 1994, Tennessee started TennCare, an innovative managed care reform program designed to avert a pending Medicare crisis. It was conceived to enlist and pay a managed care organization to assume responsibilities for general medical care and mental health and substance abuse (MH/SA) services. It never materialized because of widespread opposition. In July 1996, the TennCare Partners program was launched. It was a "carve-out" arrangement designed to consolidate all MH/SA services under a separate program. It started chaotically and soon deteriorated into a crisis. The TennCare program and its flaws are described.

TennCare Partners.—Under the TennCare Partners program, many patients did not receive care or lost continuity of care. The traditional "safety net" mental health system nearly dissolved. TennCare Partners had 3 major flaw designs: (1) it lacked a single point of accountability for patient care; (2) it spread funds previously earmarked for severely mentally ill patients across the entire Medicaid population; and (3) it used a single capitation rate with no risk adjustment for severity of illness to pay the behavioral health organizations.

Discussion/Conclusion.—Other states considering similar funds will need to protect vulnerable patients by risk-adjusting capitation payments and by focusing resources on care for persons who are severely mentally ill. States need to minimize program complexity and ensure the accountability of managed care networks for the behavioral health care needs of their patients. States considering this approach should start with a small program.

▶ One of the most closely watched "experiments" in mental health care reform is the move of the Medicaid and uninsured populations in Tennessee to managed care. Although the authors attribute the "failure" of this program primarily to the flawed design (e.g., trying to cover the entire Medicaid and uninsured population using a dollar amount previously spent for only the chronic mentally ill), there are so many other factors that doomed it from the start that their comment and lessons-learned section are almost as long as a separate article (1,500 words). From what I understand, now, 5 years later, they still haven't got it right.

J.A. Talbott, M.D.

The Effects of Public Managed Care on Patterns of Intensive Use of Inpatient Psychiatric Services
Geller JL, Fisher WH, McDermeit M, et al (Univ of Massachusetts, Worcester; Lighthouse Inst of Chestnut Health Systems, Bloomington, Ill)
Psychiatric Serv 49:327–332, 1998   5–32

Introduction.—The trend of deinstitutionalization is now more common with mental health care patients, particularly with the advent of new drugs and statutes governing the involuntary detention of patients in state hospitals and community-based care. This trend may have caused patients with previously long hospitalizations to now have multiple short admissions amid cycles of remission and decompensation. Managed care may have further magnified the problems. Under a public sector managed care program, the characteristics of frequent users of inpatient treatment were explored to determine whether their pattern of inpatient use affected their overall use of hospital days.

Methods.—A client tracking system was used to identify individuals with 5 or more admissions in 4 fiscal years. These patients were compared with other patients who did not have multiple admissions to determine their demographic and clinical characteristics and the types of hospitals they used.

Results.—Young white female patients with personality disorder and a history of substance abuse, but not a current substance use disorder, were more likely to require multiple admissions than other patients. As measured by the Georgia Role Functioning Scale, they tended to be lower functioning. As measured by the global personal distress portion of this scale, they also tended to have higher levels of distress. These patients accounted for up to 27% of all admissions in the 4 fiscal years and made up to 8% of all clients with a psychiatric admission who were enrolled in a case management program. Significantly longer lengths of stay resulted for these patients with multiple admissions when they were admitted to a hospital where they had not been previously admitted in the past 12 months.

Conclusion.—Subpopulations of persons at high risk for multiple admissions should be able to receive special attention in states setting up public-sector managed care or revising existing public-sector managed care contracts. To enable frequent users of acute care facilities to return to the same facility that previously discharged them, networks of inpatient providers should be created.

▶ Geller et al.'s findings make sense (e.g., that high-users are different and should be treated differently, especially by using the same hospital and employing networks of experts in their care). But many insurers and providers are fearful of not having a big enough risk pool and suffering adverse economic results when at risk for a disproportionate number of such patients. Their findings also remind us that not all "chronic patients" suffer from schizophrenia; here, female patients with borderline personality disorder are among those most in need of specialized services.

J.A. Talbott, M.D.

A Comparison of Clozapine and Haloperidol in Hospitalized Patients With Refractory Schizophrenia
Rosenheck R, for the Department of Veterans Affairs Cooperative Study Group on Clozapine in Refractory Schizophrenia (Yale School of Medicine, New Haven, Conn; Hines Veterans Affairs Med Ctr, Ill; Veterans Affairs Cooperative Studies Program Clinical Research Pharmacy Coordinating Ctr, Albuquerque, NM)
N Engl J Med 337:809–815, 1997   5–33

Background.—Clozapine is an expensive antipsychotic drug commonly used to treat individuals with refractory schizophrenia. Clozapine is associated with a low rate of extrapyramidal side effects, but has been known to cause agranulocytosis. There are no long-term evaluations of the effect of clozapine on symptoms, social functioning, or use and cost of heath care.

Methods.—In a 1-year, randomized, double-blind study, clozapine and haloperidol were compared at 15 Veterans Affairs medical centers. Clozapine was administered to 205 patients and haloperidol was administered to 218 patients. All patients had refractory schizophrenia and had been hospitalized for 30–364 days the previous year.

Results.—Among patients given clozapine, 117 continued their assigned treatment for the study year, but only 61 patients given haloperidol continued their assigned treatment. Using the Positive and Negative Syndrome Scale of Schizophrenia, it was noted that patients given clozapine had 5.4% lower symptom levels compared with patients given haloperidol. In intention-to-treat analysis, differences in the quality of life scale were not significant. However, these differences were significant among patients who did not cross over to the other treatment. During the 1-year study period, patients given clozapine were hospitalized for fewer days for psychiatric reasons and used more outpatient services than patients given haloperidol. The total cost per capita was about $58,150 for patients given clozapine and about $61,890 for patients given haloperidol. The cost of the antipsychotic drugs per capita was about $3,200 for clozapine and

$367 for haloperidol. Patients given clozapine had less tardive dyskinesia and fewer extrapyramidal side effects. Three patients given clozapine had agranulocytosis, but all made a full recovery.

Discussion.—In patients with refractory schizophrenia who use hospital resources frequently, clozapine was slightly more effective than haloperidol. Clozapine was also associated with fewer side effects. Although clozapine was much more expensive than haloperidol, the overall treatment costs were comparable because patients receiving clozapine spent less time in the hospital.

▶ Question: Why is this article abstracted for this section? Answer: Because the belief by state governments and managed care organizations that clozapine is more costly than standard antipsychotics (e.g., haloperidol) is not borne out by this study. Its fewer side effects and treatment efficacy should overcome bureaucrats' doubts.

J.A. Talbott, M.D.

Psychiatrists' Duties in Discharging Sicker and Potentially Violent In-patients in the Managed Care Era
Simon RI (Georgetown Univ, Washington, DC)
Psychiatric Serv 49:62–67, 1998   5–34

Introduction.—In the managed care era, the treatment of psychiatric inpatients has changed dramatically, with most units becoming short-stay acute care settings. Hospitalization is generally limited to suicidal, homicidal, or gravely disabled patients with complex major psychiatric disorders. To maintain length-of-stay statistics within predetermined limits, the hospital administration may exert pressure for early discharge of these patients. The ultimate burden of liability for treatments gone awry is often borne by the psychiatrists. With shorter patient hospital stays, psychiatrists have limited opportunity to communicate with patients. In managed care settings, psychiatrists have certain responsibilities and legal duties to their patients, including disclosure of all treatment options, exercise of appeals for patient care that has been denied, provision of emergency and acute treatment regardless of decisions regarding coverage, cooperation with utilization reviewers, and warning and protecting third parties.

Duties.—Psychiatrists must provide full disclosure of all treatment options, even those that are not covered under the terms of a managed care plan. Families or other substitute health care decision makers may need to be informed if agitated and violent psychiatric patients do not have the capacity to understand treatment options. Managed contracts that contain limitations on full disclosure to patients should not be signed by psychiatrists. Their duty to appeal involves advocating for patient care they believe is essential or advisable.

More Duties.—The psychiatrist's duty to treat involves being liable for failure to treat patients within the defined standard of care. If there are limitations imposed by a third-party payor that are in conflict with the physician's judgment, the physician who complies without protest when his medical judgment dictates otherwise cannot avoid ultimate responsibility for his patient's care. When it comes to the violence-prone patient, the psychiatrist is responsible for the patient's care and has a duty to advocate. Psychiatrists should cooperate with utilization reviewers' requests for information. It is essential to carefully document a current assessment of risk of violence, accurately describe the current clinical condition of the patient, and explain why the patient cannot be treated as an outpatient.

Conclusion.—Sicker patients and those who are potentially violent should not be prematurely discharged because of pressure from managed care organizations. By limiting the time and resources for diagnosis and the assessment of the risk of potential violence, the policies of such organizations can place psychiatrists and patients in a precarious position.

▶ We all agonize over the new ethics imposed by changing health care, but few write about it. Simon's listing of our various "duties," especially the "duty to appeal," should be read by all who practice in today's hazardous environment. It is not easy, but Simon makes our responsibilities clearer.

J.A. Talbott, M.D.

Field Test of a Tool for Level-of-care Decisions in Community Mental Health Systems
Srebnik D, Uehara E, Smukler M (Univ of Washington, Seattle; Eastside Mental Health Services, Bellevue, Wash)
Psychiatric Serv 49:91–97, 1998   5–35

Introduction.—Whenever service providers design treatment plans to meet clients' needs, levels of care are used implicitly. There is a wide variability of services provided to clients with similar needs because service providers' decisions about level of care are highly flexible and idiosyncratic. Service providers and program planners can be helped by increasing the predictability of level-of-care decisions through the use of decision-support tools. For guiding level-of-care decisions for mental health outpatient clients, few tools exist. A level-of-care decision-support tool based on clinical need was described. Its reliability and validity were tested. The relationship of the tool's level-of-care placement to sociodemographic characteristics such as age, gender, and ethnicity was also examined.

Methods.—A decision-support tool with 8 levels of care and a computerized decision-tree algorithm for level-of-care placement were developed by panels of clinical managers and administrators of mental health centers. The 8 levels are brief intervention, medication maintenance, monitoring, rehabilitation, residential care, intensive community support, assertive community treatment, and inpatient services. A package that included variables in the level-of-care model, but not the algorithm itself, was used

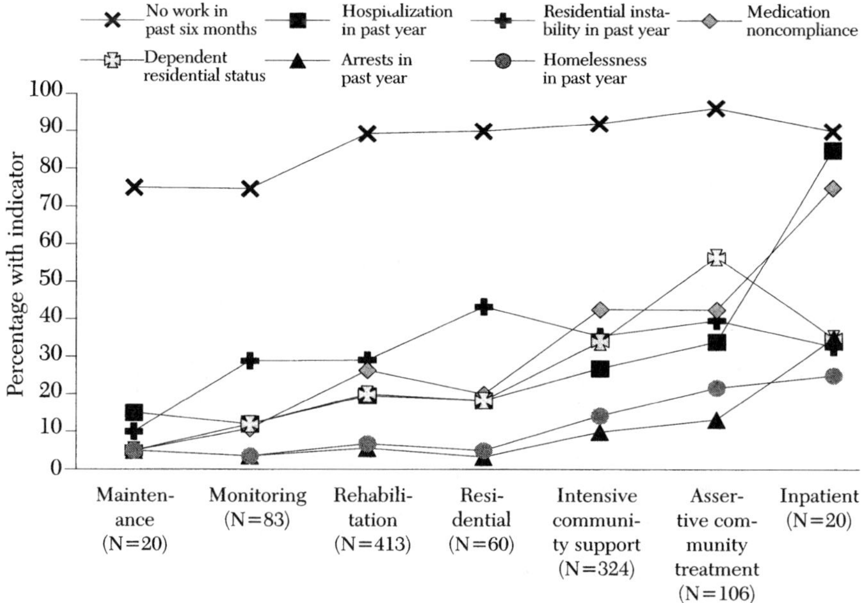

FIGURE 1.—Percentage of individuals with severity indicator placed in 7 levels of mental health care. (Courtesy of Srebnik D, Uehara E, Smukler M: Field test of a tool for level-of-care decisions in community mental health systems. *Psychiatric Serv* 49:91–97, 1998. Copyright 1998, the American Psychiatric Association. Reprinted by permission.)

by case managers to assess a random sample of 1,034 adults from 1 county mental health system. To assess the tool's concurrent validity, other variables were included.

Results.—Strong interrater reliability was found in level-of-care placements based on the decision-support tool. Each indicator of clinical severity was significantly related to the level-of-care placement (Fig 1). Functioning as measured by the Global Assessment of Functioning Scale, lack of work activity, medication noncompliance, residential independence, homeless periods, residential moves, arrests, and psychiatric care were significantly related to the expected direction of level of care, demonstrating concurrent validity.

Conclusion.—The level-of-care decision-support tool is reliable and valid according to preliminary empirical evidence. By incorporating the impact of collateral services, social supports, motivation for services, and current mental health services, it could be further refined.

▶ I have included this abstract because I think it codifies what we have needed for years: a way to determine levels of care. To date, level-of-care decisions have really been "hit or miss," and with the increasing necessity of conserving resources, an effective system can, indeed, be a useful tool.

J.A. Talbott, M.D.

Work and Rehabilitation

The Impact of Psychiatric Disorders on Work Loss Days

Kessler RC, Frank RG (Harvard Med School, Boston)
Psychol Med 27:861–873, 1997   5–36

Background.—Traditionally, the main concerns of psychiatric epidemiology have been to estimate incidence and identify risk factors. More recently, there has been interest in determining the social consequences of psychiatric disorders, especially the effects on socioeconomic status. Epidemiologists and policy analysts have estimated the financial costs and social consequences of psychiatric disorders to further the debate on universal health coverage for psychiatric problems. Studies have shown that psychiatric disorders exact significant personal costs from individuals, their families, and their communities in regard to finances, role functioning, and quality of life. From a policy perspective, the effects of psychiatric disorders on lower rates of participation in the labor force, reduced work hours, and lower earning are important issues. Work impairments have serious implications for the economy.

Methods.—Data were obtained from the US National Comorbidity Survey, a survey of respondents aged from 15–54 in the United States. This survey focuses on employed individuals. The relationships between DSM-III-R psychiatric disorders and work impairment were examined in major occupational groups.

Results.—Results are based on 4,091 respondents. There is marked variation across occupations in the 30-day prevalence of DSM-III-R psychiatric disorders. The average prevalence was 18.2% for any given disorder, with a range of 11%–29.6%. In contrast, the average prevalence of work days lost because of psychiatric reasons was not significantly different across occupations. The average number of psychiatric work days lost was 6 days per month per 100 workers, and the average number of psychiatric work cutback days was 31 days per month per 100 workers. Work impairment was higher among the 3.7% of workers with comorbid psychiatric disorders (49 work loss days and 346 work cutback days per month per 100 workers) than in the 14.5% of workers with pure disorders (11 work loss days and 66 work cutback days per month per 100 workers) or the 81.8% of workers with no disorders (2 work loss days and 11 work cutback days per month per 100 workers). The effects of psychiatric disorders on work loss were similar across all occupations, but the effects on work cutback days were greater among professionals.

Discussion.—Psychiatric disorders have negative effects on the labor force in terms of lost work productivity. The 30-day DSM-III-R psychiatric disorders were associated with significant numbers of work loss and work cutback days. The effects vary substantially depending on the disorder and occupation. These results may help the current social policy debates on national health insurance and coverage for psychiatric disorders in various societies.

▶ We have known for a couple of decades that work is 1 of the best proties for mental disability that we have and that mainstream employment is 1 of the most difficult goals for the severely and persistently mentally ill to attain. Two findings of this study are strikingly evident: (1) the devastating power of comorbidity, and (2) the economic impact of loss of product and income caused by affective disorders. These results should prompt companies to be much more supportive of psychiatric diagnosis and treatment (as they have of Employee Assistance Programs) to reduce days lost to emotional disorders.

J.A. Talbott, M.D.

A Capitated Model for a Cross-section of Severely Mentally Ill Clients: Employment Outcomes
Chandler D, Meisel J, Hu T-w, et al (Univ of California, Berkeley; Lewin-VHI; Yale Univ)
Community Ment Health J 33:501–516, 1997   5–37

Introduction.—In studies of the most successful programmatic approach to serving the seriously mentally ill in the community (the PACT Model) employment has only sometimes been an outcome. It is important to understand how employment services can be integrated with the core service team and other components of the PACT Model because of the relative success of these programs in reducing hospitalization and in improving some other outcomes. Supported employment is a more recent approach that has raised much interest and hope. A cross-section of seriously mentally ill clients was reviewed to determine 3-year client outcomes.

Methods.—In a cross-section of severely mentally ill clients, employment outcomes were examined in a 3-year controlled study of 2 Integrated Service Agencies. The models integrated supported employment and transitional employment with a core services team in the context of comprehensive, rehabilitatively oriented services.

Results.—Paid employment was obtained by significantly more Integrated Service Agency members than comparison clients. The difference was dramatic at the urban site, with 73% vs. 15% finding work during the study period and 29% of the Integrated Service Agency clients working competitively.

Conclusion.—Increased employment opportunity for all seriously mentally ill clients should be considered. It is not effective to simply provide high funding for team-based case management, without a structured employment program. If given a range of opportunities, most clients will seriously try working.

▶ Mainstream employment is a tough goal for those with chronic mental illnesses. However, the success of this program, as well as others mentioned by the authors, lends support to their conclusion that all seriously mentally ill patients can benefit from this sort of program.

J.A. Talbott, M.D.

Trauma and Posttraumatic Stress Disorder

Is Gulf War Syndrome Due to Stress? The Evidence Reexamined
Haley RW (Univ of Texas, Dallas)
Am J Epidemiol 146:695–703, 1997   5–38

Introduction.—The vague, undiagnosable illness known as Gulf War syndrome has been attributed to wartime stress, mainly on the basis of studies of posttraumatic stress disorder (PTSD). However, the idea that chronic illnesses can result from general life stress does not have a great deal of scientific support. There is evidence to suggest that veterans with Gulf War syndrome have findings associated with diffuse neurotoxic injury. The evidence linking Gulf War syndrome to PTSD was critically reexamined.

Methods.—The author reviewed 16 studies cited in the final report of the Presidential Advisory Committee on Gulf War Veterans' Illnesses. Three other studies were identified in a literature review. For each study, the observed estimates of PTSD were corrected for the sensitivity and specificity of the psychometric scale used.

Results.—In each study, the prevalence rate of PTSD was determined by critical cutpoints on psychometric scales, instead of by clinical psychiatric interviews. The mean reported prevalence was 9%, with a range of 0%–36%. However, on correction for measurement errors, the true PTSD rate was 0% in 18 of 20 cases. For all subgroups of Gulf War veterans, mean scores on the Mississippi Scale for Combat-Related Posttraumatic Stress Disorder fell in the range of scores for well-adjusted veterans of the Vietnam War, and well below those of Vietnam veterans with psychiatrically confirmed PTSD (Fig 1).

Conclusion.—Previous studies of PTSD and "stress-related symptoms" in Gulf War veterans may reflect false positive errors of measurement of nonspecific symptoms. Mean PTSD scores for Gulf War veterans do not fall into the same range as that observed in Vietnam veterans with confirmed PTSD. Until the plausible physical causes of Gulf War syndrome have been thoroughly studied, a psychological explanation for the symptoms should not be assumed.

▶ The physical symptoms that Gulf War veterans have complained of ever since that conflict have puzzled physicians, including psychiatrists and government leaders. Haley's reanalysis of some 19 studies from a methodologic point of view concludes that we must look at causes other than stress for these complaints. In a related article,[1] the authors take a similarly dim view of our ability to designate the Gulf War complaints as a new disease or

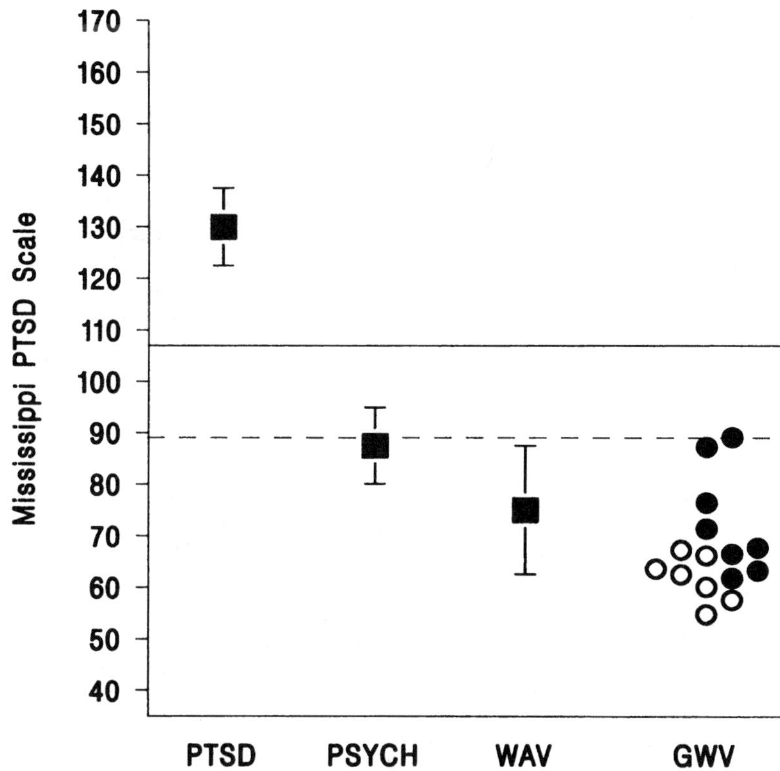

FIGURE 1.—Mean scores and standard deviations for the Mississippi Scale for Combat-Related Posttraumatic Stress Disorder (M-PTSD) by diagnosis groups in Vietnam veterans (*squares*) from Keane et al. and mean M-PTSD scores from 7 studies of Gulf War veterans (*circles*), i.e., Sloan et al., Sutker et al., Perconte et al., Wolfe et al., Ross and Wonders, and Southwick et al. *PTSD* indicates 30 Vietnam veterans with clinically confirmed post-traumatic stress disorder; *PSYCH* indicates 30 Vietnam veterans with inpatient, nonpsychotic psychiatric disorders; and *WAV* indicates 30 well-adjusted Vietnam veterans. *Solid circles* represent high-risk groups (e.g., high combat stress exposure, women) of Gulf War veterans (*GWV*), and *open circles* represent low-risk groups. The two highest values for Gulf War veterans were measured with the Mississippi Scale for Combat-Related PTSD modified for Desert Storm veterans, on which scores may be inflated by as much as 8 points. The *solid horizontal reference line* represents Keane's cutpoint for defining PTSD (sensitivity = 0.93, specificity = 0.89) and the *dashed line* represents Kulka's cutpoint (sensitivity = 0.94, specificity = 0.80). (Courtesy of Haley RW: Is Gulf War syndrome due to stress? The evidence reexamined. *Am J Epidemiol* 146:695–703, 1997.)

attribute clear causality of this "syndrome" to environmental/toxic/chemical/ etc. reasons. So the jury is still out.

J.A. Talbott, M.D.

Reference

1. Wegman DH, Woods NF, Bailar JC: How would we know a Gulf War syndrome if we saw one? (invited commentary). *Am J Epidemiol* 146:704–711, 1997.

Diseases Among Men 20 Years After Exposure to Severe Stress: Implications for Clinical Research and Medical Care
Boscarino JA (Catholic Health Initiatives-Southeast Region, Louisville, Ky)
Psychosom Med 59:605–614, 1997   5–39

Objective.—Exposure to severe environmental stress—including combat and natural disasters—is known to be associated with the onset of specific psychiatric disorders. There is some evidence that such severe stress may also be linked to the onset of chronic diseases, but outcome studies have been limited by bias and confounding. The long-term medical consequences of severe stress exposure should be detectable in combat-exposed Vietnam veterans with posttraumatic stress disorder (PTSD). A large sample of Vietnam veterans was studied to seek associations between PTSD and the onset of major disease after military service, with controls for selection bias and confounders.

Methods.—One thousand three hundred ninety-nine male Vietnam veterans were studied at a mean of 17 years after combat exposure. Three hundred thirty-two men had a lifetime diagnosis of PTSD. All these men participated in a national, random, in-person study of Vietnam veterans. Disease associations with current and lifetime PTSD were assessed. The analysis controlled for preservice, in-service, and postservice factors, including intelligence, race, region of birth, enlistment status, volunteer status, Army marital status, Army medical profile, hypochondriasis, age, smoking history, substance abuse, education, and income.

Results.—A lifetime PTSD diagnosis was more likely for veterans with lower intelligence test results, those with hypochondriasis, those with alcohol or drug dependence, and those with 10–18 pack-years of smoking. Lifetime PTSD status was significantly associated with several categories of disease, after controlling for other factors. These included circulatory disease, odds ratio (OR) 1.62; digestive disease, OR 1.4; musculoskeletal disease, OR 1.78; endocrine-nutritional-metabolic disease, OR 1.58; nervous system disease, OR 2.47; respiratory disease, OR 1.54; and nonsexually transmitted infectious diseases, OR 2.14.

Conclusion.—This study suggests a direct link between combat stress and a broad range of medical diseases. These associations are still present after adjustment for potential biases, confounders, and behavioral risk factors. Further study of the medical consequences of exposure to severe environmental stress are needed. Future explanations of disease should feature better integration of traditional biomedical models of disease pathogenesis with psychological models.

▶ In contrast to the conclusions of Abstract 5–39, this study concludes that stress does influence the development of subsequent physical symptoms, health, and medical utilization, perhaps through immunologic suppression. In addition, as we know, persistent memories are found years (in this case, about 17) after combat.

J.A. Talbott, M.D.

Reservation Card for the Year Book

Yes! I would like my own copy of *Year Book of Psychiatry and Applied Mental Health*® at the price of **$76.00** (**$84.00** outside the U.S.) plus sales tax, postage, and handling. Please begin my subscription with the current edition according to the terms described below.* I understand that I will have 30 days to examine each annual edition.

Name ____

Address ____

City _______________________________ State __________ ZIP ___________

Method of Payment

Check (in U.S. dollars, drawn on a U.S. bank, payable to *Year Book of Psychiatry and Applied Mental Health*®)

❑ VISA ❑ MasterCard ❑ Discover ❑ AmEx ❑ Bill me

Card number ________________________________ Exp. date: ___________

Signature ____

Prices are subject to change without notice.   PMC-362

An outstanding resource for your nursing colleagues!

Yes! Begin my one-year subscription to *Journal of the American Psychiatric Nurses Association* (6 issues).

Name ____

Institution ____________________________________

Address _______________________________________

City _______________________ State __________

ZIP/PC __________ Country ____________________

Specialty _____________________________________
(Students, please list Institution)

Subscription prices (through 9/30/99)

		USA	Canada*	Int'l
Individuals	❑	$50.00	$69.55	$65.00
Institutions	❑	89.00	111.28	104.00
Students (full-time)	❑	26.00	43.87	41.00

Method of payment

Enclose payment (check or credit card number) and we'll send an extra issue FREE!

❑ Check (in U.S. dollars, drawn on a U.S. bank, and payable to *Journal of the American Psychiatric Nurses Association*)

❑ VISA ❑ MasterCard ❑ Discover

❑ AmEx ❑ Bill me Exp. date__________

Card #____

Signature _____________________________________

*Includes Canadian GST

Individual/student subscriptions must be in the name of, billed to, and paid for by the individual.

Canada/Int'l prices include airmail postage.
Prices subject to change without notice.

J066991YA

---

*Your Year Book service guarantee:

When you subscribe to the *Year Book*, you will receive advance notice of future annual volumes about two months before publication. To receive the new edition, you need do nothing—we'll send you the new volume as soon as it is available. If you want to discontinue, the advance notice allows you time to notify us of your decision. If you are not completely satisfied, you have 30 days to return any *Year Book*.

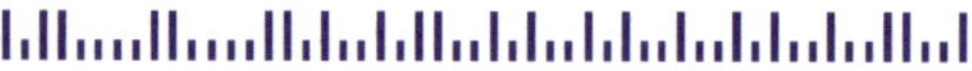

BUSINESS REPLY MAIL
FIRST-CLASS MAIL   PERMIT NO 135   ST LOUIS MO

POSTAGE WILL BE PAID BY ADDRESSEE

SUBSCRIPTION SERVICES
MOSBY, INC.
11830 WESTLINE INDUSTRIAL DRIVE
ST. LOUIS   MO 63146-9988

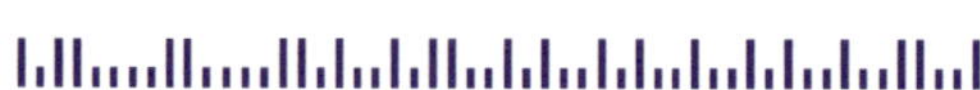

BUSINESS REPLY MAIL
FIRST-CLASS MAIL   PERMIT NO 135   ST LOUIS MO

POSTAGE WILL BE PAID BY ADDRESSEE

SUBSCRIPTION SERVICES
MOSBY, INC.
11830 WESTLINE INDUSTRIAL DRIVE
ST. LOUIS   MO 63146-9988

Want to speed up the process?

**To order a *Year Book* or *Advances*,
you also may call 1-800-426-4545**

**To subscribe to a journal today,
call toll-free in the U.S.:
1-800-453-4351
or fax 314-432-1158
Outside the U.S., call: 314-453-4351**

Visit us at: *www.mosby.com/periodicals*

Mosby, Inc.
Subscription Services
11830 Westline Industrial Drive
St. Louis, MO   63146 U.S.A.

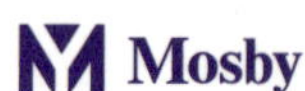 **Mosby**

Cumulative Impact of Sustained Economic Hardship on Physical, Cognitive, Psychological, and Social Functioning
Lynch JW, Kaplan GA, Shema SJ (Univ of Michigan, Ann Arbor; Public Health Inst, Berkeley, Calif)
N Engl J Med 337:1889–1895, 1997   5–40

Purpose.—Previous studies have demonstrated a link between low income and poor health. However, most of this research has assessed income at only 1 point in time, thus neglecting the long-term health effects of low income or transitions in income. Income information collected across 4 decades was used to examine the cumulative effects of sustained low-income status.

Methods.—In 1965, 1974, and 1983, as part of a prospective, population-based study of predictors of health and functioning, information was collected from a representative sample of adults in Alameda County, California. In 1994, 2,730 subjects who had participated in 1974 were studied again. The data were analyzed to determine the cumulative effects of economic hardship, defined as a household income of less than 200% of the federal poverty level.

Results.—The analysis included data on 1,081 to 1,124 respondents. The subjects' median age in 1994 was 65 years. The degree of economic hardship—ranging from 0 to 3 times less than 200% of the poverty level—was significantly associated with measures of functioning, after adjustment for age and sex. Social isolation was the only unaffected functional measure. Respondents meeting the criterion for economic hardship in 1965, 1974, and 1983 had significantly more difficulty with independent activities of daily living such as cooking, shopping, and managing money (odds ratio [OR], 3.38); activities of daily living such as walking, eating, and toileting (OR, 3.79); and clinical depression (OR, 3.24). For subjects in excellent or good health in 1965, economic hardship in that year was significantly associated with symptoms of depression and cognitive difficulties. The data suggested that illness resulted from economic hardship, rather than the other way around.

Conclusion.—Sustained exposure to economic hardship is strongly and consistently associated with reduced physical, psychological, and cognitive function. In this study, adjustment for risk factors and prevalent diseases did not significantly change the relationships, although these covariates were related to many of the functional outcomes. The health effects of low income over time could have important implications for public health, health care, and economic policy, especially in this era of welfare reform and transition to managed care.

▶ I have included this study because, although it does not mention stress or posttraumatic stress disorder, it not only confirms prior studies showing a link between poverty and poor mental and physical health, it demonstrates several other points. For instance, it shows the devastating effects of *sustained* economic hardship and the increased "odds" of being depressed or displaying "cognitive difficulties." The authors' ability to measure subjects at 3 points in time (over almost 20 years) lends strength to their conclusions that poverty contributes to poor health, rather than vice versa, and that the longer poverty goes on, the worse the subject's health.

J.A. Talbott, M.D.

Declining Prevalence of Psychiatric Disorder in Older Former Prisoners of War

Tennant C, Fairley MJ, Dent OF, et al (Univ of Sydney, Australia; Concord Hosp, Sydney, Australia; Australian Natl Univ, Canberra)
J Nerv Ment Dis 185:686–689, 1997   5–41

Background.—Previous studies have shown high rates of anxiety disorders, depressive illness, and other health problems among former prisoners of war (POWs). However, all of these studies have been retrospective; none have monitored changes in mental disorder status over time in a randomly selected group of POWs. Such a study was performed in World War II veterans who had been POWs.

Methods.—In 1982–1983, the investigators studied a random sample of Australian World War II veterans who had been captured and held by the Japanese at the fall of Singapore in 1942. A group of non-POW veterans was studied simultaneously. Both groups were interviewed by a psychiatrist, including evaluation by self-rated anxiety and depression scales. The veterans were reexamined 9 years later, when almost all were retired, to see whether their high prevalence of anxiety and depressive disorder had persisted into old age.

Results.—Two hundred eight veterans were interviewed in 1991–1992; their mean age at that time was 73 years. The prevalence of anxiety disorders had decreased from 33% in the 1980s to 17% in the 1990s. An even greater reduction was seen in the prevalence of depressive disorders: from 27%–9%. The former POWs had greater declines in the prevalence of both disorders than did non-POWs.

Conclusion.—Previous studies have shown elevated rates of anxiety and depression among World War II POWs, even 40 years after their incarceration. Further follow-up suggests that reductions in anxiety and depression occur when the former POWs reach old age. The impact of POWs' traumatic wartime experiences may finally begin to fade after they reach their 70s.

▶ It is puzzling that ex-POWs had decreased anxiety and depression compared with non-POWs of World War II. The authors wonder whether this is because POWs' symptoms were more likely to be a consequence of "external stress." I wonder whether this may be the result of the group cohesion and preparation in situ for concentration camp hardships.

J.A. Talbott, M.D.

Posttraumatic Stress Disorder in U.S. Army Vietnam Veterans Who Served in the Persian Gulf War

McCarroll JE, Fagan JG, Hermsen JM, et al (Uniformed Services Univ of the Health Sciences, Bethesda, Md; Office of Civilian Health and Med Programs of the Uniformed Services, Aurora, Colo; Univ of Maryland, College Park)
J Nerv Ment Dis 185:682–685, 1997   5–42

Introduction.—Posttraumatic stress disorder (PTSD) may be classified as acute, chronic, or delayed onset. Several types of changes later in life—possibly including repeated exposure to combat—may reactivate latent PTSD. Some reports have suggested that some Vietnam veterans who later served in the Gulf War experienced problems with PTSD and other psychiatric and medical conditions. Cases of PTSD in Gulf War veterans were reviewed, comparing those with and without previous service in Vietnam.

Methods.—The review included 136 cases of PTSD resulting from participation in Operation Desert Storm that were adjudicated by the United States Army Physical Disability Board. Thirty-four of the veterans (mean age, 44) had also served in Vietnam. They were compared with the 102 veterans who had not served in Vietnam (mean age, 30). Only men were included because there were no women for comparison in the Vietnam group.

Results.—Only about half of veterans in the Vietnam group were actually deployed to the Persian Gulf; the rest had recurrence or exacerbation of existing PTSD in anticipation of deployment. The odds ratios for PTSD among veterans with previous service in Vietnam ranged from 5 to 24.

Conclusion.—Veterans with a history of previous war stress are at increased risk of PTSD compared with persons without such experience. Recurrent or exacerbated PTSD may occur even in anticipation of future combat service. If further research confirms these findings, high priority could be placed on identification of PTSD in combat-exposed troops to provide intervention to improve the chances that they could function in future conflicts.

▶ This is the first of several articles that I included because of their relevance to risk factors for the development of PTSD. Here, the point is made that preexisting war experience predisposed veterans redeployed to the Persian Gulf War to PTSD symptoms. Anticipatory stress is an understudied phenomenon and the high rate of PTSD raised by the *threat* of return to combat understandably somewhat cripples an armed force in wartime.

J.A. Talbott, M.D.

Risk Factors for Posttraumatic Stress Symptomatology in Police Officers: A Prospective Analysis

Carlier IVE, Lamberts RD, Gersons BPR (Univ of Amsterdam)
J Nerv Ment Dis 185:498–506, 1997   5–43

Background.—A person's risk of the development of posttraumatic stress disorder (PTSD) is affected by the trauma itself, by preexisting vulnerability factors, or by a combination of the 2. Most previous studies of PTSD risk factors have focused on victims of disasters, Vietnam veterans, or crime victims. Police officers may form a unique group at risk of PTSD in that they commonly face both violent and depressing incidents. Internal and external risk factors for posttraumatic stress symptoms in police officers were studied.

Methods.—The study included 262 Dutch police officers—218 men and 44 women with mean ages of 33 and 28 years, respectively. All officers had been exposed to traumatic incidents; 69 had posttraumatic stress symptoms and 193 did not. The officers were interviewed 2 weeks after the traumatic incident and again at 3 and 12 months. Potential risk factors were selected by univariate analysis, and predictors of posttraumatic stress symptoms were identified by multiple logistic regression.

Results.—The interviews revealed PTSD in 7% of the sample overall and posttraumatic stress symptoms, or subthreshold PTSD, in 34%. The only significant predictor of posttraumatic stress symptoms at both 3 and 12 months was trauma severity. Additional predictors of symptoms at 3 months included introversion, difficulty in expressing feelings, emotional exhaustion at the time of trauma, insufficient time permitted by employers to deal with the trauma, dissatisfaction with organizational support, and an insecure job future. Additional predictors of trauma at 12 months were lack of hobbies, acute hyperarousal, subsequent trauma exposure, job dissatisfaction, brooding over work, and lack of social interaction support in private life.

Conclusion.—A 7% rate of PTSD and a 37% rate of posttraumatic stress symptoms were found among traumatized police officers. Risk factors for posttraumatic stress symptoms vary with time after the event, although the severity of the trauma was significant at all times studied. Some of the risk factors identified were organizational in nature, which could have important implications for occupational health interventions.

▶ The conclusions of this study, although centered on "risk factors," are of considerable importance in designing programs of intervention. Although some factors (e.g., introversion, difficulty in expression of feelings) are clearly brought by the individual to the stressful situation and may or may not be enduring, others (e.g., uncertainty about continued employment, brooding over work, insufficient time allowed for coming to terms with the trauma) provide guidelines for intervention.

J.A. Talbott, M.D.

Social Support and Psychopathology in the War Zone

Fontana A, Rosenheck R, Horvath T (Northeast Program Evaluation Ctr, West Haven, Conn)
J Nerv Ment Dis 185:675–681, 1997   5–44

Introduction.—Social support has long been thought to protect against the adverse effects of exposure to stress, both directly and conditionally. This so-called buffering hypothesis of support holds that social support plays an important role when exposure to stress is high and the ability to cope with it is reduced. In war, unit cohesion may aid in short-term coping with combat but may actually be detrimental in dealing with the aftermath of combat. A growing body of evidence suggests that experiences on homecoming are a critical factor in the development of chronic posttraumatic stress disorder (PTSD). The protective effects of unit cohesion and homecoming support were studied in Vietnam veterans.

Methods.—The study used data on 1,198 male Vietnam theater veterans from the National Vietnam Veterans Readjustment Study. The men's average age was 42 years; 49% were white, 27% were black, and 23% were Hispanic, reflecting minority oversampling. Diagnostic interviews for axis I affective and anxiety disorders and PTSD were performed. Social support was assessed in terms of unit cohesiveness and support from family and friends at homecoming. The data analysis paid particular attention to the possibility that unit cohesion had long-term negative effects.

Results.—Unit cohesion had no significant direct effect on PTSD or any other form of psychopathology. Contrary to the buffering hypothesis of support, the combination of high unit cohesion and high war zone stress was associated with the highest levels of PTSD and psychopathology. Homecoming support had direct negative effects on both PTSD and other forms of psychopathology. In support of the buffering hypothesis, the protective effects of homecoming support were greater for subjects with high exposure to war zone stress.

Conclusions.—In contrast to previous thinking, this study finds that unit cohesion in a combat zone may have detrimental effects in terms of PTSD and other psychiatric disorders, especially in combination with high exposure to combat stress. The findings support the suggestion that high unit cohesion may heighten the sense of loss and guilt when others in the unit are wounded or killed. Homecoming support appears to have a critical protective effect against PTSD, particularly for veterans with high levels of exposure.

▶ When I was in medical officers' training pre-Vietnam, the conventional wisdom was that group integration was, if anything, a protective element regarding PTSD. This study certainly stands that idea on its head. On the other hand, in partial explanation of this finding, I also remember that some of the "old hands" in Vietnam told me experienced combat soldiers warned new recruits *not* to get attached to others so they would not feel bad if and when they died. However, the belief that positive homecoming helps, and vice versa, does hold up.

J.A. Talbott, M.D.

Sex Differences in Posttraumatic Stress Disorder
Breslau N, Davis GC, Andreski P, et al (Henry Ford Health Sciences Ctr, Detroit; Case Western Reserve Univ, Cleveland, Ohio; Univ of Michigan, Ann Arbor)
Arch Gen Psychiatry 54:1044–1048, 1997   5–45

Objective.—In the general population, posttraumatic stress disorder (PTSD) appears to be more frequent among women than men. This epidemiologic finding may suggest that women are more vulnerable to the effects of traumatic experience, but little additional research has been done. Risk factors for PTSD have been identified and might interact with gender to increase susceptibility to PTSD. This study sought to determine whether previously identified risk factors could explain sex difference in PTSD and whether the sex difference is influenced by age at exposure to PTSD.

Methods.—A random sample of 1,007 young adults underwent a diagnostic interview to assess the presence of DSM-III-R disorders. Sex-related changes in the hazards ratio for PTSD were analyzed in a Cox proportional hazards model, including potential risk factors. The ability of these risk factors—including pre-existing psychiatric disorders, family history of anxiety disorders, and early separation from parents—to explain the greater susceptibility of women to traumatic exposures was analyzed.

Results.—The sexes were comparable in lifetime exposure to traumatic events and number of traumatic events. However, women with traumatic exposures had a higher prevalence of PTSD than did men: hazards ratio 2.3, with a 95% confidence interval of 1.5 to 3.6. This sex difference was affected by pre-existing anxiety or major depressive disorders, though not by family history of anxiety disorder or early separation from parents. The sex difference was amplified for subjects with traumatic exposures in childhood, rather than later on.

Conclusions.—With exposure to a traumatic event, females are more likely to develop PTSD than males. This sex-related difference may be more pronounced for females exposed to trauma during childhood, as opposed to after age 15 years. The observed sex difference in prevalence of PTSD may involve characteristics of both the individuals and the traumatic exposures. In both sexes, preexisting anxiety or major depressive disorders, family history of anxiety disorders, and early separation from parents are significant risk factors for PTSD.

▶ The positive clinical lesson here is that in both sexes prior anxiety and major depressive disorders, family history of anxiety disorders, and early separation were related to the later development of PTSD. The puzzling finding is why women experiencing the same rate of exposure to traumatic events have such a higher rate of PTSD. Can the explanation be that men, being more competitive, aggressive, war-like, and so on, anticipate the possibility of trauma (see Abstract 5–43) more than women, or is this a sexist stereotype?

J.A. Talbott, M.D.

Warriors as Peacekeepers: Features of the Somalia Experience and PTSD

Litz BT, King LA, King DW, et al (Boston Dept of Veterans Affairs Med Ctr; Boston Univ; Oklahoma State Univ; et al)
J Consult Clin Psychol 65:1001–1010, 1997   5–46

Purpose.—The United States military has increasingly taken on the role of international peacekeeper. This places a new and diverse set of responsibilities on combat-trained personnel: though they are generally expected to show restraint and neutrality, they must be prepared to respond to life-threatening situations. Few studies have examined the psychologic consequences of such peacekeeping missions. The relationships between the various factors involved in peacekeeping missions and the symptoms of posttraumatic stress disorder (PTSD) were examined.

Methods.—The study included 3,310 active-duty United States military personnel assigned to the Somalia peacekeeping mission between 1992

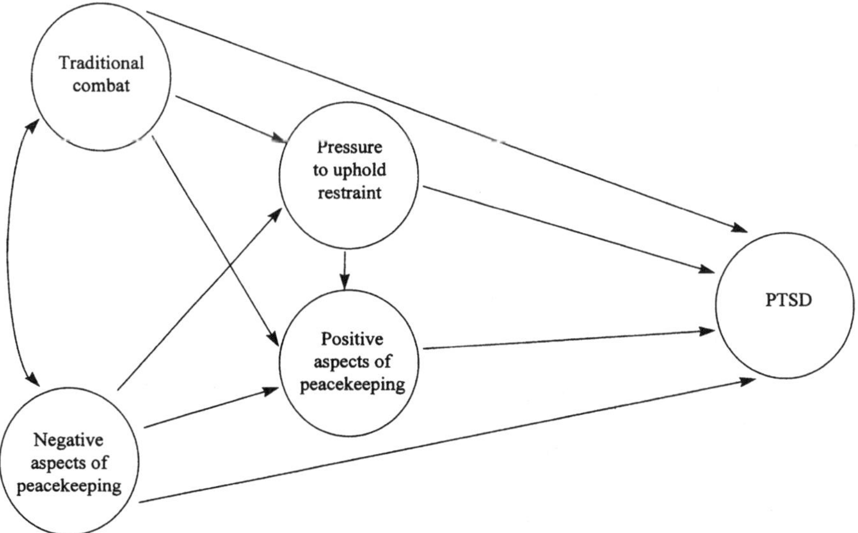

FIGURE 1.—Initial, most saturated model of relationships among exposure and appraisal variables and posttraumatic stress disorder (PTSD). (Reprinted with permission from Litz BA, King LA, King DW, et al: Warriors as peacekeepers: Features of the Somalia experience and PTSD. *J Consult Clin Psychol* 65:1001–1010, copyright 1997 by the American Psychological Association.)

and 1994. Seven percent of the subjects were female. Four variables associated with peacekeeping missions were identified: traditional combat events, negative aspects of peacekeeping, pressure to uphold restraint, and positive aspects of peacekeeping (Fig 1). The relationships of these variables to symptoms of PTSD were then examined. Racial differences were assessed by applying structural equation modeling procedures to data from subsamples of African Americans and non–African Americans.

Findings.—For both racial groups, the severity of PTSD symptoms was significantly influenced by both exposure to traditional combat and the negative aspects of peacekeeping. Also, each of these variables was directly related to pressure to uphold restraint and to the positive aspects of peacekeeping. More complex patterns of association were noted in terms of pressure to uphold restraint, positive aspects of peacekeeping, and PTSD. These complex relationships were significantly different between racial groups.

Conclusions.—The influence of military peacekeeping missions on PTSD are studied. The findings suggest that the need to show restraint in the face of potentially life-threatening circumstances may be particularly difficult for combat-trained personnel. However, frustration with the pressure to uphold restraint is not necessarily implicated in the development of PTSD. The racial differences observed emphasize the need for attention to cultural influences on the individual's experience of and adjustment to peacekeeping missions.

▶ If, as many posit, our armed forces will be more involved in small conflicts and peacekeeping in the future than in "wars," we need to know the consequences. It is ironic that restraining the use of force is "good" in peacetime but counter to what we instill in those prepared for combat (so much of which is based on the classic study by S.L.A. Marshall during World War II showing that the more an infantryman fires at the enemy, the better his "hit rate)."

J.A. Talbott, M.D.

Reference

1. Marshall SLA: *Men Against Fire: The Problem of Battle Command in Future Wars.* Gloucester, Mass, 1975.

Psychological Distress After Cancer Cure: A Survey of 459 Hodgkin's Disease Survivors

Loge JH, Abrahamsen AF, Ekeberg Ø, et al (Univ of Oslo, Norway; Norwegian Radium Hosp, Oslo, Norway; Trondheim Univ, Norway)
Br J Cancer 76:791–796, 1997   5–47

Background.—Most survivors of Hodgkin's disease (HD) are young adults. These patients may face significant physical, social, and psychological problems as a result of their disease and its treatment. Psychological distress is very common among patients with HD but is usually of short duration. Few studies have examined potential predictors of psychological distress among HD survivors. A large, nationwide sample of HD survivors was studied to examine their levels of psychological distress and identify predictors of anxiety and depression after cure.

Methods.—A mail questionnaire, including the Hospital Anxiety and Depression Scale (HADS) was sent to 557 Norwegian HD survivors. There were 459 responders—255 men and 204 women, mean age 44—for a compliance rate of 82%. The responses were used to assess anxiety and depression "caseness" after cancer cure. Information on the patients' disease and treatment was gathered from hospital records. Risk factors were identified by multiple logistic regression analysis.

Results.—Caseness scores were recorded for 27% of the sample overall: 14.5% for anxiety, 4% for depression, and 8.5% for anxiety and depression. Significant predictors of anxiety caseness were low education, odds ratio (OR) 2.07; an observation period of 7 years or longer, OR 3.07; combined radiation therapy and chemotherapy, OR 2.77; having psychiatric symptoms before HD, OR 2.55; and developing psychiatric symptoms during treatment for HD, OR 3.51. Predictors of depression caseness were age, OR 1.03, and having psychiatric symptoms before HD, OR 5.1. The prevalence of anxiety among HD survivors was higher than in the general population, particularly for 7- to 10-year survivors. Patients who received the most intensive treatment were at elevated risk of anxiety caseness, and those with distress during treatment tended to have difficulties with long-term adjustment.

Conclusions.—Anxiety appears to be a relatively common problem for survivors of HD. The risk of anxiety is elevated for patients receiving combined-modality treatment and for those with longer postcure observation periods. Attention to these predictors during treatment and follow-up may improve the long-term outcomes of HD survivors.

► Some persons object to studies examining psychological distress or posttraumatic stress disorder (PTSD) in non-disastrous circumstances, partially at the risk of trivializing them, but as with combat's relationship to PTSD, where more exposure leads to more and more severe PTSD, more intensive treatment leads to more long-term anxiety. General hospital and cancer unit psychiatrists can certainly benefit from such knowledge.

J.A. Talbott, M.D.

Treatment of Posttraumatic Stress Disorder by Exposure and/or Cognitive Restructuring: A Controlled Study
Marks I, Lovell K, Noshirvani H, et al (Inst of Psychiatry and Bethlem-Maudsley Hosp, London)
Arch Gen Psychiatry 55:317–325, 1998   5–48

Introduction.—Posttraumatic stress disorder (PTSD) investigations have not yet determined whether cognitive restructuring alone helps PTSD as much as prolonged exposure therapy alone or whether the 2 combined are better than each alone. These questions were addressed in a comparison of these 2 treatment approaches with a relaxation approach that contained neither and was largely a placebo in panic-agoraphobia and obsessive-compulsive disorder.

Methods.—Eighty-seven outpatients with PTSD of at least 6 months' duration were randomized to ten 90-minute individual sessions of either (1) prolonged exposure, (2) cognitive restructuring, (3) combined prolonged exposure therapy plus cognitive restructuring, or (4) a control group using a relaxation approach. Sessions were audiotaped. Blinded assessors (a psychiatrist or psychologist) screened and rated patients at baseline during the 11-week treatment period and throughout 2 years of follow-up.

Results.—Seventy-two (82.8%) of 87 patients completed their program. There were no between-group differences in the pattern of results, regardless of rater, statistical method, measure, occasion, or therapist. There were marked improvements in patients who participated in prolonged exposure and cognitive restructuring, both singly and combined. Improvements continued up to a 6-month follow-up and were significantly greater than the moderate improvement achieved from the relaxation approach.

Conclusion.—Both prolonged exposure and cognitive restructuring produced marked broad-spectrum improvement on their own in patients with chronic PTSD, compared with relaxation. There was no added benefit from the combination of prolonged exposure and cognitive restructuring.

▶ I've included this article because it demonstrates how complex and yet, still unresolved, are the questions about treating PTSD. In many ways, this article is concerned more with the difference between cognitive therapy and exposure than what treatment (including medication) works best for persons suffering from PTSD. I realize that such a study would be impossibly complex and this lack of clarity is not much different from the situation with other disorders, but to arrive at decisions about sequenced or simultaneous decisions, we need such comparative treatment data.

J.A. Talbott, M.D.

Violence, Homicide, and Suicide

Psychological Preparedness for Trauma as a Protective Factor in Survivors of Torture
Başoğlu M, Mineka S, Paker M, et al (Inst of Psychiatry, London; Northwestern Univ, Evanston, Ill; Psychiatric Hosp, Istanbul, Turkey)
Psychol Med 27:1421–1433, 1997   5–49

Introduction.—Mechanisms of traumatization and factors related to post trauma psychological functioning have been the focus of research in survivors of trauma. Predictors of posttrauma psychological status have been related to severity of trauma, age at trauma, education, psychiatric illness, intelligence, ability to maintain calmness and control during traumatic events, posttrauma life events, and social support. Little has been studied, however, about the psychological preparedness of being tortured and posttraumatic stress. Knowledge of torture methods, prior expectations of torture, and exposure to similar stressors during political activity leading to a sense of mastery and training in stoicism techniques may be part of psychological preparedness. Generally, predictable stressors have less of an impact than unpredictable stressors. The effects of torture on nonactivist torture survivors and activist torture survivors were compared.

Methods.—There were 34 torture survivors with no history of political activity, commitment to a political cause or group, or expectations of arrest and torture who were compared with 55 tortured political activists. The torture survivors were given structured interviews, and their levels of anxiety, depression, and posttraumatic stress were measured.

Results.—Relatively less severe torture was inflicted on nonactivists than on political activists, but the nonactivists had higher levels of psychopathology. Greater perceived distress during torture and more severe psychological problems were associated with less psychological preparedness. Between the 2 groups, there was a 4% variance in general psychopathology and 9% in posttraumatic stress disorder symptoms (Table 3).

Conclusions.—The uncontrollability and unpredictability of stressors in the effects of traumatization are affected by prior immunization to traumatic stress. The behavioral and cognitive components of psychological preparedness in traumatization should be further researched to provide more insights into treating survivors of torture.

▶ This will probably be received as terribly "politically incorrect," because all of us have trouble contemplating the idea of preparing individuals to cope with torture rather than eliminating it. But it must be said; immunization to a host of drastic circumstances, torture being about the worst, can be helpful in ameliorating its sequelae. The authors' use of political activitists as an example of more prepared victims may be true, but I would think some groups, e.g., combat pilots, would be even better. The lack of predictability of education runs counter to other studies and does not settle that issue yet.

J.A. Talbott, M.D.

TABLE 3.—Comparison of Psychological Status Between Political Activists and Non-activists

	Political Activists (N = 55)		Non-activists (N = 34)		
	Mean	S.D.	Mean	S.D.	t^*
Beck Depression	9·5	(7·4)	19	(13)	3·7†
Hamilton Depression	5·0	(4·5)	9·0	(8·0)	2·7‡
Hamilton Anxiety	7·5	(6·5)	13	(11)	2·7‡
State Anxiety	40	(11)	48	(9·0)	3·8†
PTSD-RS	70	(18)	86	(21)	3·6†
MMPI-PTSD scale	14	(8)	20	(9·5)	2·9‡
General Health Questionnaire	6·8	(7·9)	15·5	(14·5)	3·2‡
GHQ-Somatic symptoms	1·3	(1·8)	3·2	(3·4)	2·9‡
GHQ-Anxiety	1·6	(2)	3·8	(4·2)	2·8‡
GHQ-Social functioning	1·5	(2)	2·6	(2·9)	1·9§
GHQ-Depression	0·8	(0·3)	2·8	(3·4)	3·2‡
Number of PTSD symptoms	5·9	(4·4)	9·1	(4·7)	3·2‡
	N	%	N	%	χ^2
SCID Diagnoses					
Current major depression	2	4	8	24	6·5‡
Past major depression	16	29	6	18	0·9
Current PTSD	10	18	14	58	4·5‖
Lifetime PTSD	18	32	18	53	2·8§
PTSD symptoms‖					
Intrusive recollections	22	40	27	79	12†
Distress when reminded of trauma	25	46	29	85	12†
Flashbacks	20	36	16	47	0·60
Nightmares	26	47	16	47	0·00
Avoidance of trauma thoughts	12	22	20	59	11‡
Avoidance of reminders of trauma	18	33	19	56	3·7‖
Inability to recall trauma aspects	20	36	9	27	0·50
Diminished interest in activities	12	22	15	44	3·9‖
Feelings of detachment	16	29	12	35	0·14
Restricted affect	12	22	13	38	2·1
Sense of foreshortened future	16	29	15	44	1·5
Sleep disturbance	20	36	20	59	3·4
Irritability/outbursts of anger	19	35	19	56	3·1
Memory/concentration impairment	34	62	18	53	0·40
Hypervigilance	13	24	23	68	15¶
Startle reactions	21	38	19	56	0·0
Physiological reactivity	18	33	18	53	2·8

*Symptoms present at some stage following trauma.
†$P < 0.001$.
‡$P < 0.01$.
§$P < 0.1$.
‖$P < 0.05$.
¶$P < 0.0001$.
Abbreviations: PTSD-RS, Posttraumatic Stress Disorder–Rating Scale; *MMPI*, Minnesota Multiphasic Personality Inventory; *GHQ*, General Health Questionnaire; *SCID*, Structured Clinical Interview Diagnosis.
(Courtesy of Başoğlu M, Mineka S, Paker M, et al: Psychological preparedness for trauma as a protective factor in survivors of torture. *Psychol Med* 27:1421–1433, 1997. Reprinted with the permission of Cambridge University Press.)

A 2-year Longitudinal Analysis of the Relationships Between Violent Assault and Substance Use in Women
Kilpatrick DG, Acierno R, Resnick HS, et al (Med Univ of South Carolina, Charleston)
J Consult Clin Psychol 65:834–847, 1997   5–50

Introduction.—In the United States, violent assault is an ongoing problem for millions of women, with about 10.3% physically assaulted and 12.7% raped each year. Whether women's substance use–abuse leads to violent assault, whether violent assault increases risk of substance use–abuse, and whether the substance use–abuse violent assault relationship is reciprocal were determined. Also determined was whether there are different patterns with the use of alcohol, a legal substance vs. use of marijuana and hard drugs, which are illicit substances.

Methods.—There were 3,006 women with a mean age of 35.9 who were followed up for 2 years in a 3-wave longitudinal study. At each wave of the study, dependent measures were obtained. Questions concerned lifetime and new assault status, drug use, and alcohol abuse.

Results.—Women in wave 1 who reported substance use were almost twice as likely to experience an assault during the next 2 years as women without drug use. Women who used drugs and who had been previously assaulted had the greatest risk of new victimization. An assault on women who did not use drugs was associated with a high rate of progression to substance use. A vicious cycle became apparent of substance use increasing risk of future assault and assault increasing risk of subsequent substance use with illicit drugs.

Conclusions.—Reduction of drug use behaviors may reduce risk of subsequent victimization. Active substance users have a need for crime prevention and risk reduction efforts. This study demonstrated an increased risk but did not verify causation. Younger women had a greater risk of abusing alcohol and using drugs, and whites had a greater risk of using drugs.

▶ The interactive link between violence and substance abuse is certainly understandable. The authors' conclusion that no matter where it starts, the cycle of violence and substance abuse keeps repeating is rather depressing. But their recommendation that intervention needs to address not only short-term symptoms but substance abuse, prior victimization, and increasing safety is valuable.

J.A. Talbott, M.D.

The Impact of an Elementary School–based Violence Prevention Program on Visits to the School Nurse
Krug EG, Dahlberg LL, Brener ND, et al (Ctrs for Disease Control and Prevention, Atlanta, Ga)
Am J Prev Med 13:459–463, 1997   5–51

Introduction.—Violence prevention programs have been implemented across the country in schools and include conflict resolution lessons in the classroom and multifaceted community-based programs for high-risk youth. In 1994, PeaceBuilders began in elementary schools in Tucson, Arizona. The program emphasizes prosocial behavior, and activities are designed to improve daily interactions among students, teachers, administrators, parents, and support staff. Children learn to praise individuals, avoid put-downs, seek wise individuals as friends and advisors, right wrongs, and notice and correct hurts. There was anecdotal evidence that children in PeaceBuilders schools visited the nurse less often than children in other schools.

Methods.—The weekly number of nurse visits for injuries and fights and all other reasons were compared in 4 PeaceBuilders schools and in 3 control schools. Nurses' logs were examined during the assessments.

Results.—In the intervention schools, the rate of visits to the nurse per 1,000 student days decreased 12.6%, while in the comparison schools, the rate of visits remained unchanged. For injury-related visits, the same trend was noted. There was little change in fighting-related injuries in the intervention schools, but the control schools had a 56% increase. In intervention schools, injuries and visits to nurses decreased in comparison with control schools.

Conclusions.—During the 2-year period, injuries and visits to the school nurse decreased in the intervention schools. A useful tool to evaluate some types of elementary school–based violence prevention programs may be monitoring visits to the school nurse. Other methods of evaluation are student self-reports, teacher reports, playground observations, and school and law enforcement records.

▶ Prevention of violence is an intriguing issue. Obviously, given the various kinds of violence, organized and not, that seem to dominate our national and international news, we'd all like to know how to stop it. This is a small but helpful step in the right direction; clearly, preteen intervention could have a wonderful payoff. More studies need to be conducted and more types of interventions need to be tried, but this is a heartening development.

J.A. Talbott, M.D.

Suicide After Natural Disasters

Krug EG, Kresnow M-J, Peddicord JP, et al (Natl Ctr for Injury Prevention and Control, Atlanta, Ga)
N Engl J Med 338:373–378, 1998   5–52

Introduction.—Every year millions of people around the world are affected by natural and man-made disasters. Injury is experienced by about 1.5 million households in the United States as a result of floods, tornadoes, hurricanes, and earthquakes. For up to 5 years after a disaster, increased respiratory, gastrointestinal, and cardiovascular symptoms have been reported. Also reported have been posttraumatic stress disorder, insomnia, depression, substance abuse, and domestic violence. The psychological sequelae can persist for up to 5 years after a natural disaster from problems such as the death or injury of family members; loss of property, financial assets, or employment; and disruption of the social fabric of community life. There may be a relationship between suicide rates and disasters. In sites where single natural disasters occurred, suicide rates were examined.

Methods.—There were 377 counties selected; each had been affected during a 4-year period by a single natural disaster taken from a list of all the events declared by the United States government to be federal disasters. For the 36 months before and the 48 months after the disaster, data on suicides were collected and aligned around the month of the disaster. According to the type of disaster, pooled rates were calculated. In the affected counties and in the entire United States, comparisons were made between the suicide rates before and those after disasters.

Results.—In the 4 years after floods, suicide rates increased by 13.8%, from 12.1–13.8 per 100,000 persons. There was an increase of 31% in the 2 years after hurricanes, from 12–15.7 per 100,000. There was a 62.9% increase in the first year after earthquakes, from 19.2–31.3 per 100,000. There was no statistical significance in the 4-year increase of 19.7% after earthquakes. Rates computed in a similar manner for the entire United States were stable. Both sexes and all age groups accounted for the increases in suicide rates. After tornadoes or severe storms, the suicide rates did not change significantly.

Conclusion.—After severe earthquakes, floods, and hurricanes, suicide rates increase, and the need for mental health support after severe disasters is confirmed. Strategies of prevention can include providing social support and facilitating aid to victims.

▶ We are well aware of the increased psychiatric morbidity after natural disasters—from the Coconut Grove fire in the 1940s to the Buffalo Creek disaster of the 1960s—but most of the concern has focused on posttraumatic stress disorders, depression, and anxiety. This finding of increased suicides is impressive and disturbing. Many communities have natural disaster teams but not all do, and such a concrete negative consequence of disasters should galvanize us to action.

J.A. Talbott, M.D.

Violence During Pregnancy: Measurement Issues
Ballard TJ, Saltzman LE, Gazmararian JA, et al (Ctrs for Disease Control and Prevention, Atlanta, Ga)
Am J Public Health 88:274–276, 1998   5–53

Introduction.—It has been estimated that the prevalence of females experiencing violence during pregnancy is 0.9%–20.1%, compared with its prevalence at any time of 9.7%–29.7%. It is not known if pregnant females are at higher risk for violence initiated during pregnancy or whether the rate of violence increases, decreases or ceases during pregnancy in females who experience ongoing violence. Standardized quantitative methods are needed to determine the occurrence and timing of violence during pregnancy and the context in which pregnancy-related violence occurs. Described are several suggestions for enhancing investigations of violence during pregnancy.

Suggestions.—To determine whether violence occurring during pregnancy is specific to pregnancy or just part of an ongoing pattern, violence should be assessed before and during pregnancy. Four patterns of violence in relation to pregnancy have been identified: (1) no violence before pregnancy, but violence during pregnancy, (2) violence both before and during pregnancy, (3) violence before pregnancy but not during pregnancy, and (4) no violence either before or during pregnancy. Data regarding the perpetrator(s) of violence during prepregnancy and pregnancy can help to determine continuing patterns of violence. The Georgia Women's Health Survey and the Pregnancy Risk Assessment Monitoring System (PRAMS) are 2 surveys that incorporate these suggestions. These surveys may be used to address key points in the violence-during-pregnancy issue.

Conclusion.—Protecting females from violence that endangers them and their unborn children requires better measurements of the frequency of violence during pregnancy and during periods of nonpregnancy. The identification of risk factors and other psychosocial phenomena that correlate with violence during pregnancy will also assist in the formation of effective public health intervention programs.

▶ This article caught my eye because it was somewhat bizarre—later I decided to include it because I'm not sure we have communicated the high occurrence of violence to pregnant women to our primary care and obstetrical colleagues. Picking up on such episodes could help in primary (to the children) and secondary (for the children and mother) prevention efforts.

J.A. Talbott, M.D.

Miscellaneous

The Effects of Divorce and Separation on Mental Health in a National UK Birth Cohort

Richards M, Hardy R, Wadsworth M (Univ College London)
Psychol Med 27:1121–1128, 1997   5–54

Background.—The negative impact of divorce and separation on health and mental health is well known. Although there are reports of divorce and separation having a negative impact on health, it is unclear how early vulnerability, the material and social consequences of divorce, and the direct emotional effects of divorce affect individuals.

Methods.—The Medical Research Council's National Survey of Health and Development was used to measure anxiety, depression, and potential alcohol abuse in 2,085 individuals aged 43 years. Participants were married and had never divorced or separated, or had divorced or separated at least once. Analyses were done after controlling for sociodemographic features, early vulnerability factors, and current stressors.

Results.—Divorce and separation were associated with higher anxiety, depression, and abuse of alcohol, before and after adjusting for educational attainment, age at first marriage, parental divorce, childhood aggression and neuroticism, current financial hardship, lack of a confidante, and frequency of social contact with friends or family. The association between divorce and risk of alcohol abuse was nonsignificant after adjusting for risk of alcohol abuse. There were associations between divorce and psychopathology, even though 50% of individuals who had separated or divorced were remarried or reunited with their spouse during the study period. No association between these mental health measures and the time from an individual's first separation or divorce was seen.

Discussion.—Divorce and separation have a long-term negative impact on mental health. It is unclear to what extent anxiety, depression, and alcohol abuse are a cause or effect of marital breakdown and divorce.

▶ The study's premise seems so obvious and intuitive; why even write it up? Because this clears away confounding variables and shows that separation and divorce per se have powerful psychological consequences. Also, of note is the long-term impact of such events. Clearly we can no longer see separation and divorce merely as developmental, situational, or inevitable problems in everyday living.

J.A. Talbott, M.D.

Natural History of Male Psychological Health, XIV: Relationship of Mood Disorder Vulnerability to Physical Health
Vaillant GE (Harvard Univ, Boston)
Am J Psychiatry 155:184–191, 1998

5–55

Introduction.—Vulnerability to mood disorder may lie on a continuum with a negative pole on 1 end and a positive pole on the other end. Data were used from a 55-year longitudinal trial originally designed to assess positive mental health. This longitudinal trial determined that major disorder is as important an independent predictor of premature physical morbidity as cigarette or alcohol abuse. The antecedents and consequences of positive mental and physical health were assessed in adult men.

Methods.—Of 237 men followed up since attending college between 1939 and 1942, 64 (27%) undistressed men had never used mood-altering drugs or consulted a psychiatrist before the age of 50 years. The health of these men at age 70 was compared with the health of (1) 20 men classified as depressed at age 70; (2) 109 men classified as neither healthy nor depressed at age 70; and (3) 44 men classified as having alcohol dependence or abuse at age 70.

Results.—At age 70, the 64 males in the undistressed group had significantly better health than the 109 males in the intermediate group. Three (5%) of the 64 males were dead or disabled at age 70, compared with 30 (28%) of 109 males in the intermediate group and 9 (45%) of the 20 depressed males. There was a significant between-group difference in the mean age of the maternal grandfathers at death. Group differences in longevity were not able to be explained by either personality disorder; cigarette, dietary, or alcohol abuse; or longevity of the research subjects' other first-degree ancestors.

Conclusion.—Risks of affective disorder may lie along a continuum. The better physical health of undistressed males may be the result of their not seeking change in mood or state. Lifelong resistance to mood disorder may be reflected by a lifestyle that embraces self-care and many healthy, even stodgy habits.

▶ George Vaillant's treasure trove of data from the class at Harvard that included John F. Kennedy keeps turning up interesting findings as the years roll on. Here, Vaillant shows both the continuum of the risk of affective disorder as well as the specific risk factors. I like the idea that taking care of oneself and adopting healthy habits is important but not that one should, in his words, become "stodgy."

J.A. Talbott, M.D.

Loneliness
Schwartz RS, Olds J (Cambridge, Mass)
Harvard Rev Psychiatry 5:94–98, 1997   5–56

Introduction.—The problem of social isolation and loneliness is rising in this country. This is an important trend, especially because social connection is linked to physical health and mortality rates. Ways that psychotherapy can be more effective in helping patients solve problems of loneliness were suggested.

Defining the Problem.—The number of people living alone has increased dramatically in the last half of this century. In any given year, about 20% of the American population relocates. The number of Americans who socialize with their neighbors is declining annually. Participation in civic associations has declined dramatically. The pursuit of privacy and busy lifestyles has added to the problem of loneliness. A 1990 Gallup poll reported that 36% of respondents had recently felt lonely.

There is a definite relationship between social isolation and psychiatric illness. Survival of persons with metastatic disease has been shown to be prolonged by involvement in a support group. Immune function and health in human beings and primates have been shown to be compromised in several investigations.

Resolving the Problem.—Loneliness is not typically a focus of psychiatric treatment, but is an issue with many patients undergoing psychotherapy. The usual approach is psychotherapy, Prozac, or a self-help group. Loneliness is not just a problem of psychopathologic disorder. Healthy people are also lonely, particularly given the demographic and social changes in this country. The nature of the psychotherapist-patient relationship can even enhance social isolation. The therapist can assist patients in finding activities that they can join with others in a shared task on a regular basis.

Conclusion.—Loneliness can be problematic. It is a normal emotion and maybe even a necessary one. It helps preserve bonds within families and larger social groups that are crucial to human survival. In earlier times, the interdependency of community life kept lonely people involved. Today, the network of shared connections has frayed so much that people don't know how to alleviate loneliness when it takes hold. Psychotherapists can be helpful in assisting patients invent ways to link to others and to continue inventing when initial attempts fail.

▶ Loneliness, like crying, is one of those facts of life that are probably unstudied because of their ubiquitousness. The authors' belief that we can "be more effective" in handling loneliness now is interesting. Treatment of depression, increasing contacts with social networks, and increasing shared tasks are all helpful, but the authors' belief that we are experiencing an "explosion" may not be warranted.

J.A. Talbott, M.D.

Antidepressant Prescribing Practices of Outpatient Psychiatrists
Olfson M, Marcus SC, Pincus HA, et al (College of Physicians & Surgeons of Columbia Univ, NY; Western Psychiatric Inst and Clinic, Pittsburgh, Pa; American Psychiatric Association, Washington, DC; et al)
Arch Gen Psychiatry 55:310–316, 1998   5–57

Introduction.—Antidepressants are being used with increasing frequency. Reasons for the increase include development of new antidepressants, a surge of public interest in antidepressants, drug company marketing strategies aimed at the general public, and the clinical usefulness of antidepressants in an expanding range of psychiatric and general medical disorders. Changes in the demographic, patient payment, and clinical correlates of antidepressant prescription by psychiatrists in office-based practice were assessed.

Methods.—The National Center for Health Statistics annually samples a nationally representative group of visits to physicians in office-based practice via the National Ambulatory Medical Care Survey. Data from the 1985 and 1993–1994 surveys were examined for associations between the survey year and antidepressant prescription, adjusting for the presence of other variables.

Results.—The proportion of outpatient psychiatric visits in which antidepressants were prescribed increased from 23.1% in 1985 to 48.6% in 1993 to 1994. Patients with mental illness were 2.3 times more likely to receive an antidepressant in 1993 to 1994 than in 1985. Selective serotonin reuptake inhibitors were responsible for about half of the psychiatric visits with an antidepressant prescription. Increases in the rate of antidepressant prescriptions were especially noticeable for children and young adults, caucasians, and new patients in addition to patients with adjustment disorders, personality disorders, depression not otherwise specified or dysthymia, and some anxiety disorders.

Conclusion.—In less than a decade, the proportion of psychiatric outpatient visits for which a prescription for an antidepressant was written more than doubled. About half of all 1993 to 1994 visits included an antidepressant prescription. This increase was greatest for patients with less severe mental illness.

▶ I guess that the news here is good; we've become more diagnostically and psychopharmacologically sophisticated; we're using old and new medications for a broader array of illnesses, and patients are better informed and more willing to take antidepressants. I'm sure all of us, though, would like to see data on the improved quality of life, days worked, and other benefits to the economy of this increased prescribing.

J.A. Talbott, M.D.

Surviving Social Assistance: 12-month Prevalence of Depression in Sole-Support Parents Receiving Social Assistance
Byrne C, Browne G, Roberts J, et al (McMaster Univ, Hamilton, Ont, Canada; Caroline Med Group, Burlington, Ont, Canada)
Can Med Assoc J 158:881–888, 1998   5–58

Introduction.—It is well known that concurrent poverty and depression can occur among single parents receiving social assistance. Few data are available concerning the mental health status of this population and their use of health care services. The prevalence, correlates, and health care expenditures associated with depression among sole-support parents receiving social assistance were examined.

Methods.—Sole-support parents who applied for social assistance in 2 regions of southwestern Ontario, Canada were assessed using measures of adult adjustment and quality of life. Information was obtained from the parent regarding all children aged 4 to 12 years. The dollar value of lifetime use of social assistance was calculated. Health care service use was analyzed to determine direct and indirect health care expenditures.

Results.—The 12-month prevalence rate of depressive disorder among parents in this cohort was 45.5% (345 of 760). In this cohort also, 247 (32.5%) had major depressive disorder alone, 19 (2.5%) had dysthymia, and 79 (10.4%) had both major depressive disorder and dysthymia ("double depression"). Parents with major depressive disorder, particularly those with double depression, had significantly higher rates of coexisting mental illness, compared with those without depressive disorders. Parents with depressive disorder reported higher rates of developmental delay and behavior problems in their children, compared with parents without depression. Parents with depression and their children had higher expenditures for health care services than parents without depression.

Conclusion.—It is not known if depression or poverty comes first in single parents on social assistance. A little more than half of the sole-support parents have few children with problems and adequate-to-superior mental health, coping skill, and social adjustment abilities. Almost half of the remainder have coexisting problems. Initiatives targeting the latter group must address a mix of health and social circumstances.

▶ I've included this article because it's a reminder of how complicated and interconnected are social and psychiatric conditions. I'm not sure I agree with the authors that it doesn't matter what's chicken and what's egg because, I suspect, we might have more support for interventions if we knew where to put our first dollar.

J.A. Talbott, M.D.

A State-University Collaboration to Serve Persons With Developmental Disabilities and Mental Health Needs

Ryan R, Neligh GL, Aderman S (Univ of Colorado, Denver)
Community Ment Health J 33:445–454, 1997   5–59

Introduction.—There is a growing interest in state-university collaborations in mental health. A new state-university collaborative program in Colorado jointly sponsored by the Colorado Division for Developmental Disabilities, the Colorado Division of Mental Health, and the Programs for Public Psychiatry of the Department of Psychiatry of the University of Colorado Health Sciences Center has been developed.

The Program.—The emphasis of this collaborative program is the needs of adults and adolescents with developmental disabilities and mental health needs. Treatment of clients is based on accurate comprehensive diagnosis, using Diagnostic and Statistical Manual-IIIR/IV criteria. Psychiatrists in community mental health may not have received any education about appropriate psychiatric techniques for this patient population. Working with persons with dual diagnosis at the university level is ideal as there is little research regarding community populations; the university setting provides an educational and treatment opportunity. The director of this multi-agency collaboration divides time between direct clinical service and academic activities.

Program Activities.—The first task of the program was the development of a model of service that would be useful to individuals in community living. The interdisciplinary team approach resulted in improved functioning and decreased use of sedation. A traveling team was assembled that visits more than 26 sites around the state of Colorado. Team members are able to provide hands-on education regarding positive and updated techniques. Education in dual diagnosis is now part of required education in all years of psychiatric residency. Research activities are varied and are augmented by the availability of an entire state's database.

Conclusion.—The goals initially set for the program have been met. The state saves about $120,000 yearly in psychiatric consultation fees alone. The early experience with this state-university collaboration of working with people with dual diagnoses has been promising. The approach is a potential source of useful service to this otherwise underserved population.

▶ The track record for state-university collaborations in mental health is now considerable; it is helpful to hear of this translated to mental retardation/developmentally disabled. This programmatic description from one of the pioneering state-university collaborations (Colorado) is useful as a road map for those who want to address this complex task.

J.A. Talbott, M.D.

Abuse Histories of Psychiatric Inpatients: To Ask or Not to Ask?
Read J, Fraser A (Univ of Auckland, New Zealand)
Psychiatric Serv 49:355–359, 1998

5–60

Introduction.—There are significantly higher rates of childhood abuse among psychiatric inpatients than among the general population. Among female inpatients, the prevalence of childhood abuse is as high as 85%, and the rates for male inpatients are as high as 39%. Previous studies have shown that rates of abuse are reported to be higher when the patients are asked directly. Including a general question about abuse on an admission form may have an effect on disclosure rates. A review was conducted of a hospital that used such a form to determine whether staff will ask the questions if they are not trained, and whether a higher disclosure rate would occur among patients who were asked directly about abuse.

Methods.—After the introduction of a new admission form with a section inquiring about abuse, the medical records of 100 consecutive admissions were examined. Use of the new admission form was recommended to the staff, but its use was not mandatory.

Results.—Only 17 of the 53 patients for whom the new form was used had the abuse section of the new form completed. There was a prevalence rate of 32% for 1 or more of the 4 types of abuse in the review of the medical records of all 100 consecutive admissions. Of the 17 patients who were asked directly about abuse, 14 (82%) said they had experienced abuse. The probability of being asked about abuse was negatively related to male gender and being more disturbed or disturbing. If not asked directly, men may be particularly unlikely to disclose childhood abuse.

Conclusion.—In standardized admission procedures, an inquiry about abuse should be included. Inpatient staff should be provided with training in when and how to ask patients about abuse. When responses are affirmative, staff should be trained in how to follow up effectively.

▶ I placed this article here because I think its topic is a critical area for the field and not just a stress/trauma related issue. Given the enormous controversy over the very high rates of reported trauma in psychiatric patients vs. the scandalous examples of some therapists seemingly encouraging some patients to "falsely remember" child sexual abuse, we all need to have some better means of operating practically, soundly, and ethically. Certainly, routinely asking patients about abuse and using a specially trained staff makes a lot of sense.

J.A. Talbott, M.D.

6 Clinical Psychiatry

Introduction

In previous years, I have ordered the articles in the clinical section from the most common syndromes to the least common. From year to year, the literature both stays the same in this field and is radically different. This year is no exception. It also strikes me again this year that despite the multiple detractors of psychiatry and its knowledge base, this year's literature is striking in its breadth and quality. We in fact know a great deal about clinical psychiatry. One of our biggest concerns is making this knowledge available to the people who need it, and that certainly includes our primary care and general medicine colleagues. This chapter ends with a large section of articles on that topic again this year, along with articles about how we might help teach what we know to this sector of the medical community group.

The first article in the affective disorders section details an attempt to utilize a remarkably powerful large twin registry to define the diagnostic boundaries of major depression. The ability to use external objective data in this case to define our diagnostic criteria, is an example of an important goal in psychiatry. In a similar vein, the next articles concern utilization of another external criteria, functional neuroimaging, to define aspects of the affective disorders. The next article is a follow-up from last year on the interrelationship of depression and smoking, an issue of increasing importance as we try to deal with the nicotine epidemic in the United States. A set of articles carefully delineates the prognosis of the affective disorders and also modern data about suicide mortality. As we already knew, these are severe syndromes associated with terrible morbidity. The affective disorders section ends with several articles which try to come to grips with the magnitude of affective disorders in the elderly.

The next section concerns the anxiety disorders, but unlike last year there is a profusion of valuable articles in this field. The first article deals with the critical issue of the relationship of panic to the legion of patients presenting with chest pain, and others clearly document the considerable morbidity in this severe syndrome. A group of articles here represent some of the best data about the prognosis and outcome of panic disorder currently available. The section ends with an extraordinary case report of a patient who developed obsessive-compulsive disorder following an infarction of the globus pallidus, a very interesting phenomenon, to say the least.

One article on substance abuse is included this year, a critically important 1 which demonstrates through a carefully done trial the value of selective serotonin reuptake inhibitors in depressed alcoholics.

The articles on schizophrenia this year focus on high-quality studies of the outcome of schizophrenia. One important large study covered here documents how poorly most patients with this tragic disorder are currently being treated.

This is the first year that I have included a section on posttraumatic stress disorder. It's my own belief that the increase in research on these disorders reflects a growing understanding of their critical importance. The section begins with an interesting study of the triggering of posttraumatic stress disorder symptoms in World War II veterans by media coverage of the anniversary of that war. The section includes an article on the effect of natural disasters, and another on the growing recognition of the frequency of childhood physical and sexual assault histories in adult women with serious psychiatric problems. Two articles concerning the physiology of trauma reactions and the psychiatric difficulties which evolve also appear.

The next section covers the important consensus statement issued last year about the treatment of Alzheimer's. This is followed by 2 carefully performed studies on eating disorders.

The largest section is the last, and, once again, it features a discussion of the relationship of psychiatry to our primary care and general medicine colleagues. The large number of important studies and articles in this area underscore what I have for some time believed to be a "sea change" in psychiatry. I believe that in the next decade or two, perhaps half our work will be done helping our primary care colleagues to deal with psychiatric issues and in performing research in that area.

Several articles concerning the treatment of depression in HIV-positive patients, the often overlooked morbidity of insomnia, and the positive effects of carbamazepine on chronic pain begin the final section. These are followed by articles on the treatment of depression in physically ill patients including the issue of depression's interaction with anxiety. The very interesting finding that anxiety can increase physical morbidity in coronary artery disease patients is presented. An article on the presence of personality disorders in patients experienced by primary-care physicians as "difficult" is included. This is an area that has been consistently overlooked.

The next section presents a series of articles on the frequent confusing presentation of anxiety and depression in primary care. These include discussion of what we now understand to be the "usual care" of depression in primary care and the fact that a large percentage of patients are either not detected, or are treated inadequately. An excellent article by the Seattle group demonstrates that correct treatment does, in fact, make a significant difference. Reports of various attempts to improve the situation by using practice nurses who develop specialty skills in this area and other techniques to try to improve the care of these patients are included.

This section concludes with 4 articles that struggle with how we can use education methods to improve the situation. Are there things we can do in medical school, during residency, or with post-graduate training that will work? We know that the average primary care physician does not feel qualified or comfortable in dealing with the majority of psychiatric complaints of their patients, and it is clear that the care they are currently delivering is probably substandard. Education appears to be part of the issue, but a profound change in the way we educate physicians is actually required.

I hope you enjoy these articles as much as I did.

James C. Ballenger, M.D.

Affective Disorders

Boundaries of Major Depression: An Evaluation of DSM-IV Criteria
Kendler KS, Gardner CO Jr (Virginia Commonwealth Univ, Richmond)
Am J Psychiatry 155:172–177, 1998   6–1

Introduction.—The depressive syndrome is well described. Yet, the boundaries of the depressive state have received little attention. Two mutually exclusive hypotheses regarding major depression were assessed, as articulated in the *Diagnostic and Statistical Manual of Mental Disorders*, fourth edition (DSM-IV), as follows: (1) Is major depression a discrete syndrome with "points of rarity" at its boundaries? or (2) Is major depression a diagnostic convention imposed on a continuum of depressive symptoms of varying severity and duration?

Methods.—Caucasian female same-sex twins who were part of a longitudinal investigation of genetic and environmental risk factors for common psychiatric disorders were interviewed 3 times during a mean of 61.3 months. Three important features of the syndrome of major depression were assessed to determine whether they were predictive of future depressive episodes in the index twin and of risk of major depression in the co-twin. They were the number of symptoms listed under criterion A in DSM-IV for major depressive episode; level of severity or impairment required for rating individual symptoms as present; and duration of episode.

Results.—An increasing number of criterion A symptoms were predictive of a greater risk for future depressive episodes in the index twin and increased risk for major depression in the co-twin. This relationship was not observed with duration of episode. Severity predicted risk in the co-twin. The index twin with severe impairment had a significant risk for future episodes, compared with those with less impairment. There was no evidence for a discontinuity at the boundaries proposed by DSM-IV. Syndromes that met less than 5 criterion A symptoms, were less than 2 weeks in duration, or had symptoms that were mild or produced no impairment had predictive and familial validity. These subsyndromes were consistently predictive, at high levels of significance, of risk for subsequent episodes of major depression and risk for major depression in a co-twin, as defined in the *Diagnostic and Statistical Manual of Mental Disorders*, third edition, revised.

Conclusion.—There was little empirical support for the DSM-IV parameters of 2 weeks' duration, 5 symptoms, or clinically significant impairment. The current DSM-IV diagnostic conventions for major depression may be arbitrary and not reflective of a natural discontinuity in depressive symptoms.

▶ This study provides clear and excellent evidence for what most of us believe, and it underscores the difficulties with the categorical diagnostic schema utilized in the DSM-IV, in which a certain threshold was defined with the rationale that everyone above that threshold has the disorder. Unfortunately, it misses ill people below that line—and this is especially true with depression. Many of the people failing to meet the threshold have a great deal of difficulty.

Ken Kendler's excellent analysis of his twin studies documents that in fact DSM-IV requirements of 2 weeks' duration, 5 symptoms, or clinically significant impairment all failed to differentiate the risk for depression. His data suggest that, in fact, depression is a continuum of depressive symptoms, and DSM-IV places an arbitrary imposition on that continuum. There is no clear delineation between those who are well and those who are not.

J.C. Ballenger, M.D.

Neuroanatomical Correlates of Happiness, Sadness, and Disgust
Lane RD, Reiman EM, Ahern GL, et al (Univ of Arizona, Tucson; Univ of Wisconsin, Madison; Good Samaritan Regional Med Ctr, Phoenix, Ariz)
Am J Psychiatry 154:926–933, 1997   6–2

Background.—In previous studies, the universality of basic emotions such as anger, fear, happiness, sadness, surprise, and disgust was established. This universality suggests that many emotions are inherent to the human neurologic structure. To date, positron emission tomography (PET) studies of humans experiencing emotions have been rare. The PET studies allow scientists to chart brain activation sequences. This study examined happiness, sadness, and disgust, using PET to determine which brain structures are involved in these emotions.

Method.—Twelve right-handed women (mean age, 23.3 years), who were neurologically fit as determined by an MRI and who passed screening for emotional reactions, viewed silent color films designed to induce happiness, sadness, and disgust. The test subjects also viewed 3 nature films which were used as controls. Each clip was approximately 2 minutes in length, but only the 1 minute, determined to be the most emotionally intense, was monitored by a 1-minute PET study. Test subjects were also scanned during autobiographical recall sessions in which they recapitulated moments of intense and less intense emotions. They did this with their eyes closed. Subjects were told the desired emotional response previous to the showing of each clip. The order of trials was randomized. During each film clip, researchers ranked 7 emotions subjectively on an 8-point visual analogue scale. The overall brain activity during each emotion was obtained by superimposing the multiple images gained from PET scans over the MRIs for each test subject.

Results.—The 3 emotions studied were all accompanied by enhanced activity in the medial prefrontal cortex and in the thalamus. Anterior and posterior temporal structures were also shown to increase in activity, especially when the film was used. Sadness induced through recall was associated with increased activity in the anterior isula. Sadness showed less activity in the ventral mesial frontal cortex than happiness

Conclusion.—Regions of the brain that show increased electrical activity during happiness, sadness, and disgust were identified. These regions differentiate between positive and negative, and elicitor and valence emotions.

▶ Modern brain imaging techniques allow us to begin to study some of the basics of our field. In this study, PET scan images of normals experiencing happiness, sadness, and disgust demonstrated the brain structures underlying these emotions. These and similar studies with functional MRI[1] are beginning to give us fascinating information regarding the location of the basic emotions and promise much for the future.

J.C. Ballenger, M.D.

Reference

1. George MS, Ketter TA, Post RM: What functional imaging studies have revealed about the brain basis of mood and emotion, in Panksepp J (ed): *Advances in Biological Psychiatry*, ed 2. Greenwich, Conn, JAI Press, 1996, pp 63-113.

The Functional Neuroanatomy of Mood Disorders

Soares JC, Mann JJ (Univ of Pittsburgh, Pa; Columbia Univ, New York)
J Psychiatr Res 31:393–432, 1997   6–3

Introduction.—Earlier reports suggest an association between fronto-subcortical brain circuits and the pathophysiology of primary and secondary mood disorders. The 2 primary brain neuroanatomical circuits believed to be involved in mood regulation are a limbic-thalamic-cortical circuit (including the amygdala, mediodorsal nucleus of thalamus, and medial and ventrolateral prefrontal cortex) and a limbic-stiatal-pallidal-thalamic-cortical circuit (including the striatum, ventral pallidum, and regions of the other circuit) (Fig 1).

It is possible that mood disorders may result from dysfunction in various parts of these interconnected circuits. The brain abnormalities in mood disorder might be manifested by structural changes, restricted to a functional level, or related to brain development or degenerative factors. The

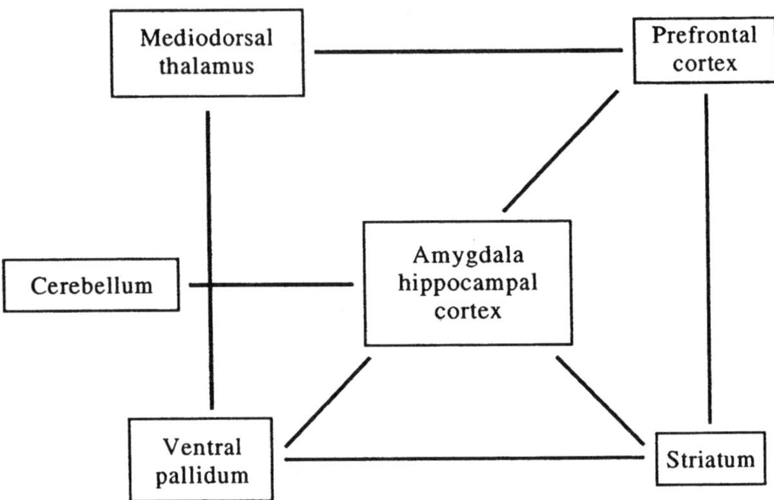

FIGURE 1.—The key brain areas participating in mood regulation are represented in the figure. They have extensive connections among themselves. The 2 main neuroanatomical circuits believed to be involved in the pathophysiology of mood disorders are a limbic-cortical circuit connecting the amygdala, the mediodorsal nucleus of thalamus, and the medial and ventrolateral prefrontal cortex, and a limbic-striatal-pallidal-thalamic-cortical circuit connecting the striatum, the ventral pallidum, and the regions of the other circuit. According to this model, mood disorders could result from dysfunction in different regions of these interconnected circuits. (Reprinted from the *Journal of Psychiatric Research* courtesy of Soares JC, Mann JJ: The functional neuroanatomy of mood disorders. *J Psychiatr Res* 31:393-432, copyright 1997 by kind permission from Elsevier Science Ltd, The Boulevard, Langford Lane, Kidlington OX5 1GB, UK.)

accumulated functional neuroimaging findings in mood disorders were reviewed to evaluate a proposed neuroanatomical model of pathophysiology.

Functional Brain Imaging Review.—Reports conflict regarding global brain functional changes. Most do not support the presence of global blood flow or metabolic abnormalities, except in late-life depression or bipolar disorder. Regional cerebral blood flow and glucose metabolism deficits have been observed and may be indicative of brain regions participating in neuroanatomical circuits involved in mood disorders. Reduced prefrontal cortex blood flow and metabolism are the most consistently replicated findings and correlate with illness severity in both unipolar and bipolar depressed individuals.

Basal ganglia abnormalities involving reduced blood flow and metabolism have been detected in depressed unipolar and bipolar patients. Temporal lobe abnormalities are present in patients with bipolar disease and may be present in those with unipolar disease. Evidence of abnormalities in other limbic regions is inconclusive. Cognitive impairment may be related to reduced metabolism in frontal and cerebellar areas.

An association between functional neuroimaging findings and clinical course—and, thus, state and trait characteristics—has not been systematically analyzed. Antidepressant medications seem to reverse some of the recognized functional brain changes in the depressed state. This has not been observed with electroconvulsive therapy.

Conclusion.—The structural, neurotransmitter, and neuropathologic correlates of functional abnormalities in patients with mood disorders have yet to be identified. Functional abnormalities in the frontal, subcortical, and limbic structures seem to be part of the pathophysiology of mood disorders.

▶ This is an excellent review of an important and rapidly emerging area of our field. Increasingly, the imaging studies of depression are finding consistent abnormalities of decreased blood flow and metabolism in both unipolar and bipolar depressed patients in the prefrontal cortex and, to a somewhat lesser extent, the basal ganglia. Antidepressant medications seem to reverse some of these brain imaging abnormalities. Unlike many areas of biological psychiatry, findings in this area seem to be replicated by follow-up studies and are emerging as 1 of the solid findings of psychiatric science.

J.C. Ballenger, M.D.

Major Depression and Stages of Smoking: A Longitudinal Investigation
Breslau N, Peterson EL, Schultz LR, et al (Henry Ford Health Sciences Ctr, Detroit)
Arch Gen Psychiatry 55:161–166, 1998   6–4

Introduction.—Recent epidemiologic trials have suggested a correlation between major depression and smoking. Among the causal explanations for this association is the idea of self-medication, i.e., using nicotine to medicate depressed mood. The role of depression in smoking progression and cessation, and the role of smoking in first-onset major depression was prospectively assessed.

Methods.—A random sample of 1,200 persons aged 21–30 years from a large health maintenance organization in southeastern Michigan were interviewed in 1989 regarding history of smoking and major depression. Follow-up interviews were conducted in 1990, 1992, and 1994. Of 1,004 persons interviewed at baseline, complete follow-up data were available for 974 (97%).

Results.—Examination of the 5-year prospective data suggested that (1) a history of major depression at baseline was correlated with a threefold increase in the risk for progression to daily smoking; (2) a history of major depression at baseline did not significantly reduce a smoker's rate of quitting during the ensuing 5 years; (3) a history of daily smoking at baseline markedly increased the risk for major depression; and (4) analysis of the combined lifetime data showed consistent results. These estimates were decreased somewhat when the history of early (before age 15 years) conduct problems was controlled.

Conclusion.—These findings that daily smoking increased the risk for first-onset major depression are congruent with earlier reports of increases in depressive symptoms and higher risk for episode of major depression in persons with a history of prior smoking. Shared causes for smoking and depression are plausible. Self-medication of depressed mood may be a factor in smoking progression; the neuropharmacologic effects of nicotine and other smoke substances on neurotransmitter systems may be linked to depression.

▶ As our society struggles to rid itself of the habit of smoking, a very interesting and provocative finding has evolved. It appears that smoking and depression have an intimate relationship, and that even the onset of first-time depression has been observed when people have discontinued smoking. This study showed that a history of depression significantly increased the risk of development of daily smoking which, itself, increased the risk of major depression. Current research actually suggests that smoking and depression may share a common etiology. Recent imaging data suggest that smoking inhibits the monoamine oxidase enzyme and, therefore, may well operate like monoamine oxidase inhibitor itself. This could make plausible what many smokers say: that smoking picks up their mood. It would appear that psychiatry has an important role in trying to understand and deal with the epidemic of nicotine addiction in our society.

J.C. Ballenger, M.D.

Twelve-month Outcome After a First Hospitalization for Affective Psychosis
Strakowski SM, Keck PE Jr, McElroy SL, et al (Univ of Cincinnati, Ohio)
Arch Gen Psychiatry 55:49–55, 1998   6–5

Introduction.—Factors affecting the course of illness in patients with affective psychosis have rarely been subjected to prospective evaluation; thus, they are are poorly defined. Findings of a 12-month, prospective outcome trial of 109 patients after their first hospitalization for affective psychosis were reported.

Methods.—Patients underwent diagnostic, symptomatic, and functional evaluations at baseline (index hospitalization) and at 2, 6, and 12 months after discharge to determine syndromic, symptomatic, and functional outcome predictors.

Results.—During the 12-month follow-up period, 56% of patients were able to achieve syndromic recovery. More frequent and rapid syndromic recovery was observed in the presence of full treatment compliance. Full compliance was seen more often in whites and in patients free of substance abuse. Symptomatic recovery and functional recovery were observed in 35% and 35%, respectively, of patients during the same 12-month interval. Symptomatic recovery was slower in patients with substance abuse and was correlated with higher socioeconomic status. Higher socioeconomic status and good premorbid function were correlated with functional recovery.

Conclusion.—Not many patients were able to achieve a favorable outcome in the year after a first hospitalization for affective psychosis. Lower rates or delayed onset of recovery were correlated with lower socioeconomic status, poor premorbid function, treatment noncompliance, and substance abuse.

▶ This study follows a cohort of 109 patients for 1 year after their first psychiatric hospitalization for affective psychosis. The outcome was poorer than hoped for, and the authors clearly documented a series of factors associated with lower rates of recovery or slower recovery. Not surprisingly, these included lower socioeconomic classes, poor premorbid functioning, treatment noncompliance, and substance abuse.

J.C. Ballenger, M.D.

Three- to 5-year Prospective Follow-up of Outcome in Major Depression
Van Londen L, Molenaar RPG, Goekoop JG, et al (Leiden Univ, The Netherlands)
Psychol Med 28:731–735, 1998   6–6

Introduction.—Major depression can be a lifelong episodic condition requiring ongoing pharmacotherapy and psychotherapy in as many as 75% to 80% of patients. Neuropeptide concentrations in plasma were followed prospectively in a 3- to 5-year longitudinal trial of a Dutch cohort of 56 patients with depression.

Methods.—All patients met the *Diagnostic and Statistical Manual of Mental Disorders*, third edition, revised criteria for major depression and were given a diagnosis by a psychiatrist. In all patients, a standardized dose of pharmacotherapy was initiated. Psychotherapy approaches varied among patients; they included cognitive behavioral therapy, group therapy, supportive therapy, and attendance at day treatment. Patients did not receive electroconvulsive therapy. Follow-ups were performed monthly for 3 years or more.

Results.—Forty-nine of 56 patients were followed for 36 to 60 months. At 9 months after start of treatment, 49% and 45% of patients were in full and partial remission, respectively. In the next 3 to 5 years, 82% of patients reached full remission. Sixteen percent of patients required 2 years or more before achieving full remission. Most relapses and recurrences occurred in the first 15 months after partial or full remission, in most cases, even in the presence of continuing pharmacotherapy. Relapses or recurrences after the first 15 months were infrequent. There was a 41% relapse or recurrence rate within the first 5 years. Patients with residual symptoms usually relapsed within the first 4 months after remission, compared with a relapse interval of 12 months for patients without residual symptoms. Previous depressive episodes and psychoticism were predictive of relapse. Psychomotor retardation at inception was predictive of a longer time to partial remission.

Conclusion.—Major depression is a seriously impairing disease, frequently with residual symptoms and an episodic remitting character. Continuing active and adequate treatment are needed for residual symptoms after remission, during the first 4 months after partial remission, and starting at 12 months after full remission.

► In this study, outpatients with depression were followed for 3 to 5 years. The results are strikingly similar to those of National Institute of Mental Health (NIMH) studies in that after 9 months, only 49% of patients had reached full remission; and after 3 to 5 years, only 82% had reached full remission. The authors also found a recurrence rate of 41% during the first 5 years; this was slightly lower than the NIMH results reported by Keller and colleagues.[1]

J.C. Ballenger, M.D.

Reference

1. Keller MB, Shapiro RW, Lavori PW, et al: Recovery in major depressive disorder: Analysis with the life table and regression models. *Arch Gen Psychiatry* 39:905-910, 1982.

Recovery From Major Depression: A 10-year Prospective Follow-up Across Multiple Episodes
Solomon DA, Keller MB, Leon AC, et al (Brown Univ, Providence, RI; Cornell Univ, New York; Univ of Iowa, Iowa City; et al)
Arch Gen Psychiatry 54:1001–1006, 1997   6–7

Background.—Repeated episodes of depression often occur in major depressive disorder. Recovery from major depression across multiple mood episodes in patients with unipolar major depression at intake was described, and the relationship between sociodemographic and clinical variables with illness duration was studied.

Methods.—Two hundred fifty-eight subjects treated for unipolar major depressive disorder were followed up prospectively for 10 years. The Longitudinal Interval Follow-up Evaluation was used to assess the course of illness. Illness duration was calculated using survival analyses for the first 5 recurrent mood episodes after recovery from the index episode.

Findings.—In 91% of the patients, the diagnosis remained unipolar major depressive disorder. Median illness duration was 22 weeks for the first recurrent mood episode, 20 weeks for the second, 21 weeks for the third, and 19 weeks for the fourth and fifth. The proportion of patients recovering by any 1 time point was similar from 1 episode to the next. The consistency of illness duration from 1 recovery to the next was low to moderate for patients with 2 or more recoveries. Illness duration could not be consistently predicted by any of the sociodemographic or clinical variables studied.

Conclusions.—The duration of recurrent mood episodes was relatively uniform in this cohort of patients treated at tertiary care centers for major depressive disorders. Mean duration was about 20 weeks.

▶ This large study followed 258 patients treated for unipolar major depressive disorder for 10 years under careful research conditions. As such, it provides some of the best information we have available about the course of major depressive disorder. Very interesting similarities across multiple episodes were documented—each seemed to average ≅5 months for recovery to occur, although most patients did recover. This type of definitive and very clear finding is useful to clinicians in working with families and patients predicting what will happen to them over time with treatment.

J.C. Ballenger, M.D.

Recurrence in Affective Disorder: I. Case Register Study

Kessing LV, Andersen PK, Mortensen PB, et al (Univ of Copenhagen; Univ of Aarhus, Risskov, Denmark)
Br J Psychiatry 172:23–28, 1998   6–8

Introduction.—Recurrence is not frequently the focus in investigations of long-term outcome in patients with affective disorders. Several trials have confirmed Kraepelin's original 1921 observation that duration of time to recurrence diminishes as a function of the number of previous episodes. Some recent trials have yielded contradictory results. The rate of recurrence was assessed in unipolar and bipolar disorders in a large patient sample from Denmark.

Methods.—All psychiatric admissions were evaluated from the nationwide register in Denmark from January 1, 1971, to December 31, 1993. Patients with unipolar and bipolar disease were followed for hospital readmissions as an expression of disease recurrence.

Results.—There were 20,350 first-admission patients discharged with a diagnosis of affective disorder—depressive or manic/cyclic type—from 1971 to 1993. The time to recurrence decreased with the number of previous episodes for both unipolar and bipolar disease. Unipolar and bipolar disease had markedly different courses. Early in the illness, patients with bipolar disease had significantly higher risk of recurrence than patients with unipolar disease. Polarity had no influence on risk of further recurrence later in the disease process. The strikingly different initial course helps demonstrate the distinction between unipolar and bipolar disease.

Conclusion.—These findings concur with those of earlier reports that describe a deteriorating course for unipolar and bipolar disease, despite treatment.

▶ I have often thought that the most important issue in the treatment of depression is not so much the resolution of the current depression as the prevention of recurrence. Much of my personal scientific work around "kindling" was based on evidence that affective disorders appear to speed up over time. This has remained a controversial area, and this study provides excellent data from more than 20,000 patients that recurrence in both unipolar and bipolar illness becomes increasingly rapid, i.e., with shorter periods between successive episodes. The authors also provide partial evidence that treatment does not prevent this progression.

J.C. Ballenger, M.D.

Suicide Mortality Among Patients Treated for Depression in an Insured Population
Simon GE, VonKorff M (Group Health Cooperative of Puget Sound, Seattle)
Am J Epidemiol 147:155–160, 1998   6–9

Introduction.—Nearly 15% of depressed patients eventually commit suicide. Few data are available for suicide risk among depressed patients not treated by specialists. Current treatment decisions are based on data from specialty and inpatient samples. Suicide mortality was assessed among an entire population of patients treated for depression in the Group Health Cooperative of Puget Sound (GHC), a large health maintenance organization in western Washington state.

Methods.—All GHC members treated for depression during 1992, 1993, and 1994 were identified by computerized discharge diagnosis, outpatient visit diagnosis, and outpatient prescription records. All deaths and deaths from suicide before January 1, 1995, were identified through computerized death certificate data.

Results.—From January 1, 1992, to December 31, 1994, 35,546 individuals were treated for depression, involving 62,159 person-years of follow-up. Of 850 deaths among persons treated for depression, 36 (4.2%) were considered as definite or possible suicides. The overall suicide mortality rate was 59 per 100,000 person-years. Suicide mortality was significantly higher among males than females (118 vs. 36 per 100,000 person-years). The risk per 100,000 person-years decreased from 224 in patients receiving any inpatient psychiatric treatment to 64 for persons receiving outpatient specialty mental health treatment, 43 for those treated with antidepressant medications in primary care, and 0 for those treated in primary care without antidepressants.

Conclusion.—The overall suicide risk among patients treated for depression is notably lower than previous estimates, based on specialty and inpatient samples. The risk of death by suicide was highest among patients treated in inpatient and specialty settings. For patients with less severe illness, the burden of depressive illness was primarily expressed through functional impairment and personal suffering.

▶ Another excellent study from the Seattle GHC of Puget Sound authors provides excellent modern data on suicide rates. They are able to demonstrate that the rate is lower than previously reported and is very different according to whether patients are treated as inpatients, in an outpatient mental health setting, or in primary care—probably relating to the obvious differences of illness severity in those settings.

J.C. Ballenger, M.D.

Temporal Profiles of the Course of Depression During Treatment: Predictors of Pathways Toward Recovery in the Elderly

Dew MA, Reynolds CF III, Houck PR, et al (Univ of Pittsburgh, Pa)
Arch Gen Psychiatry 54:1016–1024, 1997   6–10

Objective.—Although depression is known to be associated with psychosocial stress, cognitive impairment, and sleep alterations that tend to worsen with age, correlates and predictors of response to treatment of or recovery from major depressive episodes late in life are not well understood. Baseline variables that predict treatment response or recovery in the elderly have not been identified. Pretreatment psychosocial, clinical, and electroencephalographic sleep variables that predicted different temporal profiles of recovery or influenced incidence and recurrence of depression were investigated in a diagnostically homogeneous cohort of elders.

Methods.—A daily sleep-wake log was maintained by 95 depressed patients aged 60 years or older for a 14-day psychotropic drug-free and alcohol-free period before the baseline assessment. Sleep was monitored for 3 consecutive nights. All patients received nortriptyline and psychotherapy. Depressive symptoms were evaluated weekly for 12 weeks and biweekly for 6 weeks. Cluster analysis was used to identify any distinct recovery profiles.

Results.—Cluster analysis identified 4 groups of elders. The largest group (n = 29) responded quickly and sustained improvement. The second cluster included slow but sustained responders (n = 21). The third cluster (n = 23) were nonresponders. The fourth cluster (n = 22) showed fluctuating patterns over time. Baseline characteristics that predicted the type and timing of recovery included major life stressors before the onset of the initial episode, higher perceived chronic stress, lower social support, older current age, younger age at first episode, current endogenous episode, greater severity of current perceived sleep impairment, greater severity of current anxiety symptoms, and lower percentage of REM sleep.

Conclusion.—Individuals have different courses of recovery from depression. These different courses can be identified and used to predict individual recovery paths.

▶ This study from the Pittsburgh group provides excellent data documenting the course of recovery from depression in the elderly. With their large patient sample and careful methodology, they were able to identify predictors of poor response. These included high acute and chronic stress, poor social support, anxiety, being older, and poor subjective and objective (electroencephalographic) sleep profiles. Few of the patients had reoccurrence by even 4 weeks in the study. This study argues that we should be tailoring our treatments with these issues in mind.

J.C. Ballenger, M.D.

Diagnosis and Treatment of Depression in Late Life: Consensus Statement Update
Lebowitz BD, Pearson JL, Schneider LS, et al (Natl Inst of Mental Health, Bethesda, Md; Univ of Southern California, Los Angeles; Univ of Pittsburgh, Pa; et al)
JAMA 278:1186–1190, 1997   6–11

Background.—In 1991, the National Institutes of Health (NIH) Consensus Panel on Diagnosis and Treatment of Depression in Late Life concluded that depressive illness is widespread in the elderly, that such depression is a serious public health concern, and that comorbidity of depression with other illnesses is especially problematic in the elderly. Since then, considerable progress has been made in understanding the diagnosis, treatment, and design of service provision systems for late life depression. In light of new scientific evidence, the NIH has systematically reviewed these earlier conclusions.

Review.—NIH staff and experts reviewed the original consensus statement and identified areas for update.

Conclusion.—They concluded that, though the initial consensus statement is still true, important new information has been published in several areas, such as the onset and course of late-life depression; comorbidity and disability; sex and hormonal issues; and newer medications, psychotherapies, and approaches to long-term treatment. Important new information has also emerged in the areas of the impact of depression on health services and health care resource use, late-life depression as a risk factor for suicide, and the importance of heterogeneous forms of depression. Depression among the elderly continues to be an important public health problem. There is a substantial burden of unrecognized or inadequately treated depression. However, effective treatments are available. Aggressive approaches for recognizing, diagnosing, and treating depression in the elderly are needed to minimize suffering, improve overall functioning and quality of life, and limit inappropriate uses of health care resources.

▶ I found this paper both interesting and heartening. I had been a panel member of the 1991 NIH Consensus Panel on the diagnosis and treatment of depression in late life, and so this update was quite interesting. I was not aware that updates occur after a consensus statement. This article documents how useful they can be. The new group updated most of the conclusions we had reached, because a great deal of new information has been discovered since 1991. We knew then that depression in late life was a tremendously prevalent illness that was generally under-recognized and poorly treated. This article makes that all the more clear but reviews how much more we have learned in the past 6 to 7 years.

J.C. Ballenger, M.D.

Association Between Mood-stabilizing Medication and Mental Health Resource Use in the Management of Acute Mania
Sajatovic M, Gerhart C, Semple W (Cleveland Veterans Affairs Med Ctr, Brecksville, Ohio)
Psychiatric Serv 48:1037–1041, 1997   6–12

Objective.—Lithium, valproate, and carbamazine are all effective in the management of acute mania. The time course of response, compliance, and other utilization of services were examined in patients with acute mania who were treated with a variety of regimens using mood stabilizers.

Methods.—Demographic, clinical, and resource utilization information was collected on 96 (8 female) patients (75% white and 25% black) aged 23 to 83 years, with a diagnosis of bipolar mania and treated at the Cleveland Veterans Administration Medical Center between January 1, 1993, and December 31, 1995. Patients were divided into 4 treatment groups based on therapy: lithium (n = 29), anticonvulsants (n = 17), multiple mood stabilizers (n = 42), and no therapy (n = 8). Groups were compared using analysis of variance.

Results.—Patients receiving anticonvulsant monotherapy had significantly more comorbid psychiatric illnesses (mainly substance abuse or dependence) than patients taking multiple mood stabilizers. On average, those taking multiple mood stabilizers were hospitalized significantly longer (30.3 days) than those taking lithium (20.7 days), anticonvulsant therapy (17 days), or no therapy (17.1 days). Those taking lithium had a significantly shorter mean hospital stay than those taking multiple mood stabilizers. The short hospitalization period for those not taking therapy was mainly the result of their refusal to remain hospitalized. Use of seclusion or restraint in the hospital did not differ among treatment groups. Compliance after hospital discharge was poor for all groups.

Conclusion.—Agents other than lithium, in particular valproate, have changed treatment, outcomes, and utilization of resources in patients with bipolar disorder. Anticonvulsant therapy appears to be more effective than lithium for patients with other psychiatric conditions, especially substance abuse. Compliance after hospital discharge is poor.

▶ This article studies the treatment of a large number of patients with bipolar disorder and documents how modern treatment has become remarkably complicated for many patients. Only one third of these patients were treated with lithium monotherapy and 10% were taking no mood stabilizers. One group was taking an anticonvulsant, and the largest group of patients (almost half) were taking multiple mood stabilizers. Bob Post has been outspoken in asking our field to move more rapidly to the realization that many manic patients need 4 to 5 medications if we hope to manage the complex difficulties they have and that this strategy is the most effective one in many patients.

J.C. Ballenger, M.D.

Anxiety Disorders

Prevalence and Recognition of Panic States in STARNET Patients Presenting With Chest Pain

Katerndahl DA, Trammell C (Univ of Texas, San Antonio)
J Fam Pract 45:54–63, 1997   6–13

Background.—Panic disorder is a common cause of noncardiac chest pain. The prevalence of panic states in patients seeking medical care for chest pain in primary care settings was documented, along with the recognition rate of panic states by family physicians and the impact of lack of recognition on interventions and costs.

Methods.—Fifty-one patients seeking care with a new complaint of chest pain completed the panic disorder section of the Structured Clinical Interview (SCID) of the *Diagnostic and Statistical Manual of Mental Disorders, Third Edition, Revised* (DSMMD-R) before seeing the physi-

TABLE 3.—Physician Diagnoses After the Initial Visits of 51 Patients Who Presented With Chest Pain

Diagnosis	Frequency (n)
Psychiatric	
Panic	4
Anxiety/stress	12
Depression	3
Pulmonary	
Pleuritic	1
Bronchitis	1
External chest	
Costochondral	2
Thoracic outlet syndrome	1
Chest wall neuralgia	2
Musculoskeletal	4
Cardiovascular	
Coronary insufficiency	2
Hypertension	2
Gastrointestinal	
Peptic ulcer/gallstones	1
Reflux esophagitis	4
Other	
Perimenopausal	1
Viral syndrome	5
Symptomatic	
Noncardiac	1
None, chest pain	5

(Courtesy of Katerndahl DA, Trammell C: Prevalence and recognition of panic states in STARNET patients presenting with chest pain. *J Fam Pract* 45:54-63, 1997. Reprinted by permission of Appleton & Lange, Inc.)

cian. Using the SCID, diagnoses of panic disorder, infrequent panic, or limited symptom attacks were assigned.

Findings.—About half the patients met criteria for panic disorder or infrequent panic. However, physicians recognized few as having a panic state. Patients with panic disorder were more likely to be followed up or referred, which increased costs. Patients with infrequent panic underwent more testing, associated with higher testing and overall costs. Panic diagnoses were also associated with increased psychotropic and total medication costs (Table 3).

Conclusions.—Though panic states are common, they are rarely recognized in patients seeking medical attention for chest pain. The presence of panic results in more testing, follow-up, and referral, which increase costs. Failure to diagnose panic leads to increased medication prescription, higher costs, and inappropriate pharmacotherapy.

▶ We have clearly learned that patients presenting with chest pain frequently have panic attacks and panic disorder. This study carefully follows a group of new patients with complaints of chest pain and unfortunately redocuments that their panic difficulties are rarely diagnosed by their physicians; however, having panic disorder or panic attacks leads to higher follow-up costs, more and often inappropriate medications, and higher referral costs. This is consistent with the large international primary care study[1] which also demonstrated tremendous underdiagnosis. However, in that study the presence of even one panic attack was predictive of the presence of an anxiety disorder or depression difficulties in 99% of patients. I think it's time that we changed our educational patterns to strongly emphasize the recognition that a single panic attack is the "tip of the iceberg" and where the primary care physicians' attention should be directed.[2]

J.C. Ballenger, M.D.

Reference

1. Santorius N, Ustun TB, Costa E, et al: An international study of psychological problems in primary care. *Arch Gen Psychiatry* 50:819-824, 1993.
2. Ballenger JC: Comorbidity of panic and depression: Implications for clinical management. *Intl Clin Psychopharmacol*, in press 1998.

Anxiety Disorders in Elderly Patients
Banazak DA (Michigan State Univ, East Lansing)
J Am Board Fam Pract 10:280–289, 1997   6–14

Introduction.—For the primary care physician, the treatment of anxiety in an elderly patient can be clinically challenging. Anxiety disorders in elderly patients commonly coexist with other medical and psychiatric illnesses. Several effective treatments are available in this situation. A literature review of the causes and treatments—pharmacologic and non-pharmacologic—for anxiety in the elderly is reported.

Anxiety in the Elderly.—Research suggests that 10% to 20% of elderly people have clinically significant symptoms of anxiety. Late-life anxiety problems commonly encountered by primary care physicians include general anxiety disorder, phobias, panic disorder, and obsessive-compulsive disorder. These disorders may be associated with symptoms in multiple body systems; motor restlessness; and physiologic symptoms, including tachycardia or tachypnea. A variety of co-morbid conditions are commonly seen, such as depression, alcoholism, drug use, and multisystem disorders. In evaluation of the elderly patient with anxiety, the distinction between medical and psychological factors is essential. Anxiety is sometimes relieved by effective treatment for a medical condition. Certain drugs are also related to anxiety.

There have been few specific studies of treatment for anxiety in older adults. Cognitive therapy may be effective through exploring and challenging the patient's misperceptions and fears. Certain behavioral approaches may also be effective, such as diary keeping, relaxation, distraction, and role playing. Frail elderly patients with diffuse anxiety may need environmental interventions, such as home health care or case management. For patients with severe anxiety leading to functional impairment, drug treatment may be indicated. Options include benzodiazepines, buspirone, or antidepressant therapy. The initially prescribed dose should be one half the usual adult dose, and treatment should be monitored carefully.

Discussion.—The characteristics and treatment of anxiety in the elderly are reviewed. It is important to consider both psychologic and medical factors in evaluation; there are many pharmacologic and nonpharmacologic options for treatment. For patients who do not respond to treatment, referral to a mental health professional may be indicated. The author calls for clinical trials of primary care treatments for anxiety in the elderly.

▶ This study concerns 1 of the biggest gaps in our knowledge base in the anxiety field, that is, anxiety in the elderly population. This is similar to the situation in depression 10 years ago where there were almost no trials in the elderly depressed; the same can be said in the anxiety field now. We desperately need carefully performed anxiety studies in the elderly.

J.C. Ballenger, M.D.

The Quality of Life and Employment in Panic Disorder

Ettigi P, Meyerhoff AS, Chirban JT, et al (Panic, Anxiety, and Depression Ctr of Virginia, Richmond; Capitol Outcomes Research Inc, Alexandria, Va; Cambridge Hosp, Mass; et al)
J Nerv Ment Dis 185:368–372, 1997
6–15

Background.—Panic disorder is a highly prevalent condition in America that often includes psychiatric comorbidity. Panic disorder is associated with suicide attempts, major depression, and employment problems. The work productivity and quality of life of people with this condition were examined.

Method.—Researchers gathered information on 84 patients with panic disorder who were rated at least "moderately ill" on the clinician's global impression of severity scale (CGI-S). Patients were not included in the study if they exhibited marked psychiatric comorbidity. At baseline, test subjects were given a journal for documenting the occurrence and characteristics of panic attacks. At this time, researchers also estimated the duration of panic attacks. At 4 weeks, patient diaries were reviewed, CGI-S was assessed, and patients were asked to complete a survey. Among the survey questions were those from the SF-36, an 8-domain test that gauges quality of life, and from the Work Productivity and Impairment test, which gauges the effect of symptoms on work productivity. Both of these tests were scored against U.S. population norms.

Results.—Sixty-seven percent of patients exhibited no psychiatric comorbidity. Twenty-five percent of patients were unemployed and only 57% had full-time employment. Even employed patients gave themselves a low work productivity rating. The quality-of-life scores (from the SF-36) of patients were markedly lower than those of U.S. population norms (P less than 0.01). The SF-36 domains of mental and emotional well-being were scored much lower than that of physical well-being.

Conclusion.—Panic disorder causes marked impairment in ability to work and quality of life. Psychiatric comorbidity, which was present in 33% of patients, does not adequately explain these results.

▶ This study documents clearly not only the emotional morbidity associated with panic disorder but also the interference with work functioning. This is part of the growing research base regarding the interference with employment and occupational capabilities secondary to the anxiety disorders. With an unemployment rate as high as 25% in panic patients, coupled with interference with work functioning from panic disorder and other anxiety disorders, we should no longer sit by while certain parts of our society trivialize these disorders. Facing this interference with occupational capabilities is a potentially important way of de-stigmatizing these disorders.

J.C. Ballenger, M.D.

Comorbid Psychiatric Disorders in Subjects With Panic Attacks
Katerndahl DA, Realini JP (Univ of Texas, San Antonio)
J Nerv Ment Dis 185:669–674, 1997   6–16

Objective.—Whereas the association between panic disorder (PD) and other psychiatric disorders is recognized, the nature of these associations is not clear. The association between both panic disorder (PD) and infrequent panic (IP) and other psychiatric conditions was documented, and the temporal relationship between the onset of panic and other co-morbid conditions was clarified and explored.

Methods.—Randomly selected community-dwelling adults 18 or older who met DSM-III-R criteria for panic attacks and age-, sex-, and race or ethnicity-matched controls were interviewed about psychiatric co-morbid conditions. Temporal associations with disorders, onset of first attack, and duration of attack were established. Correlations were analyzed statistically.

Results.—Panic and control groups, average age 39.8, were 78% female, 56% Hispanic, and 14% African-American. Hollingshead socioeconomic status scores were 62.5% for the panic group and 59.3% for the control group. Half of the panic group and 66% of the control group were married. The panic group had significantly more co-morbid psychiatric disorders than did the control group (3.9 vs. 1). Panic disorder patients had significantly more severe phobic avoidance and significantly higher SCL-90 somatization and phobic anxiety scores. Factor analysis included PD with phobic avoidance, substance abuse, and major depression with social and simple phobias and obsessive compulsive disorder. Only individuals with phobic avoidance reported onset of panic attacks before that of avoidance. For all other co-morbid conditions, onset of panic was secondary, with co-morbid conditions usually beginning simultaneously. Age of onset correlated more frequently with co-morbid conditions than with duration of panic.

Conclusion.—Individuals with PD and IP have high rates of co-morbid psychiatric conditions. Generalized anxiety disorder does not compound the problem. Agoraphobia appears to develop after or simultaneously with panic attacks. In other co-morbid conditions, panic attacks tend to occur secondarily.

▶ This study compares patients who did meet criteria for panic disorder with those who had only infrequent panic attacks. The group of patients with isolated and infrequent panic attacks is becoming increasingly interesting in and of itself. The recent 14-country World Health Organization primary care study documented that more than 15% of the patients had a panic attack in the previous month. Of these patients, 99% had either an anxiety disorder or depressive disorder. In the reference below,[1] I suggest that we should reorient to looking for the panic attack as the "tip of the iceberg," especially in primary care.

In this study, the authors document that the patients meeting DSM-III-R full criteria for panic disorder, when compared to the infrequent panic group, were quite similar and differed only in a higher rate of phobic avoidance. This study is supportive of the DSM-IV criteria for the diagnoses of Panic Disorder and Agoraphobia, which also pleases me because I was the chair of that DSM-IV committee. We changed the criteria from a specific number of panic attacks to "recurrent attacks" with clear sequelae secondary to those attacks. We had a clear belief that it was the correct way to diagnose panic disorder but with less evidence than is currently available.

J.C. Ballenger, M.D.

Reference

1. Ballenger, JC. Cormorbidity of panic and depression: Implications for clinical management. *Intl Clin Psychopharmacol*, in press 1998.

Agoraphobia and Panic Disorder: 3.5 Years After Alprazolam and/or Exposure Treatment

Kiliç C, Noshirvani H, Başoğlu M, et al (Hacettepe Univ, Ankara, Turkey; Inst of Psychiatry, London)
Psychother Psychosom 66:175–178, 1997   6–17

Background.—There have been few studies on the long-term effect of exposure therapy in treating agoraphobia/panic. This study follows up ex-exposure and ex-relaxation patients who participated in a previous study, to determine whether these treatments result in lasting improvements.

Method.—Follow-up was performed on previous agoraphobia/panic patients who had been treated at an average of 3½ years previously during an 8-week controlled study on the effects of exposure and relaxation treatments. In the original study, psychological treatment was performed on weeks 1, 2, 3, 4, 6, and 8. In between treatments, patients performed self-exposure or self-relaxation daily and kept records of their self-treatments in a diary. Live exposure treatments lasted 2 hours, whereas relaxation treatment lasted 1 hour. The original study divided test subjects into 4 treatment groups: alprazolam plus exposure, placebo plus exposure, alprazolam plus relaxation, and placebo plus relaxation. There was a follow-up of 43 weeks after the original study. Thirty-one of the original 69 test subjects participated in this second study. The same assessor ratings were used as before: 4 phobia targets, Hamilton Depression, Hamilton Anxiety, Beck Depression, Clinician's Global Impression, Social and Work Disability, and Patient's Global Impression.

Results.—At week 8 of the original study, more improvement was detected in alprazolam patients than in placebo patients. However, after 3½ years, the drug-treated patients and those who were given placebo did not have a significant difference on any of the assessments. At baseline, the exposure patients were more ill, but they had made more progress by the eighth week. Seven of 31 patients remained improved at week 43. All 7 patients were exposure patients. For the most part, test subjects maintained gains made during the original study through 3½ years. Ex-exposure patients faired better than ex-relaxation patients. In considering survival time and disability, researchers found that ex-exposure patients did much better.

Conclusion.—Previous studies that suggested lasting improvements after exposure treatment are modestly confirmed by this study.

▶ As I mentioned earlier, outcome follow-up data are uncommon in panic disorder. This study followed patients 3½ years after they were treated with exposure or relaxation, with or without alprazolam. Certainly one of the greatest controversies in the field has been whether there is less relapse after exposure-type treatments than after medications, with proponents of exposure and other cognitive behavioral treatments arguing (often with data) that a much lower relapse rate is associated with those treatment types. The group medicated with alprazolam plus exposure clearly performed better initially in the acute trials, but at 3½-year follow-up, it appears that exposure therapy had the most potent effects. Most of the patients were better, although many continued to have significant difficulties.

J.C. Ballenger, M.D.

Predictors of Remission in Patients With Panic With and Without Agoraphobia: Prospective 5-year Follow-up Data
Warshaw MG, Massion AO, Shea MT, et al (Brown Univ, Providence, RI; Univ of Massachusetts, Worcester; Butler Hosp, Providence, RI; et al)
J Nerv Ment Dis 185:517–519, 1997   6–18

Introduction.—Many questions remain about the long-term course and associated predictive factors in patients with panic disorders. The available data suggest that panic disorder has a chronic course with periods of relapse and remission. Data from the Harvard/Brown Anxiety Research Program were used to identify factors associated with remission in panic disorder.

Methods.—The analysis included 412 patients who were in episodes of DSM-III-R-defined panic—with or without agoraphobia—at baseline. For each patient, follow-up data of 6 months to 5 years were available. Each patient underwent a comprehensive evaluation at intake, with follow-up using the Longitudinal Interval Follow-up Evaluation. For each week of follow-up, an Individual Psychiatric Status Rating (PSR) was made with separate assessments of panic and agoraphobia. Factors of time to remission were assessed by Cox regression analysis. Sixty-eight percent of the patients were women; mean age at intake was 40.

Results.—The probability of remission was 0.21 in the first year of follow-up and 0.40 in the first 5 years. Eighty-four percent of patients received somatic therapy in the 6 months after intake, most commonly benzodiazepines. On multivariate analysis, factors associated with a lower likelihood of remission were being in an episode of panic with agoraphobia, risk ratio (RR) 0.38; and reaching panic onset before age 15 years, RR 0.39. Factors associated with a greater likelihood of remission were high socioeconomic status, RR 1.75; being in an episode of social phobia at intake, RR 1.73; having previous episodes of panic disorder, RR 1.62; and being in good health, RR 1.66. Remission was less likely for patients with moderate-to-severe agoraphobia at intake, compared to those whose agoraphobia was mild or in remission.

Conclusions.—Factors associated with likelihood of remission in patients with panic disorder are identified. Lower socioeconomic status is related to poorer outcomes, whereas co-morbid social phobia is associated with a greater chance of remission. Though panic disorder appears to have a chronic course for most patients, some patients may show a more episodic course. Patients with multiple episodes of panic disorder may be more likely to have the episodic form. For patients in episodes of panic disorder with agoraphobia, panic severity is unrelated to time to remission, but agoraphobia severity is.

▶ We have made great strides in understanding and treating panic disorder. However, we have recognized for some time that we have a paucity of long-term follow-up data. We need to better understand the lifetime course of panic disorder and what happens with and without treatment. The Harvard/Brown Anxiety Disorders Research Program is a prospective study which is generating important data in this regard. This brief report provides some of the best data about predictors of outcome. Like previous research, the authors found that lower socioeconomic status was a negative predictor, as was agoraphobic severity. Surprisingly, they found that depression was not predictive of a poor outcome and that social phobia was associated with a better outcome. This study is part of a welcome group of studies filling out our knowledge about the full range of panic disorder patients. The studies usher in an era of more specifically tailored treatment for panic disorder patients.

J.C. Ballenger, M.D.

A Meta-analysis of the Treatment of Panic Disorder With or Without Agoraphobia: A Comparison of Psychopharmacological, Cognitive-Behavioral, and Combination Treatments
Van Balkom AJLM, Bakker A, Spinhoven P, et al (Vrije Universiteit, Amsterdam, The Netherlands; Leiden Univ, The Netherlands)
J Nerv Ment Dis 185:510–516, 1997   6–19

Objective.—Antidepressants and high-potency benzodiazepines and cognitive-behavioral treatment have been effective in panic attacks with or without agoraphobia (PA). Exposure in vivo has been used successfully in patients with agoraphobia. There have been few studies evaluating whether the combination of drugs with exposure in vivo is superior to either drugs or to exposure alone. A meta-analysis of 106 studies was performed to compare the short-term efficacy of benzodiazepines, antidepressants, psychological management, exposure in vivo, and combination treatments for panic disorder with and without agoraphobia.

Methods.—The pretest and posttest effect sizes Cohen's *d* were calculated within each of the 7 treatment types, high-potency benzodiazepines, antidepressants, psychological panic management, exposure in vivo, antidepressants with exposure, placebo with exposure, and psychological panic management with exposure, for conditions of panic, agoraphobia, depression, and anxiety. Treatments were compared with controls and then with each other.

Results.—There were 5,011 pretest patients and 4,016 posttest patients. High-potency benzodiazepines, antidepressants, psychological panic management, and antidepressants plus exposure were similar, and all were better than placebo for panic attacks. Exposure in vivo alone was not effective in controlling panic attacks. All 7 therapies were effective for treating agoraphobia, but antidepressants plus exposure was the most effective.

Conclusion.—The combination of antidepressants and exposure in vivo was the most effective short-term treatment for panic disorder.

▶ These authors performed a meta-analysis to attempt to provide answers to some of the most perplexing controversies in the treatment of panic disorder with and without agoraphobia. They compared the short-term efficacy of benzodiazepines, antidepressants, psychological panic management, exposure in vivo, and combination treatments in 106 studies with more than 5,000 patients. Interestingly, little difference was found between the treatments, but they were all more effective than placebo in the treatment of PAs. However, in the treatment for agoraphobia, the combination of antidepressants with exposure in vivo was superior to the other treatments and provides apparently the most effective treatment of that condition.

The first large, multicenter National Institutes of Mental Health-sponsored trial is now ready for publication and, interestingly, finds much the same thing as this meta-analysis.

J.C. Ballenger, M.D.

Delineating a Putative Phobic-Anxious Temperament in 126 Panic-Agoraphobic Patients: Toward a Rapprochement of European and US Views

Perugi G, Toni C, Benedetti A, et al (Univ of Pisa, Italy; Univ of Calif, San Diego)

J Affect Disord 47:11–23, 1998   6–20

Background.—In the United States, panic attacks are believed to be the hallmark of panic disorder, playing a major role in the development of the agoraphobic syndrome. In Europe, neurotic personality or prodromal features, such as mild depression and excessive worrying, are believed to precede the illness.

Methods and Findings.—One hundred twenty-six consecutive patients with panic disorder, with or without agoraphobia according to *DSM-III-R* criteria, were assessed by means of structured and semistructured interviews. Evidence suggested that characterologic and prodromal antecedents represent a putative phobic-anxious temperamental substrate, occurring in at least 30% of the sample. This temperament was characterized by 3 or more of the following features: increased sympathetic activity with repeated sporadic and isolated autonomic manifestations, marked fear of illness, hypersensitivity to separation, difficulty leaving familiar surroundings, substantial need for reassurance, and oversensitivity to drugs and substances. These attributes appeared to be of familial origin, resulting in illness that tended to manifest itself early.

Conclusions.—Despite the limitations of this study, the data support a pathogenic model of panic disorder, whereby genetic diathesis develops from subclinical to clinical manifestations along temperamental, panic, phobic, and avoidant patterns. Delineation of the phobic-anxious temperament will be useful for more completely charting the life course of the panic-agoraphobic spectrum. Avoidant and dependent patterns seem more distal in the pathogenetic chain and, in many patients, may be conceptualized as epiphenomenal to the disease process.

▶ This article by some of my friends in Pisa, Italy, continues the almost amusing European/American "battle" regarding the early origins of panic disorder. Probably because Don Klein pushed so hard that panic disorder evolved first with panic attacks, which is thought to then bring on the whole syndrome, the European psychiatrists and psychologists have been arguing ever since that this is overly simplistic. This group presents good data that a fair number of autonomic symptoms and personality characteristics that look like separation anxiety precede the whole onset of the panic disorder syndrome. I think that most of us recognize these observations and would agree with them. Maybe we have killed another "straw man."

J.C. Ballenger, M.D.

Illumination Perception in Photophobic Patients Suffering From Panic Disorder With Agoraphobia

Kellner M, Wiedemann K, Zihl J (Max Planck Inst of Psychiatry, Munich)
Acta Psychiatr Scand 96:72–74, 1997   6–21

Background.—In the past, it has been noted that agoraphobics sometimes exhibit an increased sensitivity to light. This study examined the relationship between agoraphobia and illumination perception and determined whether this photophobia can be corrected by cognitive behavioral therapy.

Method.—One hundred forty-four patients with panic disorder and agoraphobia were tested for altered illumination perception. Performing the illumination test on 10 normal, age-and-sex-matched subjects controlled the test. Subjects were asked to rate the illumination of a sheet of paper as "comfortable," "too dark," or "too bright." Patients who were determined to be photophobic underwent cognitive behavioral therapy. Post therapy, the illumination test was repeated to determine the effect of the therapy.

Results.—Of the agoraphobic patients, 10 were determined to be photophobic, all of them with no ophthalmologic or neurologic conditions. For the control and test groups, the illumination ratings "too bright" and "too dark" were comparable. However, the agoraphobic group specified a markedly lower level of illumination for their "comfortable" range. After cognitive-behavioral therapy, the test group had illumination test results comparable with those of the control group.

Conclusion.—Sensitivity to illumination associated with agoraphobia can be treated by cognitive-behavioral therapy. Further study needs to be done in this area to determine the role of conditioning processes, concomitant neurasthenic syndrome, and neurotransmitters in agoraphobic photophobia.

▶ I admit that this article was interesting to me for the same reasons the subject interested me when I studied this phenomenon in the early 1980s. These German investigators have again shown that patients with panic disorder, when symptomatic, have an increased sensitivity to light. We noticed early on that patients with panic disorder often wore sunglasses, choosing lighter ones, and then none at all as they got better and then well. In this study, the patients' photophobia improved with nonpharmacological treatment by cognitive-behavioral therapy, and then cleared up when their panic disorder did. The possibilities for what this situation relates to are certainly interesting, but unknown. The phenomenon remains fascinating.

J.C. Ballenger, M.D.

Obsessive-Compulsive Disorder Following Bilateral Globus Pallidus Infarction
Escalona PR, Adair JC, Roberts BB, et al (Albuquerque VA Med Ctr, NM; Univ of New Mexico, Albuquerque)
Biol Psychiatry 42:410–412, 1997   6–22

Objective.—Specific brain structures are involved in obsessive-compulsive disorder. Obsessive-compulsive disorder developed after bilateral globus pallidus infarction in 1 patient.

> *Case.*—Man, 34, with a 2-year history of major depression, was hospitalized briefly after a suicide attempt for encephalopathy and was prescribed sertraline. When his depressive symptoms disappeared, he discontinued sertraline without telling his doctor but had an uncontrollable urge to spit and to pull the hair on his legs, and began to have obsessional ideas about harming his wife and friends, sexual fantasies, and fears of contamination. He repeatedly washed his hands, checked, and counted. Results of physical and

neurologic examinations were negative. Magnetic resonance imaging revealed bilateral globus pallidus infarction from carbon monoxide poisoning. He was started on fluoxetine (20 mg/day). He never returned.

Discussion.—Injury to areas like the globus pallidus can disrupt processing in cortical and subcortical systems that are involved in obsessive-compulsive behavior. This case provides additional evidence for a neuroanatomical basis of obsessive-compulsive behavior.

▶ This is a remarkable case history of a 34-year-old-man who attempted suicide by carbon monoxide poisoning. He survived and after acute treatment, had florid obsessive-compulsive disorder for the first time with obsessions and rituals in multiple arenas. On examination, he had bilateral globus pallidus infarctions. This extraordinary case provides convincing evidence in support of imaging studies of obsessive-compulsive disorder that also implicate the basal ganglia.

J.C. Ballenger, M.D.

Alcoholism

Fluoxetine in Depressed Alcoholics: A Double-blind, Placebo-controlled Trial
Cornelius JR, Salloum IM, Ehler JG, et al (Western Psychiatric Inst and Clinic, Pittsburgh, Pa)
Arch Gen Psychiatry 54:700–705, 1997   6–23

Background.—Major depression and alcohol dependence are very common problems that frequently coexist. However, there are few data on alcoholic patients with depression. Fluoxetine is an effective treatment for major depression and may be effective in alcoholism as well; both conditions are known to be associated with low serotonergic functioning. However, there have been no studies of treatment with selective serotonergic agents in patients with both diagnoses. A trial of fluoxetine vs. placebo for depressed alcoholics is reported.

Methods.—The study included 51 patients with co-morbid major depressive disorder and alcohol dependence. Both diagnoses were made according to DSM-III-R criteria; depression was the primary diagnosis. There were 26 men and 25 women, mean age 35 years. The patients were randomized to receive 12 weeks of treatment with either fluoxetine, starting dose 20 mg/day, or placebo. Throughout treatment, weekly ratings of depression, using the 24-item Hamilton Rating Scale for Depression (HAM-D-24) and the Beck Depression Inventory (BDI), and of drinking were made.

Results.—Thirty-nine percent of patients had made a suicide attempt during their current episode. Depression outcomes on the HAM-D-24 were significantly better in the fluoxetine group than in the placebo group. There was no significant difference on the BDI, however. On within-group analyses, both measures showed significant improvements with fluoxetine. On global assessment, the improvement in depression was 3 times greater with fluoxetine than with placebo. Alcohol consumption during treatment was also significantly higher in the placebo group. Fluoxetine-treated patients avoided heavy drinking for nearly twice as long as placebo-treated patients. The level of depression was strongly correlated with change in the level of drinking in the placebo group but not in the fluoxetine group.

Conclusions.—In patients with co-morbid depression and alcohol dependence, fluoxetine effectively reduces both depressive symptoms and alcohol consumption. As in previous studies, depression is strongly related to drinking in depressed alcoholics. More research is needed to assess the results of fluoxetine treatment in alcoholic patients with lower levels of depression and suicidality.

▶ This article is an example of theoretical findings in biological psychiatry leading to a treatment trial that has, in fact, advanced our field, in this case with depressed alcoholics. Basic studies suggest that there probably is decreased serotonergic function in both depression and alcoholism, and this has led to a trial with fluoxetine. Interestingly and importantly, researchers found that not only were depressive symptoms significantly improved, but total alcohol consumption was also reduced. The general findings to date do not suggest that selective serotonin reuptake inhibitors are effective in nondepressed alcoholics, but this is open to further research. However, it is certainly important that we have a clear demonstration of a medication effect in this group of depressed alcoholics.

J.C. Ballenger, M.D.

Schizophrenia

The Evaluation and Treatment of First-Episode Psychosis
Sheitman BB, Lee H, Strauss R, et al (Dorothea Dix Hosp, Raleigh, NC)
Schizophr Bull 23:653–661, 1997   6–24

Introduction.—There have been relatively few studies of the characteristics and treatment of patients in their first episode of psychosis. These episodes are a traumatic event for patients and families. The diagnosis and treatment of patients with first-episode psychosis are reviewed.

Management of First-Episode Psychosis.—The patient should be approached with a broad differential diagnosis, including not only schizophrenia or other psychiatric conditions, but also neurologic and general medical disorders. Recent treatment and outcome studies have focused on clearly defining the onset of the illness; the end, or "offset" of the episode; and remission. Having such operational definitions permits more careful assessment of the response to treatment. There have been relatively few efficacy studies of standardized treatment for patients with first-episode psychosis. The available data strongly suggest that antipsychotic drugs should be used as both acute and maintenance therapy. However, these studies have not defined the optimal duration of maintenance therapy, nor identified those patients at low risk for relapse after treatment cessation. The typical patient is actively psychotic for 1 or 2 years before receiving treatment, and a longer duration of untreated psychosis is associated with a reduced response to treatment. Early treatment may lead to better outcomes. The newer antipsychotic agents have improved efficacy and reduced side effects; their use in patients with first-episode psychosis may lead to greater medication compliance and reduced relapse-associated morbidity.

Summary.—The available data on first-episode psychosis are reviewed. The differential diagnosis should include neurologic and general medical conditions. Antipsychotic medications constitute effective treatment in the acute and maintenance phases, but more study is needed. The authors identify some important areas for further research in first-episode psychosis, including the natural history of disease before presentation; the pattern of symptom development; the best medication regimen, including duration of treatment; indicators of outcome after drug discontinuation; and the effects of early treatment.

▶ I am pleased to see the increased recent focus on the first episode of schizophrenia. This article reviews some of those issues and underlines how much we still need to know about how long to treat patients with antipsychotics after clinical remission. However, it does underscore clearly the important clinical points that first-episode patients typically experience—1 to 2 years of psychosis before any treatment. We now know that a longer duration of untreated psychosis is associated with a poorer response. This research pushes us to increase efforts to identify psychosis as soon as possible in all individuals.

J.C. Ballenger, M.D.

Patterns of Usual Care for Schizophrenia: Initial Results From the Schizophrenia Patient Outcomes Research Team (PORT) Client Survey
Lehman AF, and the Survey Co-Investigators of the PORT Project (Univ of Maryland, Baltimore)
Schizophr Bull 24:11–20, 1998   6–25

Background.—The Agency for Health Care Policy and Research/National Institute of Mental Health Schizophrenia Patient Outcomes Research Team (PORT) has published treatment recommendations summarizing knowledge of current treatment efficacies. Conformance of current patterns of usual care for schizophrenic patients were investigated.

Methods.—The PORT surveyed a stratified random sample of 719 schizophrenic patients in 2 states. Acute inpatient programs and continuing outpatient programs in urban and rural locations were represented. Data were obtained from medical records and patient interviews to assess conformance of care with 12 treatment recommendations.

TABLE 2.—Rates of PORT Treatment Recommendation Conformance for Inpatients and Outpatients

Recommendation	Conformance Rates (%)	
	Inpatients	Outpatients
Acute neuroleptic	89.2	NA
Acute CPZ dose	62.4	NA
Maintenance neuroleptic	NA	92.3
Maintenance CPZ dose	NA	29.1
Anti-Parkinson	53.9	46.1
Depot	50.0	35.0
Adjunctive depression medications	32.2	45.7
Adjunctive anxiety medications	33.3	41.3
Adjunctive psychosis medications	22.9	14.4
Psychotherapy	96.5	45.0
Family	31.6	9.6
Vocational rehabilitation	30.4	22.5
ACT/ACM	8.6	10.1

Abbreviations: CPZ, chlorpromazine; *ACT*, assertive community treatment; *ACM*, assertive case management; *PORT*, Patient Outcomes Research Team; *NA*, not available.

(Courtesy of Lehman AF, and the Survey Co-Investigators of the PORT Project: Patterns of usual care for schizophrenia: Initial results from the Schizophrenia Patient Outcomes Research Team (PORT) client survey. *Schizophr Bull* 24:11-20, 1998.)

Findings.—The rates of conformance were, in general, less than 50%. Conformance rates were greater for pharmacologic treatment than for psychosocial ones and greater in rural than in urban areas. Conformance rates were lower for ethnic minorities than for whites. In addition, patterns of care differed between the 2 states studied (Table 2).

Conclusions.—Current usual treatment practices for schizophrenic patients generally fall far short of the recommendations based on best evidence on treatment efficacy. Better efforts are needed to ensure that results of treatment research are translated efficiently into practice.

▶ As if we needed another study showing how poorly our best recommended treatments are provided in actual practice! This study documents the poor treatment of schizophrenia in several states. It documents that conformance with current recommendations was "modest at best" and usually below 50%. The article, accompanied by a lively commentary and discussion of these findings by experts in the area, is worth reading. Among other things, they call for a real change in our approach to the diffusion of research findings into clinical practice. I certainly support this, because our traditional efforts just are not working.

J.C. Ballenger, M.D.

Natural Course of Schizophrenic Disorders: A 15-year Followup of a Dutch Incidence Cohort
Wiersma D, Nienhuis FJ, Slooff CJ, et al (Univ of Groningen, The Netherlands)
Schizophr Res 24:75–85, 1998   6–26

Background.—There have been many longitudinal studies of schizophrenia, resulting in a confusing picture of the disease course, outcomes, functional status, and associated predictors and risk factors. Data on the 15-year course of a cohort of patients with schizophrenia and other nonaffective functional psychoses from one area in the Netherlands were analyzed in the current study.

Methods.—Eighty-two first-contact patients with functional psychosis were studied. Psychopathosis, psychological impairments, negative symptoms, social disability, and the use of mental health care services were evaluated by standardized assessments.

Findings.—A pattern of chronicity and relapses with a high risk of suicide was evident. Two thirds of the patients had at least 1 relapse. After each relapse, 1 in 6 patients did not remit, 1 in 10 committed suicide, and 1 in 7 had at least 1 episode with affective psychotic symptoms that began a mean 6 years after the onset of schizophrenic disorder. The diagnoses of 5 patients were reclassified to bipolar disorder, according to *DSM-III-R* criteria. Demographic, illness, and treatment variables at onset of illness had very limited power to predict duration of psychosis and partial or full remission. Insidious onset and delayed mental health treatment predicted a longer duration of the first or subsequent episodes (Tables 2 and 3).

Conclusions.—An adequate relapse-prevention program should be a mental health priority. The importance of mental health treatment in

TABLE 2.—Course of Nonaffective Functional Psychosis Over 15 Years
(n = 82)

Course	*n* (%)
One episode followed by complete remission	10 (12.2)
Two or more episodes followed by complete remission	12 (14.6)
One episode followed by partial remission (anxiety/depression	5 (6.1)
Two or more episodes followed by partial remission (anxiety/depression)	9 (11.0)
One episode followed by negative syndrome	3 (3.7)
Two or more episodes followed by negative syndrome	24 (29.3)
Chronic psychotic all the time (one episode)	9 (11.0)
Course unknown (refused or untraceable)	10 (12.2)

(Reprinted from Wiersma D, Nienhuis FJ, Sloof CJ, et al: Natural course of schizophrenic disorders: A 15-year followup of a Dutch incidence cohort. *Schizophr Res* 24:75-85, 1998, with permission from Elsevier Science.)

TABLE 3.—Chronicity of Psychosis: No Remission (Chronic Psychosis) or Partial Remission (Negative Symptoms)

Course of Psychotic Episodes	Persisting Psychotic Symptoms (%)	Negative Symptoms (%)
First episode ($n = 82$)	12	15
Second episode ($n = 49$)	8	25
Third episode ($n = 27$)	19	22
Fourth episode ($n = 15$)	27	20

(Reprinted from Wiersma D, Nienhuis FJ, Sloof CJ, et al: Natural course of schizophrenic disorders: A 15-year followup of a Dutch incidence cohort. *Schizophr Res* 24:75-85, 1998, with permission from Elsevier Science.)

outcomes is probably variable, as an early warning and interventions strategy may prevent further damage and deterioration.

▶ This study follows a group of patients with schizophrenia over a 15-year period. Not surprisingly, it documented that two thirds of the subjects had at least 1 relapse and that approximately 1 in 6 did not recover at each 1 of these relapses. We have observed this in depression as well; that is, the prevention of relapses in patients with depression and now schizophrenia is of critical importance. In my comments on another article, I commented that the treatments we provide to try to prevent relapse and recurrence are probably more important than those we are now using to treat each individual episode. We should worry whether our current policies are not, in fact, moving away from these truths by limiting the follow-up of these patients. If we are, in fact, to follow our science, we would expend the resources to prevent these very damaging and costly recurrences of depression and schizophrenia.

J.C. Ballenger, M.D.

Predictors of Relapse and Rehospitalization in Schizophrenia and Schizoaffective Disorder

Doering S, Müller E, Köpcke W, et al (Univ of Innsbruck, Austria)
Schizophr Bull 24:87–98, 1998
6–27

Background.—Many researchers have attempted to determine the factors that predict the outcomes of schizophrenia. In the current study, the technique of classification and regression tree (CART) analysis was used for the first time to determine predictors of relapse and rehospitalization in patients with schizophrenia and schizoaffective disorder.

Methods and Findings.—Data were obtained from a German multicenter treatment study, which included 354 patients followed up for 2 years. According to CART analysis, significant predictors of relapse and rehospitalization were neuroleptic treatment; onset and previous course of disease, including precipitating factors, first manifestation, hospitalization in the preceding year, and suicide attempts; psychopathology, specifically residual-type schizoaffective disorder; social adjustment, reflected by marital status, employment, intensity of life, and Phillips score; previous life experiences, including trauma and psychiatric or developmental disturbances in childhood; and gender and age.

Conclusions.—This study confirms the value of neuroleptic treatment in schizophrenia and schizoaffective disorder. It also supports the notion of a multifactorial cause and the vulnerability stress model of schizophrenia.

▶ In this German multicenter study, more than 350 patients with schizophrenia and schizoaffective disorder were followed up for 2 years. The study used a new technique for CART analysis to predict relapse and rehospitalization. The investigators were, in fact, able to define predictors of relapse that were consistent with considerable previous work and included neuroleptic treatment, some factors of the onset and previous course and issues in psychopathology, issues of marital status and employment, previous life experience, age, and gender. This study found clear support for the stress lability model of schizophrenia and the value of neuroleptics.

J.C. Ballenger, M.D.

Posttrauma Syndromes

Media Triggers of Post-traumatic Stress Disorder 50 Years After the Second World War
Hilton C (Salford Mental Health Trust, Manchester, England)
Int J Geriatr Psychiatry 12:862–867, 1997   6–28

Purpose.—Posttraumatic stress disorder (PTSD) can be acute, chronic, or of delayed onset. It can even occur in elderly people many years after a traumatic event. Two elderly patients with symptoms of PTSD brought on by media reports related to WW II are reported.

Patients.—The patients were men, aged 72 and 76, who had been exposed to combat action and wounded during service in WW II. Both had also been present at the liberation of a Nazi concentration camp. One had no history of previous psychiatric problems, whereas the other had had difficulties with alcohol abuse, gambling, and depression. Both men developed distressing symptoms—including reexperiencing the traumatic event, avoidance symptoms, and increased arousal—in response to media commemorations of the fiftieth anniversary of the end of WW II. One patient briefly mentioned his war experiences but denied that his distress was related to them. He avoided further reminders of the war. The other patient agreed to further evaluation, which confirmed the diagnosis of PTSD. After receiving an additional war pension, he dropped out of therapy.

Discussion.—Delayed onset or chronic PTSD or both appear to have been activated in these patients by media reminders of their traumatic experiences during service in WW II. Elderly patients with PTSD may avoid talking about past traumatic experiences because of the distress it engenders. In this situation, the diagnosis of posttraumatic symptoms may be missed unless a military and trauma history is taken.

▶ This article documents something that I have had to deal with repeatedly with a patient of mine who has PTSD from World War II. This article presents 2 cases of elderly patients who had marked PTSD triggered by the media coverage of the fiftieth anniversary of the end of World War II. Unfortunately, it's a poorly appreciated fact that a large number of WW II PTSD patients continue to have difficulties.

J.C. Ballenger, M.D.

Suicide After Natural Disasters

Krug EG, Kresnow M-J, Peddicord JP, et al (Natl Ctr for Injury Prevention and Control, Atlanta, Ga)
N Engl J Med 338:373–378, 1998   6–29

Introduction.—The short-term and long-term physical sequelae after natural and man-made disasters are well known. The effects of disasters on mental health are under debate. Posttraumatic stress disorder and depression have been reported after disasters. Less is understood about suicide. With the link between disasters and depression and the link between depression and suicide, it is reasonable to suspect a relationship between disasters and suicide rates. Suicide rates were investigated in U.S. counties where single natural disasters had occurred.

Methods.—Of all U.S. counties with single natural disasters identified by the Federal Emergency Management Agency during the period 1982–1989, 377 were followed for data on suicide during the 36 months before and 48 months after the disaster. Data were aligned around the month of the disaster. Pooled rates were calculated according to type of disaster. Suicide rates before and after the disaster were compared for the affected counties and the entire United States.

Results.—Suicide rates increased 13.8% (12.1% to 13.8% per 100,000) in the 4 years after flood disasters. In the 2 years after hurricanes, suicide rates increased 31.0% (12.0% to 15.7% per 100,000). There was a 62.9% (19.2% to 31.3% per 100,000) increase in the year after earthquakes. At 4 years after earthquakes, there was a nonsignificant 19.7% increase in suicides. Rates remained stable during this time for the remaining United States. Increases in suicide rates were observed for both sexes and all age groups. There were no significant changes in suicide rates regarding tornadoes or severe storms.

Conclusion.—Suicide rates rise after severe earthquakes, floods, and hurricanes. Much can be done through mental health support to prevent or diminish the impact of natural disasters, thus possibly reducing the number of disaster-related suicides.

▶ This study looks at suicide r‌ċ .es after the natural disasters of floods, earthquakes, and hurricanes. Frankly, I chose this article because of my own experience in running a large psychiatric service in a city hit by a disastrous hurricane. We saw an increased rate of depression and posttraumatic stress disorder, as had previous communities hit by disasters. In this study, suicide rates increased almost 14% in the 4 years after floods, 31% in the couple of years after hurricanes, and almost 63% in the first year after earthquakes. We learned in a hurry that mental health services are needed to deal with the aftermath of these types of disasters, and this study underscores that fact.

J.C. Ballenger, M.D.

Physical and Sexual Assault History in Women With Serious Mental Illness: Prevalence, Correlates, Treatment, and Future Research Directions
Goodman LA, Rosenberg SD, Mueser KT, et al (Univ of Maryland, College Park)
Schizophr Bull 23:685–696, 1997   6–30

Objective.—In women with serious mental illness (SMI), the prevalence of sexual or physical abuse ranges between 51% and 97%. The prevalence, correlates, and treatment of physical and sexual assault among women with schizophrenia and other types of major mental illness were reviewed, as well as the role of trauma in the lives of women who have schizophrenia and other serious mental illnesses (SMIs). A research strategy for illuminating the relationship between trauma, the course of illness, and the treatment of schizophrenia in women is presented.

Correlates of Physical and Sexual Victimization.—Correlates in women with SMI include sexual delusions, depression, major medical problems, somatization, interpersonal sensitivity, anxiety, paranoid ideology, and psychoticism. In 1 study, victims of child abuse were significantly more likely to have schizophrenia. In another study of adult abuse, 40% of female inpatients who had been physically abused within the past year had posttraumatic stress disorder. Abused female inpatients remain hospitalized longer, have histories of suicide or suicidal ideation, are significantly more likely to be substance abusers, and have compulsive sexual behavior.

Treatment of Trauma Correlates.—There are few validated treatments for women with SMI. Treatment difficulties are compounded by distrust or fear of the service provider and inability to keep appointments because of continued abuse. Some women with schizophrenia may benefit from a gradual form of traditional exposure-based psychotherapy, but others may experience substantial stress when asked to recall disturbing memories.

Hypothesized Relationships Between Traumatic Victimization and Schizophrenia.—Schizophrenia may be a risk factor for adult abuse, abuse may trigger schizophrenia, or abused women may receive a misdiagnosis of schizophrenia when they actually have posttraumatic stress disorder. Abuse is also a risk factor for homelessness and HIV infection.

Research Directions.—The extent and nature of victimization of women with SMI; the interrelationship of schizophrenia and abuse; and the effects of poverty, substance abuse, homelessness, and stigma need to be investigated, and trauma treatment models need to be developed.

▶ One of the most powerful recent research areas is the documentation of the very high prevalence of physical and sexual assault in our patients. Although the issues of causation remain complex, the negative implications are being increasingly documented. In this study, seriously mentally ill women were again shown to have high rates of abuse with serious implications for their treatment and outcome of their schizophrenia. I hope this work focuses attention on this important area.

J.C. Ballenger, M.D.

Cholinergic Nerves Mediate Stress-induced Intestinal Transport Abnormalities in Wistar-Kyoto Rats
Saunders PR, Hanssen NPM, Perdue MH (McMaster Univ, Hamilton, Ont, Canada)
Am J Physiol 36:G486–G490, 1997   6–31

Objective.—Whereas the relationship between stress and gastric ulceration has been established, the effect of stress on gastrointestinal mucosa has not been well studied. Stress-induced changes in intestinal physiology in Wistar-Kyoto rats were compared with those in the parent Wistar strain, and the role of cholinergic nerves and muscarinic or nicotinic receptors in mediating the responses was examined.

Methods.—A 20-cm segment of jejunum was removed from a group of control rats injected intraperitoneally with saline and from a group of stressed rats injected intraperitoneally with either atropine sulfate, atropine methyl nitrate (a peripheral muscarine antagonist that does not cross the blood-brain barrier), or hexamethonium (a nicotinic antagonist) and then restrained for 2 hours before the procedure. Mucosa was scraped from the distal 5 cm of the excised jejunum. Cholinesterase activity was determined in intestinal mucosal homogenates. One-way and 2-way analyses of variance were used to compare groups.

Results.—Stressed rats had significantly larger stress-induced changes in ion secretion and permeability. The changes were almost twice as great in tissue from the Wistar-Kyoto rats as in tissue from the parent Wistar strain. Tissue from the Wistar-Kyoto strain had a significantly increased response to acetylcholine compared to the parent Wistar strain, suggesting a decreased breakdown of acetylcholine in intestinal mucosa. Atropine sulfate had no effect on transport in control Wistar-Kyoto rats but significantly inhibited transport in stressed rats.

Conclusion.—Stress-induced changes in ion secretion and permeability are mediated by acetylcholine.

▶ It may seem odd that I picked this article for inclusion in this year's YEAR BOOK, but for me it is this type of basic physiologic research that is helping to document the issues involved in many of the problems we see in psychiatry and general medicine. This group studied the stress-induced ulcer type changes and was able to demonstrate clearly that the stress effects are mediated by acetylcholine. It is a fairly straightforward finding that can easily be understood by clinicians and patients alike.

J.C. Ballenger, M.D.

Pain From Rectal Distension in Women With Irritable Bowel Syndrome: Relationship to Sexual Abuse

Whitehead WE, Crowell MD, Davidoff AL, et al (Univ of North Carolina, Chapel Hill; Johns Hopkins Univ, Baltimore, Md)
Dig Dis Sci 42:796–804, 1997
6–32

Objective.—Several studies have reported an increased prevalence of sexual or physical abuse in women with irritable bowel syndrome (IBS). To determine whether increased sensitivity to pain during rectal distention is a reliable indicator of IBS and not the result of psychological influences, perceptual sensitivity was measured in sexually abused and nonabused women with IBS, using the ascending method of limits, tracking, and signal detection.

Methods.—Women with IBS and controls completed an abuse interview and 2 questionnaires (Cornell Medical Index and Trauma Symptom Checklist). Rectal muscle tone and sensory thresholds were measured by the barostat technique. Three sensory threshold tests for moderate pain followed the barostat procedure. The threshold was determined using the ascending method and confirmed using the tracking technique at each of 3 distention pressures.

Results.—There were 17 sexually abused women and 15 nonabused women with IBS and 13 sexually abused women and 14 nonabused women without IBS. Although distention volume pain thresholds were significantly lower in nonabused women with IBS than in nonabused women without IBS, these thresholds were associated with levels of anxiety or somatization. Distention volume pain thresholds were similar among abused women with and without IBS. This interaction approached significance. Distention pressure pain threshold results were similar for the groups. These patterns were confirmed by the tracking method. There was a significant relationship between abuse and IBS. The perceptual response to pain was similar between groups.

Conclusion.—It appears that the lower pain thresholds measured in patients with IBS are related to levels of anxiety or somatization rather than increased sensitivity.

▶ The IBS is 1 of the most common conditions in general medicine and gastroenterology. It is an extremely costly and problematic condition. The field is developing a better and better understanding of this condition and beginning to involve psychiatry more. We have followed these issues in previous YEAR BOOKS and have documented the high prevalence of sexual victimizations in these patients, as well as the issue that there appears to be increased pain sensitivity to rectal distention in these patients. This article struggles with whether these 2 issues are correlated and finds that they were not in this study.

J.C. Ballenger, M.D.

Geriatrics

Diagnosis and Treatment of Alzheimer Disease and Related Disorders: Consensus Statement of the American Association for Geriatric Psychiatry, the Alzheimer's Association, and the American Geriatrics Society
Small GW, Rabins PV, Barry PP, et al (Univ of California, Los Angeles; Johns Hopkins Univ, Baltimore; Boston Univ; et al)
JAMA 278:1363–1371, 1997
6–33

Objective.—Early diagnosis and treatment of Alzheimer's disease (AD) are crucial to controlling the cost of expensive treatments and allowing patient and family time to prepare. A consensus conference on AD and related diseases was convened to examine the prevalence and risk factors for AD, its impact on society, the different forms of dementia and their characteristics, safe and effective treatments for AD, indications and contra-indications for specific treatments, management strategies for the primary care physician, availability of medical and community resources, important policy issues and increased access to care for patients with dementia, and promising areas of research.

Prevalence, Risk Factors, and Societal Impact of AD.—The prevalence of AD in individuals older than 65 is 6% to 8% and in individuals older than 85 is almost 30%. Only 40% of primary care physicians are aware that AD is the primary cause of dementia in older individuals. The main risk factors are age and family history. Genetic predisposition to AD is rare. The annual cost of medical care, long-term care, home care, and lost productivity as a result of AD approaches $100 billion. The toll on caregivers is inestimable.

Forms and Characteristics of Different Dementias.—Dementia, an acquired form of cognitive decline, includes AD, which affects about 67% of dementia patients; vascular dementia, which accounts for 15%; and dementia associated with Lewy bodies (DLB), which accounts for about 25%. Onset is gradual and progressive, initially affecting cognition. Changes in behavior and mood are common. Motor and sensory functions decline in the later stages. Delirium or depression can also be present. A diagnosis includes a comprehensive physical examination and a neurological and mental status evaluation.

Safe and Effective Treatment for AD and Indications and Contraindications for Specific Treatments.—Cholinesterase inhibitors can be used to treat cognitive impairment. Estrogen, nonsteroidal anti-inflammatory drugs, and botanical agents such as ginkgo biloba are being evaluated for ability to improve cognitive function. Antioxidants or selective monoamine oxidase inhibitors appear to slow functional decline. Antidepressants can be used to treat depression, and antipsychotic drugs can be used to improve symptoms of agitation or psychosis.

Management Strategies for Primary Care Physicians.—Patient management recommendations include scheduling regular surveillance and office visits every three to six months, working closely with family and caregivers to exchange information, setting up regular exercise routines to improve mood and behavior, encouraging families to provide a stimulating but not over-stimulating environment that maximizes the patient's cognitive functions and provides a sense of security, and warning families of the hazards of wandering and driving.

Medical Specialties and Community Resources.—Medical specialists are sometimes necessary. Locations of community services that provide help in independent living, skilled nursing care, and respite for family caregivers should be made available to families.

Policy Issues.—There is a need for comprehensive and integrated medical and psychiatric care for AD patients. Referral and access programs for AD patients and caregivers and reimbursement programs should be developed and expanded. The national health care delivery system needs to understand that whereas AD is a progressive disease, many of its symptoms can and should be treated.

Promising Areas for Future Research.—Some areas for future research are physician knowledge of AD, physician and societal attitudes toward AD, fiscal barriers, demographic and socioeconomic factors, disease complexity, role of specialists, accuracy of diagnosis, current and new therapies, the cost-effectiveness of long-term care and therapy, caregiver interventions, and the best ways to maintain the safety and independence of AD patients.

Conclusions and Recommendations.—Physicians need to be educated about the prevalence, diagnosis, and treatment of AD. Physicians should be aware that the diagnosis of AD is primarily one of inclusion and that AD symptoms can and should be treated. Education, support, and counseling is imperative for caregivers. Better delivery and reimbursement systems must be established, and long-term research into physician and societal beliefs, cost-effectiveness of treatment, and treatment strategies need to be conducted.

▶ This important article summarizes the consensus conference held in January 1997, on Alzheimer's disease. The primary audience was primary care physicians, and they argue that most cases can be managed in primary care settings. However, they do underscore that cases with atypical presentations, severe impairment, or complex comorbidity benefit from referral from specialists, including psychiatrists. This is a particularly important issue for psychiatry in another way because 50% of caregivers become depressed.

J.C. Ballenger, M.D.

Eating Disorders

Family and Individual Therapy in Anorexia Nervosa: A 5-year Follow-up
Eisler I, Dare C, Russell GFM, et al (Inst of Psychiatry, London; Maudsley Hosp, London)
Arch Gen Psychiatry 54:1025–1030, 1997   6–34

Background.—Specific psychological treatments appear to be effective in patients with eating disorders. The current controlled trial determined whether psychological treatments previously reported to be effective in anorexia nervosa have lasting benefits.

Methods.—Participants in a previous trial of family therapy for anorexia and bulimia nervosa were followed up at 5 years. Family or individual supportive therapy had been provided to 80 outpatients for 1 year beginning at hospital discharge after weight restoration. The patients had been divided into 4 prognostically homogeneous groups, the 2 most important being patients with early onset and short history of anorexia nervosa and those with late-onset anorexia nervosa. At 5 years, treatment efficacies were assessed by weight maintenance and by categories of general outcome and dimensions of clinical functioning, defined by the Morgan-Russell scales.

Findings.—The group as a whole showed significant improvements, mostly attributed to the natural outcome of anorexia nervosa. Improvements were most evident in the early-onset and short-history groups. Significant benefits attributable to the previous psychological treatments were still evident in 2 prognostic groups, favoring family therapy for patients with early onset and short history of anorexia and favoring individual supportive therapy for patients with late-onset anorexia nervosa.

Conclusions.—In these patients, much of the improvement documented at the 5-year follow-up could be attributed to the natural outcome of anorexia nervosa. However, the long-term benefits of psychological treatments completed 5 years earlier were still evident.

▶ Knowing what does and does not work in the treatment of anorexia nervosa is gradually becoming clear. A series of studies documenting the long-term efficacy of various treatments are available, and we have followed this issue for several years in the YEAR BOOK. This study from the Maudsley Hospital in London followed 80 patients over a 5-year period. A general improvement in the group as a whole, probably secondary to the natural history of anorexia nervosa was documented. However, the authors are able to clearly document favorable and lasting results of psychological treatments, particularly in certain subgroups.

J.C. Ballenger, M.D.

The Prevalence of High-level Exercise in the Eating Disorders: Etiological Implications
Davis C, Katzman DK, Kaptein S, et al (Toronto Hosp; Univ of Toronto; Hosp for Sick Children, Toronto; et al)
Compr Psychiatry 38:321–326, 1997   6–35

Background.—Increasing evidence suggests that physical activity may play a central role in the pathogenesis of some eating disorders. The physical activity history of patients with anorexia nervosa (AN) and bulimia nervosa (BN) during and before the onset of these disorders was investigated.

Methods.—Two patient groups were studied. The first consisted of 127 women enrolled in an eating disorder program; the second, 40 hospitalized adolescent girls diagnosed as having AN. Each patient underwent a detailed structured interview.

Findings.—A large proportion of these patients were exercising excessively during an acute phase of the disorder. Overexercising was significantly more common among those with AN than among those with BN. Premorbid activity levels significantly predicted excessive exercise comorbidity.

Conclusions.—Physical activity appears to be central in the development and maintenance of some eating disorders. These findings have important clinical implications because many people combine dieting and exercise in an attempt to lose weight and because strenuous physical activity in malnourished persons can have adverse effects.

▶ Anyone who works in the eating disorders field knows the pressure many of these patients feel to exercise. This study documents clearly that overexercise appears to be central in the development *and* maintenance of these disorders, particularly anorexia nervosa. This takes on added importance when you consider the number of people in the United States, particularly women, who are exercising and dieting.

J.C. Ballenger, M.D.

Psychiatry, Primary Care, and General Medicine

Treatment of Depressive Symptoms in Human Immunodeficieny Virus–Positive Patients
Markowitz JC, Kocsis JH, Fishman B, et al (Cornell Univ, New York)
Arch Gen Psychiatry 55:452–457, 1998   6–36

Introduction.—Few data are available regarding psychotherapy for depressive symptoms in patients with HIV. Some clinicians doubt whether psychotherapy could help patients with HIV as such patients "have reason to be depressed." The effectiveness of treating depressive symptoms with either interpersonal psychotherapy, cognitive behavioral therapy, supportive psychotherapy, or supportive psychotherapy with imipramine were compared in 101 research subjects who were HIV seropositive.

Methods.—Patients with known HIV seropositivity for at least 6 months were randomized to 16 weeks of treatment for depressive symptoms. Treatment manuals, treatment teams, and team leaders were used to encourage uniform treatment by therapists. All patients had a score of 15 or higher on a 24-item Hamilton Depression Rating Scale, had been given a diagnosis of clinical depression, and were physically healthy enough to attend outpatient therapy sessions. Patients were monitored for treatment adherence.

Results.—Significantly greater improvements on depressive measures were observed in patients randomized to interpersonal psychotherapy and supportive psychotherapy with imipramine, compared with those randomized to supportive psychotherapy and cognitive behavioral therapy.

Conclusion.—This is the first known trial of individual antidepressant psychotherapy for patients who are HIV-positive. Patients who are HIV-positive warrant and respond to specific antidepressant treatments, just like other medically ill patients with depressive symptoms. Interpersonal psychotherapy seems to be a particularly beneficial psychotherapy for patients with HIV and depressive symptoms.

▶ This article reports on the ambitious and important study of treatment of depression in HIV-positive patients with depressive symptoms. The authors found that interpersonal psychotherapy and supportive psychotherapy with imipramine were particularly effective, more effective than supportive or cognitive behavioral therapy. It would seem logical that interpersonal psychotherapy would be more effective in this population because it focuses on practical solutions to difficult situations. The study also makes it clear that treatment is effective for patients who, it is said, "have reason to be depressed." They argue with good data that treatment is appropriate because it is quite effective.

J.C. Ballenger, M.D.

The Morbidity of Insomnia Uncomplicated by Psychiatric Disorders
Weissman MM, Greenwald S, Niño-Murcia G, et al (Columbia Univ, New York; New York State Psychiatric Inst; Sleep Medicine and Neuroscience Inst, Palo Alto, Calif; et al)
Gen Hosp Psychiatry 19:245–250, 1997   6–37

Introduction.—There is a known association between insomnia and psychiatric symptoms (usually depression and anxiety), emotional distress, and impaired functioning. It is not known how much of the morbidity of sleep problems can be accounted for by associated psychiatric and sub-

TABLE 3.—First Onset of a Psychiatric Disorder Over the Subsequent Year in Individuals With Insomnia and No Psychiatric Disorder as Compared With Individuals With Neither

| | At First Interview | | | |
| | Insomnia and No Psychiatric Disorder | No Insomnia and No Psychiatric Disorder | | |
Number at Risk	414	4826	Odds Ratio*	95% CI
First onset in following year	Rate/100			
Major depression	2.7	0.5	5.4†	2.6–11.3
Panic disorder	1.0	0.1	20.3†	4.4–93.8
Obsessive-compulsive disorder	1.6	0.7	2.2	0.9–5.1
Alcohol abuse	3.3	1.8	2.3†	1.2–4.3
Drug abuse	0.6	0.3	1.9	0.5–7.2

*Odds ratio adjusted by age, sex, and site.
†*p* less than 0.05.
Abbreviations: CI, confidence interval.
(Reprinted from Weissman MM, Greenwald S, Niño-Murcia G: The morbidity of insomnia uncomplicated by psychiatric disorders. *Gen Hosp Psychiatry* 19:245-250, 1997, with permission from Elsevier Science.)

stance abuse disorders vs. the sleep problem itself. Sleep problems can be an early sign of a psychiatric problem. Data from a large community epidemiologic survey was used to evaluate the independent effects of insomnia and describe treatment used and subsequent first onset of psychiatric disorders in individuals with insomnia uncomplicated by psychiatric disorders or substance abuse.

Methods.—Data was used from an epidemiologic community survey of over 10,000 adults living in 3 U.S. communities. Individuals with insomnia in the past year without any psychiatric disorder ever (uncomplicated insomnia), with a psychiatric disorder (complicated insomnia), and with neither insomnia nor psychiatric disorders ever were compared for treatment use and first onset of a psychiatric disorder in the following year.

Results.—Eight percent, 14.9%, and 2.5%, respectively, of individuals with uncomplicated insomnia, complicated insomnia, and neither underwent treatment from the general medical sector for emotional problems in the 6 months before the interview. The rates for seeking help from the psychiatric specialty sector were 3.8%, 9.4%, and 1.2%, respectively. Persons with insomnia and no psychiatric disorder, compared with those who had neither were at significant risk for first onset of major depression, panic disorder, and alcohol abuse in the subsequent year (Table 3).

Conclusion.—Uncomplicated insomnia is associated with increased use of medical and mental health care for emotional problems and subsequent first onset of certain psychiatric disorders in the following year. It would be helpful if uncomplicated insomnia could be diagnosed and treated early.

▶ Insomnia is 1 of the most common but difficult complaints for physicians to treat. Excellent scientific methodology was used to determine some of the core issues of insomnia. The authors documented that uncomplicated insomnia is itself associated with increased use of medical and psychiatric treatment resources for emotional problems. They also documented that these patients have an increased risk of first-onset in the next year of several psychiatric problems, particularly depression. The authors argue that early diagnosis of uncomplicated insomnia should be a goal, but clearly is not one, in most medical settings at this point in time.

J.C. Ballenger, M.D.

Effect of Carbamazepine on Pain Scores of Unipolar Depressed Patients With Chronic Pain: A Trial of Off-On-Off-On Design

Kudoh A, Ishihara H, Matsuki A (Univ of Hirosaki, Japan)
Clin J Pain 14:61–65, 1998

6–38

Background.—About half of patients with depression experience different types of somatic pain, such as facial pain, headache, and cervical, abdominal, back, and lower limb pain. The mechanisms responsible for such pain are unclear, but physiologic disorders such as changes in amine metabolism or partial neurogenic dysfunction have been associated with pain. The efficacy of carbamazepine (CBZ), commonly used to treat neurogenic pain, was investigated in depressed patients with chronic pain.

Methods.—Fifteen patients were included. In all cases, antidepressant therapy had failed to relieve depression or pain. Initially, patients were given 450 mg CBZ, in doses of 150 mg 3 times a day. The dose was increased until the patients had satisfactory pain relief. This dose was continued for 3 weeks, at which time CBZ was stopped and a lactose

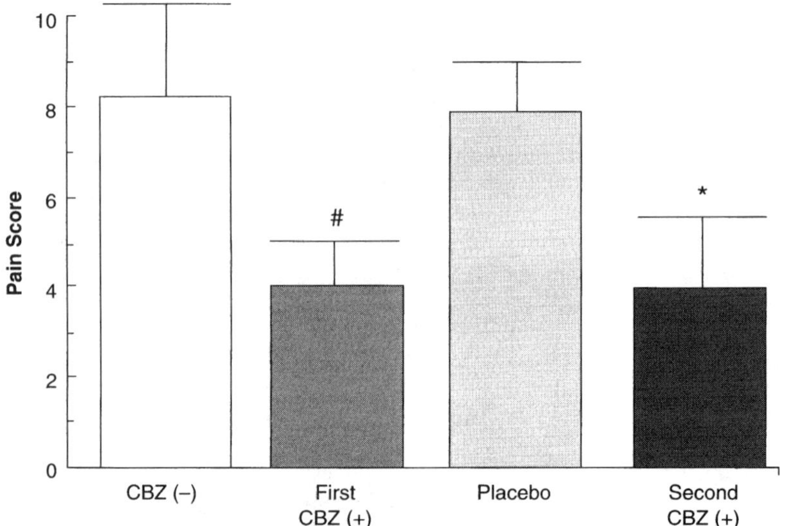

FIGURE 1.—Pain score before and after the first and second carbamazepine (CBZ) treatments. Data are expressed as mean ± SD. #*P* < 05 vs. CBZ(-). **P* < 0.05 vs. placebo. (Courtesy of Kudoh A, Ishihara H, Matsuki A: Effect of carbamazepine on pain scores of unipolar depressed patients with chronic pain: A trial of off-on-off-on design. *Clin J Pain* 14:61-65, 1998.)

placebo was administered orally 3 times a day for 3 weeks. Thereafter, CBZ was administered for another 3 weeks at the dose that previously provided satisfactory pain relief.

Findings.—Carbamazepine significantly reduced mean pain score, from 8.2 to 4 after the initial treatment. After CBZ cessation, the pain score rose significantly to 8 and then declined to 4.1 after initiation of the second treatment. Hamilton scores also decreased significantly with CBZ therapy, from 27.4 to 20.2 (Fig 1).

Conclusions.—Carbamazepine appears to have both analgesic and antidepressive effects in patients with depression and chronic pain. Alternatively, the relief of pain may result in the relief of depressive symptoms.

▶ This Japanese group documents that carbamazepine is effective in decreasing chronic pain in unipolar depressed patients who have not responded to antidepressants. Interestingly, this group's study was performed by a Japanese anesthesiologist. Many times, these very difficult patients do, in fact, end up in anesthesiology and are very difficult to treat. They often undergo many procedures in an attempt to deal with their chronic pain, and carbamazepine appears to be a clear and effective alternative.

J.C. Ballenger, M.D.

Placebo-controlled Treatment Trial of Depression in Elderly Physically Ill Patients

Evans M, Hammond M, Wilson K, et al (Wirral and W Cheshire Community Healthcare NHS Trust, Bebington, England: Univ of Liverpool, England)
Int J Geriatr Psychiatry 12:817–824, 1997   6–39

Objective.—Depression is related to physical illness in elderly people, particularly in patients with chronic progressive illness and in patients over age 75. However, studies of treatment for depression usually exclude patients with physical illness or cognitive impairment. This randomized, placebo-controlled trial examined the effects of drug treatment for hospitalized elderly patients.

Methods.—The study included 82 elderly medical inpatients with depression, 62 women and 20 men, mean age 80. Most of the patients had at least 1 acute and 1 chronic health problem. Patients with cognitive impairment were not excluded. The patients were randomized in double-blind fashion to receive 8 weeks of treatment with fluoxetine 20 mg/day or placebo. Responses were evaluated using the 17-item Hamilton Depression Rating Scale. The efficacy analysis included 62 patients who completed at least 3 weeks of treatment. Twenty-one patients in each group completed the full 8 weeks of treatment.

Results.—Among patients completing treatment, the response rate was 67% with fluoxetine vs. 38% with placebo, though the difference was insignificant. For patients taking fluoxetine, the results tended toward continued improvement with time. Analysis of 37 seriously physically ill patients who completed at least 5 weeks of treatment suggested a significant improvement in mood with fluoxetine. Fluoxetine treatment was well tolerated.

Conclusions.—In depressed elderly patients with physical illness, treatment with fluoxetine approximately doubles the chances of recovery, compared with placebo. Even with severe or multiple physical illnesses or both, fluoxetine is an effective treatment for depression in the elderly. More research is needed to confirm the better response to treatment among patients with serious physical disease. Psychological support also plays an important role in the management of depression in the elderly.

▶ As we fill in the gaps of treatment of depression in the elderly, this article provides data about the subgroup of patients who are not only elderly but also physically ill. The researchers report the welcome result that these patients did respond to fluoxetine and that severe physical illness did not interfere with that response. We find this again and again with the demonstration that antidepressants work in patients with heart disease, stroke, cancer, and other serious illnesses. However, most general physicians do not operate as if they know that fact. This is another situation of what we know not being generally utilized, especially in general medicine.

J.C. Ballenger, M.D.

Functional Status in Coronary Artery Disease: A One-year Prospective Study of the Role of Anxiety and Depression
Sullivan MD, LaCroix AZ, Baum C, et al (Univ of Washington, Seattle; Ctr for Health Studies, Seattle)
Am J Med 103:348–356, 1997   6–40

Objective.—Depression and anxiety have been implicated in the development and progression of, or death from, heart disease. Depression has been shown to affect the functional status of patients with or without chronic medical illnesses. The influence of depression and anxiety on functional status of patients with coronary disease was studied prospectively.

Methods.—Between December 1991 and February 1993, 198 patients (34 female) aged 45 to 79 years in 2 HMOs in Washington, undergoing elective cardiac catheterization for suspected coronary artery disease, were interviewed after the procedure to obtain sociodemographic information, to assess physical functioning and activity interference (repeated at 6 and 12 months), and to measure severity of anxiety and depression on the Hamilton Rating Scales for Depression and Anxiety. When possible, the patient's spouse completed the spousal version of the Multidimensional Pain Inventory. Patients were divided into 4 groups depending on their anxiety and depression scores. Using analysis of covariance, baseline, and

6- and 12-month physical function and activity interference measures were compared and correlated with baseline variables.

Results.—Physical function at all time points was significantly related to the number of coronary arteries stenosed 70% or more at baseline. Physical function scores at baseline and 12 months were significantly correlated to anxiety quartiles at baseline and to depression quartiles at baseline. Changes in physical function and activity interference scores at 12 months were significantly correlated with baseline anxiety quartiles and with baseline depression quartiles but not with the number of occluded arteries at baseline or with age, sex, education, social class, chronic disease score, or medical vs. surgical management.

Conclusion.—Although this was an observational study using self-reported measures of physical function and activity interference, these measures at baseline and 12 months were significantly and consistently related to both baseline anxiety and depression quartiles and not to the number of occluded arteries at baseline.

▶ This remarkable study is from the research group in Seattle in the Center for Health Studies of the Group Health Cooperative of Puget Sound, a large HMO. A group of patients who had coronary artery disease documented on cardiac catheterization were studied for 1 year. At baseline, physical function was correlated with the number of vessels stenosed and measures of anxiety and depression. At 1 year, decreases in physical functioning were no longer associated with the number of main coronary vessels that were demonstrated to be stenosed at baseline, but were still significantly associated with anxiety and depression. This is the kind of study that our field needs to integrate into its thinking and its lobbying and action on local medical fronts. This essentially says that the critical issue in the treatment of people with coronary artery disease is to treat their anxiety and depression. How we change this type of situation is 1 of the primary challenges for our field.

J.C. Ballenger, M.D.

Personality Disorders Among Difficult Patients
Schafer S, Nowlis DP (Univ of California, San Francisco)
Arch Fam Med 7:126–129, 1998   6–41

Background.—Although problems in a physician-patient relationship should not be attributed solely to a psychiatric disorder in the patient, some problems may stem from an unrecognized personality disorder. The association between the "difficult patient" status and personality disorder was investigated in this study.

Methods.—The study included 21 patients subjectively experienced as "difficult" by 9 family physicians. Twenty-two patients who were not considered difficult made up a control group. The subjects underwent the Diagnostic Interview for Personality Disorders.

Findings.—Personality disorders were present in 7 of the difficult patients and in only 1 of the control subjects. Five of the 7 difficult patients with personality disorder were found to have dependent personality disorder. None of the family physicians had realized that these patients had personality disorders.

Conclusions.—Unrecognized personality disorders, especially dependent personality disorder, may underlie difficult physician-patient relationships. Physician awareness of this may enhance understanding and treatment of difficult patients.

▶ I have always wondered how nonpsychiatric physicians deal with patients with some of the personality disorders that are so difficult for psychiatrists, who are trained to deal with them. In this study, family medicine physicians identified patients they experienced as difficult, and a large percentage of these pateints did, in fact, have undetected personality disorders. They argue that it would be helpful if family medicine physicians learn about personality disorders. I would agree with that.

J.C. Ballenger, M.D.

The Nature and Prevalence of Anxiety Disorders in Primary Care
Nisenson LG, Pepper CM, Schwenk TL, et al (Univ of Michigan, Ann Arbor)
Gen Hosp Psychiatry 20:21–28, 1998   6–42

Background.—Anxiety disorders are among the most common psychiatric problems in the community, with reported prevalences of 12.6% to 24.9%. The current study determined the prevalence, nature, and correlates of anxiety disorders in primary care practices and assessed their comorbidity with major depressive disorder.

Methods.—Four hundred twenty-five patients were recruited from the waiting rooms of primary care physicians. These patients were assessed by means of standard structured interviews, self-ratings, and physician ratings.

TABLE 1.—Prevalence Estimates of SCID Anxiety Disorder Diagnoses

Anxiety Disorder	Lifetime N (%)	Current N (%)
Any anxiety disorder	102 (23.9)	62 (14.6)
Panic disorder	29 (6.7)	13 (3.1)
Agoraphobia w/o panic	10 (2.4)	3 (0.7)
Social phobia	35 (8.2)	11 (2.6)
Simple phobia	42 (9.8)	27 (6.3)
Obsessive/compulsive disorder	10 (2.3)	9 (2.0)
Generalized anxiety disorder	NA	17 (4.1)

(Reprinted from Nisenson LG, Pepper CM, Schwenk TL, et al: The nature and prevalence of anxiety disorders in primary care. *Gen Hosp Psychiatry* 20:21-28, 1998, with permission from Elsevier Science.)

Findings.—The prevalence of current anxiety disorders was 14.6%. The lifetime prevalence was 23.9% (Table 1). Anxiety disorders were relatively mild. Thirty percent of the patients with anxiety disorder had only simple phobias. Anxiety disorders were often comorbid with depression, which aided physicians in their diagnosis of depression. However, physicians tended to misdiagnose anxiety disorders as depression.

Conclusions.—Anxiety disorders appear to be common in a primary care population. However, because of their relative mildness, such disorders may not require primary care physicians' increased attention to detection and treatment. Efforts should instead be focused on more severe cases of anxiety disorder.

▶ Although much of our attention in the primary care setting has been focused on depression, these authors point out that anxiety is at least as common and perhaps even more so. This study goes beyond previous studies by using the Structured Clinical Interview of DSM-III-R (SCID) to diagnose patients. They found anxiety disorders to be very prevalent, with 14.6% of the sample having a current anxiety disorder. They confirm what we already knew, that these patients also have high rates of depression, substance abuse, somatic symptoms, and eating disorders, and that these patients do poorly. They were able to test previous questions of whether anxiety helped with the diagnosis and detection of depression and found that it did, but only somewhat.

Unfortunately, they return to a frequent bias of family medicine and state that "given the ... other important potential uses of physician time" detection of mild anxiety should not be a priority in this "new age of increasing demand on primary care physicians." I would agree that if we demonstrate that mild anxiety is not much of a disability, then certainly we should focus on severe cases of anxiety. However, if this is used as an excuse (as it seems) to not detect and treat psychiatric illness in primary care, then I certainly disagree.

J.C. Ballenger, M.D.

Depressive and Anxiety Disorders in Patients Presenting With Physical Complaints: Clinical Predictors and Outcome
Kroenke K, Jackson JL, Chamberlin J (Indiana Univ; Uniformed Services Univ, Bethesda, Md)
Am J Med 103:339–347, 1997   6–43

Objective.—Recognition of depressive and anxiety disorders by primary care physicians is hampered by stigmatization, short visit times, somatization, and a physical disease diagnosis agenda. The relationship between mental disorders and physical symptoms has not been well studied. Quickly and easily recognized predictors of depressive or anxiety disorders were identified and the impact of these mental disorders on patient outcome was determined.

TABLE 3.—Independent Predictors of Mood or Anxiety Disorders

Predictor	Odds Ratio	[95% C.I.]	P
Stress recently (past week)	4.9	[3.0–8.0]	<0.001
Symptom count 6 or greater*	3.1	[1.9–5.2]	<0.001
Self-rated health only poor to fair*	2.7	[1.4–5.0]	0.002
Patient perceived as difficult by clinician*	2.4	[1.3–4.4]	0.006
Severity of symptom 6 or greater*	2.0	[1.2–3.3]	0.005
Age under 50	1.6	[1.0–2.7]	0.045

*Symptom count was from PRIME-MD 15 physical symptom checklist. Self-rated health was in response to question asking patient to rate overall health as excellent, very good, good, fair, or poor. Difficulty was defined as a score of 30 or greater on DDPRQ-10. Severity of symptom rated on a 0 (none) to 10 (unbearable) scale.

(Reprinted by permission of the publisher, from Kroenke K, Jackson JL, Chamberlin J: Depressive and anxiety disorders in patients presenting with physical complaints: Clinical predictors and outcome. *Am J Med* 103:339-347, Copyright 1997 by Excerpta Medica, Inc.)

Methods.—Before seeing a physician for physical symptoms, 500 patients (50% female, 49% white, 45% black, 6% other), average age 54.7 years, completed the depression, anxiety, and somatoform sections of the PRIME-MD self-administered Patient Questionnaire. Those who had a positive score had a psychiatric interview. Outcomes were assessed at the first visit and at the 2-week and 3-month follow-up visits. Patients completed a follow-up questionnaire evaluating symptom outcome, unmet expectations, functional status, satisfaction with care, and health care utilization and costs.

Results.—PRIME-MD detected a depressive or anxiety disorder in 29%, with 11% having more than 1 disorder. There was a highly significant dose-response relationship between the number of symptoms and the likelihood of a psychopathologic disorder. The logistic regression model identified 6 independent predictors of psychiatric status (Table 3). Four clinical predictors were especially powerful predictors of depressive or anxiety disorders. As the number of clinical predictors increased, the likelihood of psychiatric disorders increased substantially from a likelihood of 0.2 for 0 predictors to a likelihood of 36.3 for 4 predictors, including recent stress, 6 or more symptoms, patient-rated severity of symptoms of 6 or more on a 0–10 scale, and self-rated overall health of poor or fair on a 5-point scale.

Conclusion.—Patients with numerous undiagnosable physical symptoms may warrant further evaluation for depressive or anxiety disorder. These patients are more likely to report unmet expectations after the visit, be perceived by physicians as difficult, and have persistent psychiatric symptoms and stress.

▶ The principal author of this article (Kurt Kroenke) and his colleagues have contributed important understanding about the very high rate of patients who are seen by general medicine physicians with nonspecific physical complaints. Almost 90% of these patients still fail to have an organic diagnosis after a year of diagnostic workup. In this study, he examines these patients with the PRIME-MD to diagnose depressive and anxiety disorders, and not surprisingly finds that 29% of these patients have an anxiety or depressive disorder. Interestingly, these patients are predicted in this study by having more than 6 symptoms and when the physician perceives the clinical encounter as difficult. It is an interesting wrinkle that these factors lead to both the patient and the provider being frustrated and dissatisfied with the clinical interaction.

J.C. Ballenger, M.D.

The 'Usual Care' of Major Depression in Primary Care Practice
Schulberg HC, Block MR, Madonia MJ, et al (Univ of Pittsburgh, Pa; State Univ of New York, Stony Brook)
Arch Fam Med 6:334–339, 1997   6–44

Purpose.—Depression is commonly treated by primary care physicians, and current guidelines of the Agency for Health Care Policy and Research (AHCPR) suggest that most episodes of major depression can be managed effectively by a family physician or general internist. In this situation, it is important to determine whether primary care physicians' management of depression is consistent with AHCPR guidelines and achieves good outcomes. There is evidence that the pharmacotherapy and counseling interventions offered by primary care physicians may be inadequate. This study assessed the routine management of major depression by primary care physicians, including whether such management produces the outcomes expected with AHCPR-recommended interventions.

Methods.—The study used data from a randomized, controlled trial of treatment for major depression. The study was performed at a number of affiliated ambulatory family practice and internal medicine clinics serving an urban, largely lower socioeconomic class population. Included in the analysis were 92 patients with major depression diagnosed in 1 of these primary care practices. The diagnosis was made according to the Diagnostic Interview Schedule and confirmed by a psychiatrist. All 92 patients were assigned to "usual care" (UC), which was given at the discretion of the treating physician. Information on the nature of UC was collected, and the patients' clinical course was evaluated with the Hamilton Rating Scale for Depression and the Beck Depression Inventory. The relationship between treatment type and clinical course was evaluated.

Results.—In the 8 months after assignment to UC, 73% of patients received specific therapy for depression. Fifty-nine percent of patients received antidepressant medication, and counseling was recommended to about one third of these. Only about one third of patients to whom treatment was recommended received continuous treatment during follow-up, however. Treatment was unexplained by patient variables, though family physicians were more likely than internists to prescribe medication plus counseling. Sixty-three percent of prescriptions written were for tricyclic antidepressants.

Even though the physicians had been informed that the patients were depressed, the physicians reported that only about two thirds of patients were depressed at any time during follow-up. Still, the physicians claimed that they provided depression-specific treatment for approximately 80% of patients. At follow-up, 20% of patients were asymptomatic, with a Hamilton Rating Scale for Depression score of 7 or less. The clinical outcome was not clearly related to the treatment given—there was no difference in the level of improvement between patients who were prescribed adequate medication versus those who received no depression-specific treatment.

Conclusions.—For patients with major depression receiving UC in primary care practice, the results of treatment are not as good as expected for treatments that meet AHCPR guidelines. Even with "adequate" medication, outcomes are no better than for patients who receive no depression-specific treatment. More research is needed to define the aspects of care leading to effective pharmacotherapy for depression in primary care practice.

▶ Schulberg and his Pittsburgh colleagues provide an invaluable study demonstrating that, if properly conducted, depression in primary care can be treated by the primary care physician effectively. This is in contrast to most of the "usual care" studies that find that patients generally do very poorly in "usual care." This article begins to struggle with what is wrong with the treatment of depression by primary care physicians. The answers remain complicated, but 1 is that not enough patients receive antidepressants or counseling, and if they do, they receive too little and for too short a time. How we fix these problems is both important and difficult as I have said in comments about other related research findings.

J.C. Ballenger, M.D.

Treatment of Depression by Obstetrician-Gynecologists: A Survey Study
Schmidt LA, Greenberg BD, Holzman GB, et al (Univ of Maryland; Natl Insts of Mental Health, Bethesda, Md; American College of Obstetricians and Gynecologists, Washington, DC)
Obstet Gynecol 90:296–300, 1997   6–45

Background.—Women are 2 to 3 times as likely as men to experience severe depression, the lifetime prevalence for females is 10% to 21%. Most patients with psychiatric illnesses seek care from their primary physician (including their gynecologist), rather than a psychiatrist. Thus, gynecologists are often presented with cases of depression. The way the gynecologists manage patients with depression was examined.

Method.—A total of 1,370 fellows of the American College of Obstetricians and Gynecologists were surveyed. The survey presented questions dealing with drugs prescribed for depression, referrals, and the amount of training in depression the physician had received. There was a 60% survey response rate.

Results.—On the average, 4 cases of depression were diagnosed each month. Those who considered themselves primary care physicians diagnosed more cases than those who considered themselves specialists. The drug of choice prescribed for depression (74% of the time) was a selective serotonin reuptake inhibitor antidepressant. Of those surveyed, 95% reported referring patients with severe depression to a mental health care provider. Most respondents had not attended residency (80%) or continuing education (60%) courses on the treatment of depression in women.

Conclusion.—Further studies of the management by gynecologists of patients with depression are needed to meet the needs for professional education suggested by this study.

▶ As obstetrician/gynecologists increasingly ask to function as primary care physicians, many of us have wondered about their basic knowledge of psychiatric problems. This study shows very clearly that these physicians see a large number of depressed women—on average 4 new cases a month—and they utilize selective serotonin reuptake inhibitors predominantly. However, very few of these physicians have received any training during their residency, and 60% have never even completed a continuing education course on the treatment of depression. As we try to treat these disorders when they occur, and as we move toward a predominantly primary care model, we have a seemingly mammoth task before us if we are to see even a small minority of psychiatric patients well treated.

J.C. Ballenger, M.D.

Persistently Poor Outcomes of Undetected Major Depression in Primary Care
Rost K, Zhang M, Fortney J, et al (Univ of Arkansas for Med Sciences, Little Rock; Univ of Michigan, Ann Arbor)
Gen Hosp Psychiatry 20:12–20, 1998   6–46

Introduction.—Early reports indicate that primary physicians fail to detect major depression in about half of their patients with this disorder. Ninety-eight persons with current major depression who made 1 or more visits to a primary care physician were followed to (1) identify the proportion of primary care patients in routine care settings whose current episode of major depression remained undetected for up to 1 year, (2) characterize impairment and remission rates in undetected patients over 1 year, and (3) examine quality of depression treatment and remission rates in detected patients over 1 year.

Methods.—Of 636 adults identified by first-stage depression screening during telephone interviews, 162 underwent a 3-hour face-to-face baseline interview within 1 month of the telephone interview. Patients were reinterviewed at 6 and 12 months. A nondepressed comparison group was taken from 9,900 screen-negative persons who completed the telephone interview.

Results.—At 6-month follow-up, 103 of 153 research subjects made 1 or more visits, for any reason, to a family practitioner, general practitioner, or general internist. Patients who made a primary care visit within 6 months of baseline were significantly more likely to be older (50.1 vs. 36.4 years of age), less likely to be high-school educated (35.7% vs. 68.1%), and more likely to report more physical co-morbidities (3.8 vs. 1.9), compared with persons who did not make a primary care visit within 6 months of baseline. Five patients who received depression treatment from a mental health provider during the year after baseline were excluded. Of the remaining 98 patients, depression was detected by the primary care physician in 66 (67.5%). Patients who were detected were significantly more likely than their undetected counterparts to be older. The probability of depression being detected dropped dramatically after the first visit. Undetected depressed patients reported significantly more role limitations and suicide ideations (almost half) and continued to meet criteria for current major depression within the last 2 weeks at 6- and 12-month follow-up (37.5% at both follow-ups, compared with 51.3% of patients with detected current major depression).

Conclusion.—Quality improvement efforts limited to screening probably will do little to enhance outcomes in routine primary care settings. Screening efforts must be accompanied by or preceded by interventions that educate primary care physicians regarding use of efficacious courses of treatment in these patients.

▶ For regular followers of this section of the YEAR BOOK, I think it should be clear that 1 of the major areas in which psychiatry needs to focus attention is primary care, especially regarding the most common psychiatric syndrome in primary care, depression. This study from the excellent group in Little Rock, Arkansas, followed 98 adults with current major depression for a year. Strikingly, a third of those with major depression remained undetected for that year, and in almost half of them, suicidal ideation developed. Most did not visit a doctor and even if they were symptomatic when they did, they remained undetected. Some critics, trying to avoid the implications of some of these obvious truths, have stated that these patients do not need treatment. This study, again, demonstrates that these patients do very poorly and deserve effective treatment.

J.C. Ballenger, M.D.

Impact of Improved Depression Treatment in Primary Care on Daily Functioning and Disability
Simon GE, Katon W, Rutter C, et al (Univ of Washington, Seattle)
Psychol Med 28:693–701, 1998   6–47

Introduction.—Earlier trials have shown that improvement in depression is associated with improvement in function and lower disability. Few data are available that analyze the impact of depression treatment on daily functioning and productivity. Data from 2 closely related randomized trials were used to assess the impact of improved depression treatment in primary care on somatic distress, overall health, disability, and lost productivity.

Methods.—Both trials evaluated multifaceted collaborative management programs that included patient education, physician training, on-site mental health consultation, adjustment of antidepressant medication, behavioral activation, and more intensive follow-up care. Patients initiating antidepressant treatment were randomized to either usual care or to the collaborative management program. Patients were evaluated at baseline and at 4- and 7-month follow-up for several measures of impairment, daily functioning and disability: self-rated overall health, number of bodily pains, number of somatization symptoms, work changes related to health, reduction in leisure activities related to health, number of disability days, and number of restricted activity days.

Results.—In both trials, average data from 4- and 7-month assessments showed that patients randomized to the intervention group had significantly fewer somatic symptoms and more favorable overall health, compared with the usual-care group. The intervention group did nonsignificantly better on other measures of functional impairment and disability.

Conclusion.—Patients with acute depression who received improved depression treatment experienced decreased somatic distress and improved self-rated overall health. The absence of a significant intervention effect on other disability measures may be the result of a short treatment and follow-up period, coupled with the influence of other individual and environmental factors on disability.

▶ One of the groups that has contributed most significantly to our understanding of the treatment of psychiatric disorders in primary care (especially depression) is Seattle group in the Puget Sound Group Health Cooperative. In this study, they followed a series of functional measures in a group of depressed patients in primary care who were treated by usual care or by a collaborative management program that included patient education, on-site mental health treatment, medications, behavioral treatment, and monitoring of medication compliance. At both 4 and 7 months, the intervention patients had fewer somatic symptoms and had overall better health. This can be added to the growing literature underscoring the importance of treating this population adequately.

J.C. Ballenger, M.D.

Clinical Practice Guidelines on Depression: Awareness, Attitudes, and Content Knowledge Among Family Physicians in New York

Feldman EL, Jaffe A, Galambos N, et al (State Univ of New York, Stony Brook; Case Western Reserve Univ, Cleveland, Ohio)
Arch Fam Med 7:58–62, 1998   6–48

Introduction.—Clinical guidelines designed to improve quality of care are only useful if physicians are aware of their existence, have read and accepted the contents, and have a positive attitude regarding guidelines. In 1989, the U.S. government mandated that the Agency for Health Care Policy and Research (AHCPR) appoint expert panels to create clinical practice guidelines to define standards for the provision and quality of health care. Physician awareness and attitudes regarding guidelines have not been adequately assessed. The clinical practice guidelines on depression in primary care were surveyed. For comparison, the respondents were also questioned regarding guidelines for urinary incontinence and pressure ulcers.

Methods.—A random sample of 992 of the 1,752 members of the New York State Academy of Family Physicians were sent a survey instrument designed to evaluate their attitudes toward and awareness and knowledge of the content of the AHCPR clinical practice guidelines on depression in primary care. The response rate was 53.2% (519 respondents). Most respondents were aged 45 years or younger, white, male, board certified, and had had 3 or more years of a family practice residency.

Depression was treated in the primary care practices of 90.5% of respondents. Only 33.6% were aware that guidelines on depression existed, even though the guidelines had been published for 1 year. Of responding physicians, only 13.1% had a copy of the guidelines. Respondents were slightly less aware of the guidelines for urinary incontinence and pressure ulcers (30.0%). Most physicians were knowledgeable regarding the diagnosis and treatment of depression. Board certification was associated with increased knowledge of depressive illness. Physicians most likely to have positive attitudes about guidelines were those of female gender, those living in larger communities, and those with 3 or more years of residency in family practice.

Conclusion.—The AHCPR guidelines reached a small proportion of their targeted audience. It is important to find more effective methods for disseminating important evidence-based medical information to physicians.

▶ John Rush and his excellent group produced guidelines for treatment of depression in primary care for the AHCPR. Despite the excellence of these guidelines, a question remains regarding how well they are used in primary care. This study shows that only one third of surveyed family physicians were even aware of the guidelines, and approximately 13% possessed a copy. This confirms what many of us have feared. It is another example of how complicated it will be to improve the treatment of depression and other psychiatric disorders in primary care.

J.C. Ballenger, M.D.

A Diagnostic Aid for Detecting (DSM-IV) Mental Disorders in Primary Care

Weissman MM, Broadhead WE, Olfson M, et al (Columbia Univ, New York; Duke Univ, Durham, NC; Univ of South Florida, Tampa; et al)
Gen Hosp Psychiatry 20:1–11, 1998   6–49

Background.—Primary care physicians increasingly need rapid, accurate methods for assessing patients with mental and addictive disorders. A new computerized version of the Symptom-Driven Diagnostic System for Primary Care (SDDS-PC) was developed, and its validity and feasibility in primary care practice were tested.

Methods.—A total of 1,001 patients, aged 18 to 70, seeking routine care at 1 center underwent screening, which included a self-administered symptom scale for major depression, alcohol and drug dependence, generalized anxiety, panic and obsessive compulsive disorders, and suicidal behavior. After this screening, a nurse administered a brief diagnostic interview, which yielded a 1-page summary of positive symptoms and a provisional computer-generated diagnosis for the physician. Physicians then reviewed the summary and made a diagnosis. Both the nurse and the physician were unaware of the results of screening. Within 96 hours, the patients were interviewed again by a mental health professional (MHP) who was unaware of previous findings.

Findings.—Nurse and physician diagnoses showed excellent to moderate agreement. Disagreement usually resulted from physicians' ruling out major mental disorders in favor of subsyndromal or medical causes. Physicians rarely diagnosed disorders not detected by the nurse's interview. For a screened positive diagnosis, the nurse interviews required 1½ to 3½ minutes. Physician and MHP diagnoses showed moderate agreement. Most physician diagnoses made with use of the SDDS-PC were confirmed by the independent assessment of the MHP.

Conclusions.—The SDDS-PC may facilitate primary care physicians' recognition of psychiatric disorders. The use of this system can minimize the amount of time physicians spend gathering information.

▶ This study is part of the development of a computerized version of the SDDS-PC to detect mental disorders in primary care. It involves a very brief (1½ to 3½ minutes) nurse interview after self-administered screens. This then leads to a 1-page summary and a provisional computer-based generated diagnosis for the physician. It represents 1 of the potential systems that might actually be picked up by busy primary care physicians.

J.C. Ballenger, M.D.

Management of Patients With Depression by Rural Primary Care Practitioners

Hartley D, Korsen N, Bird D, et al (Univ of Southern Maine, Portland)
Arch Fam Med 7:139–145, 1998   6–50

Introduction.—Few trials have addressed how primary care physicians (PCPs) in the rural setting deal with depressed patients they have identified. Rural PCPs were surveyed by telephone to determine how they manage adult patients with depression and how their referral patterns and treatment approaches vary by practitioner, practice, and service area.

Methods.—Primary care practioners in Maine participated in a 41-item telephone survey. There were 267 respondents composed of family and general practice doctors of medicine and doctors of osteopathy, general internists, nurse practitioners, and physician assistants. The degree to which PCPs themselves treated patients with depression, rather than referring them to a mental health specialist, was assessed.

Results.—There was no significant difference between urban and rural settings in the number of patients with depression seen as a percentage of total patient volume. The PCPs reported that the greatest barriers to referral to a mental health provider were long wait for an appointment, lack of available services, patients' unwillingness to use such services, and reimbursement issues. About two thirds of respondents reported that they had had special education in depression. The only exception was nurse practitioners; only one third reported having had this education. Multivariate analyses revealed that PCP characteristics measuring knowledge and attitudes and lack of available services were significantly related to treatment and referral patterns. Practice characteristics and mental health provider supply were not significantly related to treatment and referral patterns.

Conclusion.—Individual practitioner characteristics were primary determinants in PCPs' decisions to treat or refer patients, not the availability of mental health specialty providers. Those PCPs most likely to treat patients themselves were the ones who believed themselves capable of treating depression effectively.

▶ This study is relatively typical in the family medicine literature in that the authors reached the conclusion that the best way to improve care is to increase the educational efforts of the PCP. I think this is an excellent idea. However, the authors reached this conclusion after exercising the usual antipsychiatry bias. They base a significant amount of their conclusions on the fact that PCPs in Maine do not like to refer to mental health settings, and patients do not like the referrals. Although this is undeniably true, I hope we can improve that situation while we try to improve the PCP's ability to treat depression.

J.C. Ballenger, M.D.

An Evaluation of Practice Nurses Working With General Practitioners to Treat People With Depression
Mann AH, Blizard R, Murray J, et al (Inst of Psychiatry, London; Royal Liverpool Univ, England)
Br J Gen Pract 48:875–879, 1998   6–51

Introduction.—General practitioners (GPs) frequently handle diagnosis and treatment of depression. An earlier trial has suggested that the practice nurse may make a significant contribution to the care of patients with depression. Two trials were run in parallel to assess an extended role for practice nurses in improving the outcome of depression.

Methods.—A sample of 577 depressed patients were recruited from practices of 56 GPs and 21 practice nurses participating in the Medical Research Council General Practice Research Framework in England. Patients were randomized to concurrent 4-month trials of either study 1, which evaluated the effectiveness of standardized psychiatric assessment by a practice nurse and feedback of information to the GP, or study 2, which examined the same assessment and feedback combined with nurse-assisted follow-up care. Patients treated according to GPs' usual practice formed the control group. Both groups were followed for changes in the Beck Depression Inventory (BDI) and changes in the proportion of patients fulfilling *Diagnostic and Statistical Manual of Mental Disorders*, third edition (DSM-III) criteria for major depression.

Results.—Of 577 patients, 516 were rated as depressed on the BDI and 474 met criteria for DSM-III major depression. Ninety-one percent (524 patients) were available for 4-month assessment. Patients in the study 1, study 2, and control groups all improved, with no difference in the rate of improvement for the nurse intervention groups. In study 1, mean BDI scores dropped from 18.54 to 11.53; in study 2, the mean scores dropped from 21.01 to 10.62. In study 1, the proportion of patients fulfilling criteria for DSM-III major depression fell from 80% to 30%; in study 2, it went from 80% to 27%. In both trials, the prescription rate was higher than expected, ranging from 63% to 76%.

Conclusion.—Nurse intervention did not make significant changes in short-term outcome of patients with major depression. It is not known why antidepressant medication was prescribed more often by GPs for patients in the nurse intervention groups. It may be that awareness of the severity of depression was raised by discussions between practice nurses and GPs.

▶ One of the more logical suggestions that many of us have made for improving treatment of depression in primary care has been to have a specially trained nurse assist in the care of these patients. This study, like several others, actually found this intervention disappointing. In this study, the only finding was that the prescription rates of antidepressant medications were higher (63% to 76%). Perhaps this was related to the nurse intervention.

J.C. Ballenger, M.D.

Achieving Guidelines for the Treatment of Depression in Primary Care: Is Physician Education Enough?
Lin EHB, Katon WJ, Simon GE, et al (Group Health Cooperative of Puget Sound, Seattle; Univ of Washington, Seattle)
Med Care 35:831–842, 1997   6–52

Background.—The treatment of depression in primary care varies greatly. Research suggests that a minority of depressed patients receive optimal care in everyday clinical practice. The effects of physician education on the treatment of depression were investigated.

Methods and Findings.—Data were obtained on depressed patients initiating antidepressant treatment in primary care clinics of a staff model HMO. Process of care and outcomes were investigated in quasi-experimental and before-and-after comparisons of physician practices, supplemented with patient surveys. The intervention was a year-long, extensive physician education program including case-by-case consultations, didactics, academic detailing, and role-play of optimal treatment. Quasi-experimental samples included antidepressant medication selection and adequacy of pharmacotherapy. Survey samples included intensity of follow-up, physician-delivered educational messages about depression treatment, patient satisfaction, and depression outcomes. Analysis indicated no lasting, consistent effects of education on any outcome measures.

Conclusions.—This intervention did not improve the treatment of depression in primary-care patients. However, depression treatment guidelines were achieved, suggesting that continuing programs of reorganized service delivery to support the role of a primary-care physician, along with physician training, are essential for successful guideline implementation.

▶ Over the past several years, we have closely followed the issues of psychiatric patients in primary care. This is an excellent article summarizing the important work that the group from the Center for Health Studies of the Group Health Cooperative of Puget Sound in Seattle have completed over the last few years. They have explored a number of methods to try to improve the treatment of depression in primary care. In this study, they asked the question "Is physician education enough?" and actually conclude that it is definitively not enough. They found what I have believed for some time—that we will need to change the organization of service delivery in primary care to accomplish these goals, principally by being on-site and by structuring closer follow-up of these patients.

J.C. Ballenger, M.D.

Does a Teaching Programme Improve General Practitioners' Management of Depression in the Elderly?
Butler R, Collins E, Katona C, et al (St Charles Hosp, London; St Georges Hosp, London; Univ College London)
J Affect Disord 46:303–308, 1997   6–53

Introduction.—Most trials of continuing medical education have shown that interactive teaching methods involving feedback are more effective than the traditional lecture format. These methods have not been analyzed for management of depression in the elderly. The effect that a half-day postgraduate program incorporating this educational approach had on views and knowledge of a group of general practitioners (GPs) regarding the management of depression in the elderly was assessed.

Methods.—After viewing 3 vignettes of cases of elderly patients with depression, GPs completed questionnaires regarding their choice and prescription of antidepressants, diagnosis and treatment of depression, psychological treatments, their views on depression in the elderly, and details about the GP's practice.

Results.—Of 21 GPs attending the course, 15 completed the questionnaire before and 6 weeks after completion of the course. Significant improvements were observed at 6-week follow-up in the GPs' knowledge regarding antidepressant treatment and their preference for cognitive behavioral therapy out of a range of psychological treatments.

Conclusion.—These findings indicate that a teaching program on depression in the elderly may improve GPs' management knowledge and attitudes. Future trials should assess ways to encourage GP participation, practice-based individual instruction, and which aspects of a teaching program are most useful.

► This study demonstrated that a half-day educational program did, in fact, increase the knowledge base of a group of GPs. In particular, the GPs increased their knowledge of antidepressant treatments and cognitive behavioral therapy. The authors correctly point out that it is as yet unclear whether increased education and knowledge lead to differences in practice patterns or outcomes. Most studies find that these programs are actually insufficient to significantly change outcomes, and structural changes in the practice of the GP need to be made. These probably include on-site mental health consultation and treatment and changes in the way patients are seen and followed up.

J.C. Ballenger, M.D.

Calibrating the Physician: Personal Awareness and Effective Patient Care

Novack DH, for the Working Group on Promoting Physician Personal Awareness, American Academy on Physician and Patient (Allegheny Univ, Philadelphia; Univ of Rochester, NY; Midcoast Hosp, Bath, Me; et al)

JAMA 278:502–509, 1997   6–54

Objective.—Many personal factors affect a physician's effectiveness in using communication skills. Awareness of their own personal characteristics, past experiences, values, attitudes, and biases can help physicians to enhance communication with patients. However, physicians have few educational opportunities for an organized approach to promoting personal awareness. Drawing on their experience in promoting personal awareness to enhance communication skills, the authors propose a curriculum for physician personal awareness.

Core Curriculum.—The authors present their recommendation in terms of a core curriculum in personal awareness, including topics for discussion and self-exploration. The curriculum is organized into 4 topic areas: physicians' attitudes and beliefs, their feelings and emotional responses, challenging clinical situations, and self-care. Physicians' attitudes and beliefs include core beliefs and personal philosophy, which explain why things happen, define right and wrong, and characterize one's responsibility toward others. These attitudes and beliefs may affect how physicians listen to and judge patients' stories and the extent to which they empathize with and counsel patients. Beliefs and attitudes are greatly affected by several different contexts, including family of origin issues, sex, and sociocultural milieu. Feelings and emotional responses focus on the core emotions of love and anger. Though physicians' love and caring for patients can be healing, they are only beneficial if they include clear boundaries. Understanding their emotional reactions to patients can help physicians to set appropriate boundaries, allowing them to be objective while maintaining a connection to patients. The physician's relationship to anger and conflict often affects patient care. Skills in conflict resolution affect the physician's attitude toward conflict. Physicians should be encouraged to examine what sorts of patients and situations make them angry and where they learned their responses to anger.

Certain challenging clinical situations can help physicians to understanding their attitudes toward and emotional responses to patients. All physicians have patients that they find difficult to deal with. Personal biases may make it difficult for physicians to acquire the skills they need to help certain types of patients. Discussing their feelings may help physicians to overcome their biases and gain new perspectives on dealing with various kinds of "difficult" patients. Problems in communicating with dying patients may be related to experiences with death and fears of vulnerability. Attitudes toward and beliefs about medical mistakes may have a profound impact on patient care; many physicians expect themselves to be perfect. Learning or emotional healing is especially difficult if physicians cannot discuss their mistakes with others. Some suggestions for productive discussion of mistakes with other physicians are presented. Finally, physician self-care is important, because personal issues can detract from the physician's ability to provide effective care for patients. Physicians can achieve a better balance between their personal and professional activities through reflection and increased self-awareness. Imbalance in these areas is just one of many contributors to stress in the physician's life. Monitoring their level of stress and coming up with adaptive responses are important steps toward preventing burnout.

Discussion.—Physicians' attitudes and beliefs, feelings and emotional responses, challenging clinical situations, and self-care are proposed as a core curriculum for helping physicians to enhance their personal awareness for effective patient care. Several types of activities can help to promote personal awareness, such as support groups, Balint groups, and talking about meaningful experiences in medical practice. The authors' experience with these and other approaches suggests that they can help lead physicians to better patient care and increased personal and professional satisfaction.

▶ Again, I have chosen an article about changes in the curricula in medical training. This, too, is prompted by changes in the climate of medical care, specifically the growing demand from patients for sensitive and personalized care. This is coupled with increasing recognition of the distressingly high prevalence of physicians who are not effective in the "art" of medicine, specifically, being able to elicit a patient history, promote good rapport, assist good patient decision making, and promote compliance with treatment recommendations. These authors present a series of ideas about how we might increase these qualities in future physicians, and I welcome both the suggestions and the emphasis.

J.C. Ballenger, M.D.

Medical Training in Psychiatry Residency: A Proposed Curriculum
Kick SD, Morrison M, Kathol RG (Univ of Colorado, Denver; Univ of Pennsylvania, Philadelphia; Univ of Iowa, Iowa City)
Gen Hosp Psychiatry 19:259–266, 1997   6–55

Objective.—In the future, psychiatrists must assume more responsibility for the physical evaluation and treatment of patients with behavioral or emotional problems. However, current psychiatric training programs do not emphasize physical assessment, questioning psychiatry's claim that it can integrate medical causes of psychiatric symptoms. The authors propose a new medical training curriculum for psychiatric residents.

Need for Medical Skills.—Physical illness is common among psychiatric inpatients and outpatients alike. Identifying organic vs. functional disease is a key patient assessment skill for psychiatrists, although their most advanced training takes place away from settings where physical disease is a concern. Despite their obvious role in providing medical care, many psychiatrists are reluctant to perform physical assessments, or even discouraged from doing so. The influence of psychoanalysis, boundary issues, and other barriers have encouraged psychiatrists to cede assessment and treatment of physical illness to other physicians.

Proposed Curriculum.—To overcome these barriers, the authors propose a reviewed curriculum for psychiatric residency programs to help trainees include a medical assessment, differential, and treatment in their psychiatric evaluations. The curriculum includes key attitude objectives of understanding the need for medical evaluation of psychiatric patients, and recognizing the psychiatrist's role in coordinating and supervising mental health teams in primary care settings. Knowledge objectives include the medical differential diagnosis for various psychiatric conditions, recognition and treatment of common medical disorders, and inclusion of a medical history in the psychiatric assessment. Psychiatric trainees should also understand the psychiatric manifestations of medical disorders, the medical manifestations of psychiatric disorders, and the psychiatric manifestations of psychiatric and nonpsychiatric medications. Skill objectives include performing the physical evaluation in a psychiatric setting, using laboratory and x-ray procedures, performing medical evaluations before psychiatric procedures, and properly using consultations and referrals.

Discussion.—These proposed curriculum changes will help prepare psychiatric trainees to manage the medical aspects of psychiatric disease. The psychiatrist is not meant to replace the primary care physician, but should be able to use his or her medical background to assist other medical care providers. Attitude, knowledge, and skill objectives for the new curriculum are presented, along with necessary changes in the educational setting and resident evaluations.

▶ It may seem odd to include an article on curriculum reform in psychiatric residencies in the clinical section of the YEAR BOOK. However, this proposal for increased medical training of psychiatry residents reflects a growing sense among many of us as the healthcare system evolves that psychiatrists should be increasingly involved in the care of at least routine medical problems in their patients. Because many of us think direct on-site involvement of psychiatrists in primary care settings and increased medical care of psychiatric patients in psychiatric care are clear waves of the future, many of us who are responsible for training curricula are looking in this direction. This article makes the point that we should be trained to take on management of at least some aspects of the routine medical care of our patients.

J.C. Ballenger, M.D.

7 Biological Psychiatry

Introduction

This year's selections represent, in my view, some of the most interesting recent advances in our understanding of schizophrenia, depression, obsessive-compulsive disorder, and various other psychiatric disorders. A group of articles appear on Cognition, which is central to our understanding of schizophrenia and mood disorders and neuro-degenerative disorders. A series of articles on schizophrenia show the importance of separating familial and nonfamilial schizophrenia to identify key biological and genetic deficits for the familial subtype. Without this strategy, false negatives for genetic-based deficits are likely to occur. There were no breakthroughs last year in understanding the neurochemistry of schizophrenia. More evidence for neuronal loss in schizophrenia has been found, but it is still not clear that the findings are specific to schizophrenia. The failure of L-745,870, a D_4 antagonist, to treat schizophrenia was a blow to Seeman's D_4 hypothesis, while the report by Gurevich et al. on elevated D_3 receptors in ventral forebrain and striatum of schizophrenics should revive flagging interest in that receptor. Kapur et al.'s finding that olanzapine produces full 5-HT_{2a} receptor occupancy at a subtherapeutic dose of 5 mg/kg helps to clarify that there is only a limited benefit for EPS and perhaps negative symptoms which come from blocking that receptor. Amperozide is a promising new drug for schizophrenia and alcohol abuse based on 5-HT_{2a} receptor pharmacology.

Perhaps the most interesting article on the topic of cognition is that of Jentsch et al., who provide convincing evidence in primates for the phencyclidine hydrochloride based model of schizophrenia. They found 2-week administration of phenocyclidine hydrochloride produced a chronic deficit in working memory which was due, in part, to diminished dopaminergic activity, and could be reversed by clozapine treatment. This line of research can be helpful in refining our understanding of the cognitive deficits in schizophrenia and how to treat them.

A promising new approach to treating mood disorders is described by Murphy et al., who report that various inhibitors of glucocorticoid synthesis improved depression by 50% or more in 13 of 20 (65%) depressed patients who were resistant to a variety of antidepressant drugs. Because it is an open trial, it has to be replicated in controlled studies. Glucocorticoids play an important part in social role functioning and chronic fatigue syndrome, as well as in neurotransmitter function and in neurotosic events. A pharmacologic method of regulating glucocorticoid output and responsivity in the normal range, with the appropriate diurnal rhythms, and capacity to respond to stressors of various kinds, would be a great boon in a variety of neuropsychiatric disorders.

Herbert Y. Meltzer, M.D.

Schizophrenia

Neuronal and Glial Somal Size in the Prefrontal Cortex: A Postmortem Morphometric Study of Schizophrenia and Huntington Disease
Rajkowska G, Selemon LD, Goldman-Rakic PS (Univ of Mississippi, Jackson; Yale Univ, New Haven, Conn)
Arch Gen Psychiatry 55:215–224, 1998   7–1

Introduction.—Decreased neural size has been reported for pyramidal neurons in the hippocampus, substantia nigra, and locus ceruleus in patients with schizophrenia. No size differences between the schizophrenic and the normal prefrontal cortex have been reported. Neurodegeneration of large pyramidal cells is a well-known feature of the cortical abnormalities in late-stage Huntington's disease (HD). A comparison of morphometric abnormalities observed in schizophrenia and those found in HD may give insight into cellular changes in schizophrenia. Neuronal and glial cell bodies were examined in the postmortem brains of 9 patients with schizophrenia, 7 patients with HD, and 10 normal controls.

Methods.—The perimeters of 10,722 neuronal and 19,913 glial profiles in Brodmann areas 9 and 17 were examined using a 3-dimensional image analyzer. The neurons and glia were classified by size and layer to determine specific vulnerabilities with respect to cortical architecture and circuitry.

Results.—In the schizophrenic brain, the prefrontal cortex was characterized by a downward shift in neuronal size, accompanied by a 70% to 140% per layer rise in the density of small neurons. A significant decrease in mean neuronal size was correlated with a significant reduction in the density of very large neurons in sublayer IIIc. There was no decrease in neuronal size in occipital area 17 or glial size in the prefrontal or occipital cortexes. In the prefrontal cortex of patients with HD, neuronal degeneration was confirmed by diminished neuronal size, decreased density of large neurons, and notable elevation in density of large glia.

Conclusion.—Neuropathologic changes were an ongoing process in the HD brain, but not the schizophrenic brain. In schizophrenia, there were significant reductions in neuronal size in the prefrontal cortex. A downward shift in neuronal size was detected in all layers, with a significant reduction in layer III.

▶ This study represents 1 of the most meticulous quantitative examinations of the size and density of neurons and glia ever conducted in schizophrenics. Its most serious limitations are the small sample size and the absence of a nonschizophrenic disease control group. We do not yet know whether the decrease in neuronal size in the prefrontal cortex is specific to schizophrenia. Neurons seem to be shrinking rather than disappearing. The authors suggest that a possible explanation is cytoplasmic atrophy stopping short of total degeneration in the early stages of the illness. This would be compatible with the findings of Gur et al. and Nair et al. (Abstracts 7–2 and 7–3).

H.Y. Meltzer, M.D.

A Follow-up Magnetic Resonance Imaging Study of Schizophrenia: Relationship of Neuroanatomical Changes to Clinical and Neurobehavioral Measures

Gur RE, Cowell P, Turetsky BI, et al (Univ of Pennsylvania, Philadelphia)
Arch Gen Psychiatry 55:145–152, 1998

7–2

Introduction.—Reduced brain volume has been noted on cross-sectional CT and MRI trials of patients with schizophrenia. Abnormalities in patients with first-episode (FE) schizophrenia suggest a neurodevelopmental origin, because brain dysfunction predates clinical manifestation. Reported are longitudinal findings that integrate anatomical, clinical, and neurobehavioral measures with MRI findings in 40 patients with schizophrenia.

Methods.—Of 40 patients, 20 had FE and 20 were previously treated (PT) for schizophrenia. Seventeen healthy research participants acted as controls. All research participants underwent brain MRI and neurobehavioral studies at baseline and at a mean of 30.63 months' follow-up. Volumes of whole-brain, cerebrospinal fluid, and frontal and temporal lobes were calculated. Patients were assessed for severity of negative and positive symptoms, monitoring of medications, and neurobehavioral functioning in 8 domains.

Results.—At baseline, FE and PT patients had smaller brains and frontal and temporal lobes than controls. Decreases in frontal lobe volume were observed longitudinally in patients with schizophrenia. Decreases in temporal lobe volumes were also observed in controls. The correlation between volume reduction and symptom changes varied between patient groups. However, volume reduction was correlated with diminished neurobehavioral function in both patient groups. The neuroleptic dose effect was significant for both frontal and temporal volumes in FE patients, but not in PT patients.

Conclusion.—Findings of neuroanatomic and neurobehavioral abnormalities in patients with FE schizophrenia establish that brain dysfunction occurs before clinical manifestation. There is also evidence of progression of structural changes in some patients. It is possible that anatomic changes can affect some clinical and neurobehavioral features of the illness.

▶ This study and the next (Abstract 7–3) indicate progressive enlargement of ventricles and loss of brain tissue in schizophrenia after its onset. Gur et al. demonstrate that this is true for FE patients and that the loss of brain volume correlates with progressive worsening of cognitive function. It is not clear how this progressive change relates to the concept of schizophrenia as a neurodevelopmental disorder. Although the findings are not necessarily incompatible, they do indicate that there is an ongoing morbid process that, conceivably, can be arrested.

H.Y. Meltzer, M.D.

Progression of Cerebroventricular Enlargement and the Subtyping of Schizophrenia

Nair TR, Christensen JD, Kingsbury SJ, et al (Dallas Veterans Administration Med Centre; Univ of Texas, Dallas)
Psychiatry Res 74:141–150, 1997   7–3

Introduction.—Cerebral ventricular enlargement is the most commonly observed anatomic finding in patients with schizophrenia. The timing of the development of this abnormality and its association with the evolving morbidity of schizophrenia are undefined. It is not known whether cerebral ventricular enlargement is the consequence of some early neurodevelopmental event or whether the enlargement is progressive and continuous during the course of illness. Serial volumetric MRIs of the cerebral ventricles were obtained in 18 patients with schizophrenia to determine if separate populations of schizophrenia exist.

Methods.—Patients underwent baseline MRI and repeat scan about 2 years later. Measurements of ventricular volumes were examined by an investigator blinded to each patient's age, sex, clinical characteristics, and scan date. The reproducibility of the volumetric analysis was ascertained by repeating the analyses of 4 of the images 5 times. The analyses were performed blindly and were distributed among other patients' images.

Results.—Repeated blind measurements of total ventricular volume demonstrated a less than 2% error of the segmentation method. During a 2 to 3 year follow-up, the rate of ventricular expansion (RVE) was 2.2 cm³/yr in patients with schizophrenia and 0.8 cm³/yr in controls. The RVEs in the patient group were clustered into 2 groups: 1 similar to the control group and 1 with a significantly greater rate of expansion (RVE 0.8 and 3.9 cm³/yr, respectively).

Conclusion.—These findings indicate that there are at least 2 subpopulations within schizophrenia: 1 with relatively static ventricles and 1 with progressively enlarging ventricles. At least 2 diverse etiologic processes may underlie the clinical presentation of schizophrenic symptoms. Between-group differences in neuroleptic compliance, alcohol and recreational drug abuse, and certain clinical correlates could not explain differences in ventricular expansion.

▶ In agreement with the report by Gur et al. (Abstract 7–2), this study finds a progressive increase in total ventricular volume over the course of a 2 to 3 year period. What is intriguing about this study was that there appeared to be 2 distinct groups of patients: 1 with an increase of about 5 times the rate in normal controls and the other with the same rate as the normal controls.

The group with the high rate of expansion of ventricles had a shorter duration of illness, suggesting that this process may be greater during the earlier stages of the illness. The study by Rajkowska et al. (Abstract 7–1) suggests ventricles might be increasing because of neuronal shrinkage or loss.

H.Y. Meltzer, M.D.

First-episode Schizophrenic Psychosis Differs From First-episode Affective Psychosis and Controls in P300 Amplitude Over Left Temporal Lobe
Salisbury DF, Shenton ME, Sherwood AR, et al (McLean Hosp, Belmont, Mass)
Arch Gen Psychiatry 55:173–180, 1998   7–4

Introduction.—Several trials have demonstrated that schizophrenia is related to sagittal midline decreases in P300 cognitive event-related potential and tomographic asymmetry of P300, with diminished left temporal voltage. The asymmetry observed in P300 is linked to tissue volume asymmetry in the posterior superior temporal gyrus. It is not known whether P300 asymmetry is specific to schizophrenia; whether central and lateral P300 abnormalities are the result of chronic morbidity, neuroleptic medications, and/or hospitalization; or whether the abnormalities exist at illness onset. Patients hospitalized for first-episode schizophrenia or affective psychosis underwent event-related potentials to determine whether topographic abnormalities and midline reductions of P300 voltage were present at initial onset.

Methods.—Fourteen patients with first-episode schizophrenia, 14 patients with first-episode affective psychosis, and 14 healthy controls underwent event-related potentials for the recording of P300. Participants silently counted binaurally presented target tones (97 dB, 1.5 kHz, 50-msec duration, 10–msec rise and fall times, 15% of trials) among standard tones (97 dB, 1.0 kHz) against a background of 70-dB white noise, at an interstimulus interval of 1.2 secs. Averages were calculated from brain responses to target tones.

Results.—The peak amplitude of P300 and integrated voltage over 300–400 msecs varied significantly between first-episode schizophrenics and controls over the posterior sagittal midline of the head. Smaller amplitudes were observed over the left temporal lobe in first-episode schizophrenics than in patients with first-episode affective psychosis or in controls. There were no among-group differences observed over the right temporal lobe.

Conclusion.—Observations of left-sided P300 abnormalities in first-episode schizophrenics, but not in first-episode affective psychotics or controls, indicate that P300 asymmetry is specific to schizophrenic psychosis and is present at initial hospitalization. It is likely that left temporal lobe dysfunction is present at onset in patients with schizophrenia.

▶ The authors provide evidence for an interesting marker of left temporal lobe abnormality in first-episode schizophrenic patients. The authors suggest that the abnormal symmetry in the P300-evoked response in the temporal lobe may reflect the cognitive impairment of schizophrenia, but no specific data were offered to show that the asymmetry correlated with cognitive impairment. Unlike the case in many findings of this type, specificity for schizophrenia was found, as the manic patients were not different from normal subjects. Future studies in individuals at risk for schizophrenia or in the prodrome will be of great interest.

H.Y. Meltzer, M.D.

Absence of Neurodegeneration and Neural Injury in the Cerebral Cortex in a Sample of Elderly Patients With Schizophrenia
Arnold SE, Trojanowski JQ, Gur RE, et al (Univ of Pennsylvania, Philadelphia)
Arch Gen Psychiatry 55:225–232, 1998   7–5

Introduction.—Clinical and neurobiological trials disagree regarding neurodegeneration in late-life schizophrenia. If accumulated degenerative pathology occurs, it should be more evident in older age. Postmortem examinations were performed in elderly patients with poor-outcome schizophrenia to assess neurodegeneration or neural injury.

Methods.—Autopsies were performed on 23 prospectively accrued elderly patients who were diagnosed and rated clinically before death, 14 elderly controls with no neuropsychiatric disease, and 10 controls with Alzheimer's disease. Common neurodegenerative lesions (neurofibrillary tangles, amyloid plaques, and Lewy bodies) and cellular reactions to a variety of noxious stimuli (ubiquitinated dystrophic neurites, astrocytosis, and microglial infiltrates) in the ventromedial temporal lobe and the frontal and calcarine (primary visual) cortices were quantified by immunohistochemistry and unbiased stereologic counting methods.

Results.—There were no significant between-group differences in densities of neuropathologic markers in patients with schizophrenia and controls without neuropsychiatric disease. These 2 groups had fewer lesions than did controls with Alzheimer's disease. There were no significant associations between cognitive and psychiatric ratings and densities of any neuropathologic markers in patients with schizophrenia.

Conclusion.—There was no significant postmortem evidence of neurodegeneration or ongoing neural injury in the cerebral cortex of elderly patients with schizophrenia. There was no relationship between behavioral and cognitive degeneration in late life and age-related degenerative phenomena.

▶ Despite the evidence for an ongoing morbid process in the early stages of schizophrenia as noted in the previous 3 studies, this study failed to find evidence of neurodegeneration or neural injury in the cerebral cortex of elderly patients with schizophrenia, many of whom were demented before death. These results are not necessarily incompatible with the structural imaging or neuropathologic processes previously mentioned. These results indicate that any pathologic process occurring during the early stages of the illness does not lead to frank cell death and signs of neurodegeneration, as occurs with Huntington's disease. The deficit in cognition noted in schizophrenia must, then, be related to more subtle pathologic changes, functional abnormalities in connectivity, or both.

H.Y. Meltzer, M.D.

Reduction of Synaptophysin Immunoreactivity in the Prefrontal Cortex of Subjects With Schizophrenia: Regional and Diagnostic Specificity
Glantz LA, Lewis DA (Univ of Pittsburgh, Pa)
Arch Gen Psychiatry 54:943–952, 1997   7–6

Introduction.—Multiple lines of evidence suggest that the prefrontal cortex (PFC) is a site of dysfunction in schizophrenia. The conspicuous absence of gross structural abnormalities in the PFC indicates that the pathophysiological characteristics of schizophrenia may involve more subtle disturbances in cortical circuitry, such as alterations in synaptic connectivity and transmission. Synaptophysin is a 38-kd integral membrane protein of small synaptic vesicles that appears to be vital to calcium-dependent synaptic transmission. The integrity of cortical synaptic circuitry in schizophrenia was assessed using immunocytochemical techniques and optical density measurements.

Methods.—The synaptophysin immunoreactivity in PFC areas 9 and 46 and area 17 (the primary visual cortex) was assessed in postmortem tissue specimens of 10 patients with schizophrenia and 10 controls matched for age, sex, race, and postmortem interval. A second trial was performed with postmortem tissues from 5 patients with nonschizophrenic psychiatric illness and 5 healthy controls with no history of neurologic or psychiatric disease.

Results.—Synaptophysin immunoreactivity in areas 46 and 9, but not 17, was significantly diminished across all cortical layers in patients with schizophrenia. There were no between-group differences in levels of synaptophysin immunoreactivity in areas 46, 9, and 17 in tissue from persons with nonschizophrenic psychiatric illness and from normal controls.

Conclusion.—Disturbances in the level of synaptophysin transmission in the PFC may be observed specifically in patients with schizophrenia. These findings do not reveal which neural systems are altered in the PFC of patients with schizophrenia. Additional study is needed to determine which mechanisms cause reductions in levels of synaptophysin immuno-reactivity.

▶ Synaptophysin, a key membrane protein of small synaptic vesicles, was found to be selectively low in the PFC of schizophrenics. This could easily lead to functional impairment. Further data are needed to determine which neurons are deficient in synaptophysin and what, if any, clinical correlates are associated with it. Classical and conditional knock-out mice with deficient synaptophysin would be interesting models for determining the relevance of this membrane protein to behavior.

H.Y. Meltzer, M.D.

Neurological Abnormalities in Familial and Sporadic Schizophrenia

Griffiths TD, Sigmundsson T, Takei N, et al (Newcastle Univ, England; Inst of Psychiatry, London; Natl Hosp for Neurology, London)
Brain 121:191–203, 1998   7–7

Background.—Sporadic schizophrenia may be a manifestation of prenatal environmental factors instead of the rare expression of a lower genetic risk. This may be reflected in phenotypic differences between patients with sporadic and with familial disease. The existence of neurologic abnormalities in schizophrenia and the pattern of neurologic abnormality in familial and sporadic schizophrenic patients were investigated.

Methods.—The 214 individuals studied included patients with schizophrenia from multiply affected families, the first-degree relatives of these patients, patients with schizophrenia but no family history, the first-degree relatives of these patients, and healthy controls. A systematic assessment was used to classify abnormalities as primary or integrative signs. Primary signs, elicited on standard clinical neurologic evaluation, included signs of focal damage to nuclei and tracts. Integrative signs reflected distributed brain function.

Findings.—Only the patients with sporadic schizophrenia had an excess of primary signs compared with controls. The familial schizophrenics and their first-degree relatives, but not the sporadic schizophrenic patients or their relatives, had an increase in integrative signs.

Conclusions.—The presence of neurologic abnormalities in these schizophrenic patients supports the concept of underlying brain disorder in schizophrenia. The different pattern of abnormalities found in patients with familial and sporadic schizophrenia suggests different mechanisms of underlying brain dysfunction in these 2 groups.

▶ The concepts in this article have an appealing surface validity (i.e., that there would be neurologic signs indicative of birth-related abnormalities in sporadic schizophrenia and signs of structural brain damage that might reflect neurodevelopmental abnormalities in patients with familial schizophrenia and their first-degree relatives). The results are moderately consistent with the hypothesis, but there are many patients with neither type of abnormality, and the effect is rather weak at best. Between 25% and 50% of these patients will have mainly integrative abnormalities when conservative criteria of abnormality are used.

H.Y. Meltzer, M.D.

Association Between Central Nervous System Infections During Childhood and Adult Onset Schizophrenia and Other Psychoses: A 28-year Follow-up

Rantakallio P, Jones P, Moring J, et al (Univ of Oulu, Finland; Univ of Nottingham, England; Helsinki Univ Central Hosp)
Int J Epidemiol 26:837–843, 1997   7–8

Background.—Exposure of pregnant women to influenza during epidemics may increase the risk of schizophrenia in their children. The association of CNS infections defined prospectively to age 14 years, with subsequent onset of schizophrenia and other psychosis, was studied.

Methods.—A 1966 birth cohort in Northern Finland, covering 96% of all births in the area in that year, was studied. The occurrence of CNS infections between 1966 and 1980 was documented, and registered diagnoses of psychoses between 1982 and 1993 were validated on DSM-III-R criteria.

Findings.—One hundred forty-five of 11,017 children had a CNS infection during childhood. Infections were viral in 102. Seventy-six individuals received a diagnosis of schizophrenia, and 53 had other psychoses diagnosed. Four patients with schizophrenia had had viral CNS infection, and 2 patients with other psychoses had had bacterial infection. After adjustment for neurologic abnormalities and the father's social class, the odds ratio (OR) of schizophrenia developing after viral CNS infection was 4:8. Other significant risk factors were IQ of less than 85, perinatal brain damage, and male sex. Epilepsy was not a significant risk factor. After similar adjustments, the OR of other psychoses was 6:9 after bacterial CNS infection. Other significant risk factors were IQ of less than 85 and severe hearing defect. Two of the 5 viral infections were caused by coxsackievirus B5 during an epidemic that infected 16 neonates together.

Conclusions.—Central nervous system infections during childhood are associated with an increased risk of adult-onset schizophrenia or other psychoses. Viral infections, especially coxsackievirus B5 during the newborn period, are important in the subsequent development of schizophrenia.

▶ This is the first investigation of a large, general population birth cohort with definite viral infections and controls designed to determine the relationship of the infection to schizophrenia. The rate of schizophrenia in the 145 patients with viral infections was 2.8% (4/145), which is 4 times higher than that of the control group. The period of infection was between 9 days and 87 months in the affective cases, with age at onset in the expected range of 16 to 27 years. Coxsackie B appears to be particularly dangerous in this regard (12.5% incidence). Careful assessment of such infections should be part of the workup of a psychotic patient. This nonfamilial schizophrenia needs to be carefully identified for clinical research studies of the genetics of schizophrenia, the neurodevelopmental hypothesis, etc. Whether such cases respond differently to medication needs to be studied carefully.

H.Y. Meltzer, M.D.

Neuropsychological Deficits in Probands From Multiply-affected Schizophrenic Families
Sautter FJ, McDermott BE, Cornwell J, et al (Tulane Univ, New Orleans, La; NIH, Baltimore, Md; New Orleans Veterans Affairs Med Ctr, La)
J Psychiatr Res 31:497–508, 1997   7–9

Background.—Although previous research suggests that genetic factors play an etiologic role in schizophrenia, studies using sophisticated statistical and molecular genetic methods often fail to yield replicable data identifying the gene or genes that predispose individuals to this disorder. Whether schizophrenic patients from families with more than 1 psychotic relative have more severe neuropsychologic deficits than schizophrenic patients with only 1 psychotic relative, nonfamilial schizophrenic patients, and healthy individuals was determined.

Methods and Findings.—Eighty-one schizophrenic-spectrum patients were divided into 3 groups based on the presence of psychotic disorders among first- and second-degree relatives. Results of a brief neuropsychological testing battery were compared among the 3 schizophrenic groups and the healthy control group. Significant differences were noted in a multivariate analysis. Patients from multiply-affected families had significantly greater neuropsychologic dysfunction on measures of abstract concept formation, visuomotor coordination, and attention than those from families with only 1 psychotic relative. Schizophrenic patients from low-density families had more severe deficits in fine motor control than nonfamilial schizophrenic patients.

Conclusions.—The extent of neuropsychological deficit in schizophrenic probands on tasks thought to partly measure frontal systems may be associated with the degree of genetic liability to psychosis. These deficits are seen on neuropsychological tests thought to measure functioning in frontal systems that mediate fine motor control and abstract concept formation.

▶ This is another study showing the difference between familial and nonfamilial schizophrenia. The greater deficit in cognitive functioning in schizophrenic patients with a high density of cases within the family suggests that the deficit in cognition is genetically programmed and that those families with more severe cognitive impairment are more likely to have the full-blown syndrome. The presence of a moderate cognitive deficit in first-degree relatives is an indication that there is a threshold relationship between cognitive impairment and the development of a diagnosable form of schizophrenia.

H.Y. Meltzer, M.D.

L-745,870, a Subtype Selective Dopamine D$_4$ Receptor Antagonist, Does Not Exhibit a Neuroleptic-like Profile in Rodent Behavioral Tests
Bristow LJ, Collinson N, Cook GP, et al (Merck, Sharp and Dohme Research Labs, Harlow, England)
J Pharmacol Exp Ther 283:1256–1263, 1997   7–10

Introduction.—The high-affinity, selective dopamine D$_4$ receptor antagonist, L-745,870, was analyzed in rodent behavioral models to predict antipsychotic effects and adverse reactions in humans.

Findings.—In mice, L-745,870 did not antagonize amphetamine-induced hyperactivity. In rats, L-745,870 did not impair conditioned avoidance responding at doses selectively blocking D$_4$ receptors. Both these findings were in contrast to the classic neuroleptic, haloperidol, and the atypical neuroleptic, clozapine. L-745,870 did not reverse the deficit in prepulse inhibition of acoustic startle response induced by apomorphine, a nonselective dopamine D$_{2/3/4}$ receptor agonist; this effect was eliminated in rats pretreated with the D$_{2/3}$ receptor antagonist, raclopride. In rats, L-745,870 did not affect apomorphine-induced stereotypy, but it induced catalepsy in mice at a high dose of 100 mg/kg. Such high doses are likely to be found in dopamine D$_2$ receptors in vivo. High doses of L-745,870 significantly decreased spontaneous locomotor activity in rats and reduced time spent on a rotarod revolving at 15 rpm in mice.

Discussion.—These results indicate that dopamine D$_4$ receptor antagonism does not contribute to the ability of clozapine to decrease amphetamine-induced hyperactivity and conditioned avoidance response in rodents. The lack of effect of L-745,870 in this study is consistent with its inability to relieve psychotic symptoms in humans.

▶ D$_4$ receptor antagonism was postulated by Seeman as the basis for the remarkable therapeutic advantages of clozapine. This led to a search for selective D$_4$ antagonists, the first of which to be developed was L-745,870. This study established that blockade of this receptor does not produce any of the usual effects associated with an antipsychotic. Some studies suggest that D$_4$ antagonists may enhance cognition in rodents. L-745,870 has had no effect in schizophrenia. It appears unlikely that D$_4$ antagonism may still contribute in a small way to the action of drugs like clozapine.

H.Y. Meltzer, M.D.

Reference

1. Seeman P: Dopamine receptor sequences: Therapeutic levels of neuroleptics occupy D_2 receptors, clozapine occupies D_4. *Neuropsychopharmacology* 7:261–284, 1992.

Neutrophil Cytotoxicity of the Chemically Reactive Metabolite(s) of Clozapine: Possible Role in Agranulocytosis

Williams DP, Pirmohamed M, Naisbitt DJ, et al (Univ of Liverpool, England)
J Pharmacol Exp Ther 283:1375–1382, 1997   7–11

Introduction.—Clozapine is associated with 0.8% incidence of agranulocytosis. The nitrenium ion, an unstable protein-reactive metabolite, has been implicated in the pathogenesis of agranulocytosis. A novel in vitro assay in which the in situ generation of the reactive metabolite was coupled with an assessment of polymorphonuclear leukocyte and mononuclear leukocyte viability and chemical characterization of the metabolism of clozapine was examined to determine if the reactive metabolite is cytotoxic.

Findings.—Horseradish peroxidase and water were used to generate the metabolite in situ. In the absence of these full metabolizing systems, clozapine (0–100 µM) and its stable metabolites were not cytotoxic. With either full metabolism system, both clozapine (30 µM) and demethylclozapine demonstrated cytotoxicity toward polymorphonuclear and mononuclear leukocytes. Clozapine N-oxide was not cytotoxic. Exogenous glutathione (GSH), N-acetylcysteine, and ascorbic acid were protective of cells. Bioactivation of clozapine and demethylclozapine, but not N-oxide, was paralleled by depletion of intracellular GSH. [^{14}C]Clozapine was metabolized to previously identified C6 and C9 glutathionyl conjugates and GSH conjugates, when demethylclozapine and clozapine N-oxide were bioactivated by horseradish peroxidase and water.

Conclusion.—Clozapine and its stable metabolites are not cytotoxic, but may be bioactivated to cytotoxic metabolites. The cytotoxic metabolite of clozapine is analogous to the protein-reactive metabolite that may be key in the pathogenesis of clozapine agranulocytosis.

▶ Clozapine is still a uniquely effective antipsychotic for many patients who fail to respond to any of the typical neuroleptics or the newer atypicals. Despite this fact, the drug is underused because clinicians unduly fear the risk of agranulocytosis (mortality rate: 1 in 10,000), and some patients grow weary of the weekly blood drawing. Most evidence suggests that toxic metabolites rather than an autoimmune phenomenon is the mechanism of action. This study provides important evidence that a highly charged nitrogen ion of clozapine or its metabolites (called a nitrenium ion) may be the offending agent. It is interesting that reducing agents such as ascorbic acid appear to be protective. This needs to be tested clinically.

H.Y. Meltzer, M.D.

Interaction of the Novel Antipsychotic Drug Amerpozide and Its Metabolite FG5620 With Central Nervous System Receptors and Monoamine Uptake Sites: Relation to Behavioral and Clinical Effects
Svartengren J, Pettersson E, Björk A (Kabi Pharmacia AB, Malmö, Sweden)
Biol Psychiatry 42:247–259, 1997   7–12

Background.—Behavioral, biochemical, and electrophysiologic studies of the atypical antipsychotic drug, amperozide, indicate that it affects neurotransmission of mesolimbic and mesocortical dopamine. In a previous report, it was shown that amperozide showed high affinity for serotonin 5-HT$_{2A}$ receptors and moderate affinity for striatal dopamine D$_2$ and cortical α_1-adrenergic receptors.

Findings.—In an animal model, amperozide showed low affinity for various serotonin receptor subtypes and the dopamine D$_4$ receptor transfected in COS7 cells. Amperozide displayed very weak or no interaction with other receptor species including adrenergic, histaminergic, muscarinic, benzodiazepine, γ-aminobutyric acid, amino acid, opiate, and calcium channels. Amperozide was seen to compete for [^{3}H]paroxetine binding for the serotonin transporter in the nanomolar range. In vitro and in vivo binding potency of amperozide showed the best correlation with behavioral effects, suggesting 5-HT$_{2A}$ antagonism, although serotonin uptake inhibition may have a role in the effects of amperozide on the neurotransmission of dopamine. FG5620, a metabolite of amperozide, showed 5 to 10 times less pharmacologic activity than did amperozide.

Discussion.—These findings suggest that 5-HT$_{2A}$ receptors mediate the antipsychotic effects of amperozide. 5-HT uptake inhibition and α_1-adrenergic receptor-mediated effects may also be involved, especially at higher doses.

▶ Amperozide is one of the more interesting compounds that may or may not make it to the clinic. It has shown promise in curbing cravings for alcohol and cocaine as well as being an effective antipsychotic. Thus, the drug could be of great value in the many schizophrenic patients who are co-morbid for substance abuse. It lacks any direct antidopaminergic activity, suggesting that it will not produce significant extrapyramidal side effects or tardive dyskinesia.

H.Y. Meltzer, M.D.

Mesolimbic Dopamine D$_3$ Receptors and Use of Antipsychotics in Patients With Schizophrenia: A Postmortem Study
Gurevich EV, Bordelon Y, Shapiro RM, et al (Univ of Pennsylvania, Philadelphia)
Arch Gen Psychiatry 51:225–232, 1997   7–13

Introduction.—Elevated levels of D$_2$-like receptors in the striatum modulate symptoms of schizophrenia. Direct examination of the concentration and distribution of a recently cloned member of the dopamine D_2 receptor subfamily, the D_3 receptor, could help determine its involvement both in schizophrenia and with pharmacologic actions of antipsychotic drugs. The conditions for selective binding of the radioligand iodine 125-labeled (R)-*trans*-7-hydroxy-2[Npropyl-*N*-(3'-iodo-2'propenyl)-amino]tetralin([^{125}I]*trans*-7-OH-PIPAT) to the human D_3 receptor were characterized in brain tissue from patients with schizophrenia to quantify D_3 receptors. Concentration of D^3 receptors in the caudal and rostal basal ganglia regions was measured using quantitative autoradiography in patients with schizophrenia and compared with the concentration in healthy controls.

Results.—A nearly 2-fold increase in the number of D_3 receptors was observed in the basal ganglia and ventral forebrain of 7 patients, hospitalized long-term for schizophrenia, who received no antipsychotic drugs for at least 1 month before dying. There were 15 healthy matched controls. Eight patients with schizophrenia who received antipsychotic drugs less than 72 hours before death had D_3 levels similar to those of controls. Binding characteristics and affinity of [^{125}I]*trans*-7-OH-PIPAT binding to D_3 receptors did not differ between patients with schizophrenia and controls.

Conclusion.—Levels of D_3 receptors were increased in the rostal and caudal basal ganglia structures of patients with schizophrenia who were free of antipsychotic drugs, when these levels were compared with levels in matched controls and in schizophrenic patients being treated with antipsychotic drugs.

▶ Since the discovery of the D_3 receptor by Schwarcz and colleagues, there has been little progress in defining its importance for schizophrenia, other than some evidence that stimulation of D_3 receptors may be responsible for the effect of some novel antipsychotics in increasing early gene expression in rat frontal cortex. Some basic studies have also suggested that increasing D_3 receptor stimulation may have an antipsychotic-like action. Therefore, the finding of increased numbers of D_3 receptors in the basal ganglia and ventral forebrain of unmedicated schizophrenics may be indicative of an upregulation of these receptors as the result of too little stimulation. However, many antipsychotic drugs which are D_2 antagonists are also D_3 antagonists. Therefore, clinical trials with specific D_3 agonists and antagonists are needed to clarify what, if anything, is the importance of this dopamine receptor for schizophrenia.

H.Y. Meltzer, M.D.

Lack of Enhanced Response to Repeated d-Amphetamine Challenge in First-episode Psychosis: Implications for a Sensitization Model of Psychosis in Humans

Strakowski SM, Sax KW, Setters MJ, et al (Univ of Cincinnati, Ohio)
Biol Psychiatry 42:749–755, 1997   7–14

Introduction.—Behavioral sensitization is a process in which intermittent stimulant exposure creates a time-dependent, enduring, and progressively greater or more rapid behavioral response. This model is used to examine the development of psychosis. It has rarely been used in humans. Amphetamine-induced psychosis is regarded as a model for schizophrenia and as a clinical manifestation of behavioral sensitization. Responses to a second amphetamine challenge in patients with new-onset psychosis were compared in a double-blind, placebo-controlled trial with responses of normal controls to determine if the patient group would demonstrate more, less, or similar behavioral enhancement.

Methods.—Of 13 patients evaluated, 4 had a diagnosis of schizophrenia and 9 had bipolar disorder. All participants received 2 daily doses of d-amphetamine 0.25 mg/kg, separated by 48 hours, that alternated with 2 daily doses of placebo. Patients and normal controls were measured at baseline and hourly for 5 hours all 4 days after amphetamine/placebo administration for: mood, level of activity/energy rate, and amount of speech, severity of psychosis, and eye-blink rate. Vital signs were taken hourly.

Results.—Enhanced behavioral responses were observed in normal volunteers. However, participants in the patient group did not exhibit greater or more rapid behavioral effects after a second amphetamine dose.

Conclusion.—Patients with a first episode of psychosis did not exhibit a progressive enhancement in behavioral response to repeated amphetamine challenges. It is possible that patients with psychosis are already maximally sensitized and are, thus, unable to exhibit progressive behavioral enhancement after repeated stimulant challenges. It may be that patients with psychosis do not sensitize.

▶ Repeated administration of amphetamine challenges failed to produce signs of sensitization in first-episode manic or schizophrenic patients, as it did in normal controls. Although the negative results could be interpreted as evidence that the patients already were sensitized to dopamine, it seems more likely that these data should be understood as the patient's ability to be sensitized (i.e., diminished response to excessive dopaminergic stimulation). What relationship, if any, this has to the psychopathology of schizophrenia associated with dopaminergic function—positive and negative symptoms or deficits in working memory—remains to be determined.

H.Y. Meltzer, M.D.

5-HT₂ and D₂ Receptor Occupancy of Olanzapine in Schizophrenia: A PET Investigation

Kapur S, Zipursky RB, Remington G, et al (Univ of Toronto)
Am J Psychiatry 155:921–928, 1998   7–15

Introduction.—Olanzapine is a new atypical antipsychotic that is chemically similar to clozapine and shares several features of clozapine's in vitro pharmacological profile. Olanzapine also has stronger affinities for the 5-HT₂, muscarinic, and histaminic receptors than for the dopamine D₂ receptor. But not all atypical antipsychotics are alike. Risperidone is not especially effective in patients who have not responded to clozapine, yet clozapine can be effective in up to 50% of patients who have not responded to risperidone. Patients with schizophrenia were randomly assigned, prospectively, to receive a fixed multiple-dose regimen of a clinically relevant dose of olanzapine to determine a valid estimate of olanzapine's effect on the dopamine D₂ and serotonin 5-HT₂ receptors.

Methods.—Twelve patients with schizophrenia were prospectively randomized to 5, 10, 15, or 20 mg/day of olanzapine. Three patients taking 30 to 40 mg/day also were included. When steady-state plasma levels were achieved, dopamine D₂ and serotonin 5-HT₂ receptors were estimated using [¹¹C]raclopride and [¹⁸F]setoperone positron emission tomography imaging, respectively. Clinical status, extrapyramidal side effects, and prolactin levels were studied.

Results.—Olanzapine induced near saturation of the 5-HT₂ receptors at all doses, with greater than 90% 5-HT₂ occupancy in all patients. Average D₂ occupation varied according to dose: 55% with 5 mg/day, 73% with 10 mg/day, 75% with 15 mg/day, 76% with 20 mg/day, 83% with 30 mg/day, and 88% with 40 mg/day. Two patients who did not respond satisfactorily at clinical doses of 5 and 15 mg/day, respectively, had doses systematically increased to 30 and 40 mg/day, without further benefit. Two of 3 patients with doses above 20 mg/day had akathisia requiring antiparkinsonian drugs. Two of 3 patients with doses greater than 20 mg/day had abnormal elevations of prolactin.

Conclusion.—Olanzapine saturated 5-HT₂ receptors, with a higher 5-HT₂ than D₂ occupancy at all doses. Its D₂ occupancy was higher than that of clozapine and that reported earlier for typical neuroleptics and risperidone. Unlike clozapine, olanzapine probably does use the typical D₂ mechanism for inducing clinical response. At doses higher than 20 mg/day, olanzapine may have a greater prevalence of extrapyramidal side effects and prolactin elevation. Olanzapine is a well-tolerated, atypical antipsychotic in the 10 to 20 mg/day dose range. It may lose some of its atypical clinical effects when administered at higher doses.

▶ This study provides further insight into the value of 5-HT₂ₐ receptor blockade. It shows that olanzapine, at 5 mg/day, which was not an optimal dose for these patients, provides nearly complete 5-HT₂ₐ receptor blockade, along with modest D₂ receptor blockade. Multicenter trials with this low dose indicate that it was effective in significantly fewer patients than was 10 to 20 mg/day. This suggests that this combination of pharmacologic effects is not sufficient to produce an antipsychotic effect in most schizophrenic patients. Other features of olanzapine may decrease the efficacy of this combination. It may be, as I have suggested since 1989, that the combination of low D_2 receptor occupancy and high $5-HT_{2a}$ recptor occupancy is mainly related to extrapyramidal function, negative symptoms, and cognition, not control of positive symptoms.

H.Y. Meltzer, M.D.

Reversal of Isolation Rearing–induced Deficits in Prepulse Inhibition by Seroquel and Olanzapine
Bakshi VP, Swerdlow NR, Braff DL. et al (Univ of California at San Diego, La Jolla)
Biol Psychiatry 43:436–445, 1998   7–16

Background.—The acoustic startle reflex is subject to various forms of plasticity, one of which is prepulse inhibition. This refers to the normal inhibition of the startle response when an intense startling stimulus is immediately preceded by a weak stimulus. Prepulse inhibition provides an operational assessment of sensorimotor gating, whereby an organism screens the large flow of information from its surroundings. Sensory overstimulation and cognitive fragmentation are features of schizophrenia, and deficits in sensorimotor gating are seen in individuals with schizophrenia who are receiving medication but who are still ill. There is evidence that antipsychotic treatment can reverse prepulse inhibition deficits in individuals with schizophrenia.

Methods.—The ability of quietiapine and olanzapine to reverse isolation-induced deficits in prepulse inhibition was assessed in a rat model. Quetiapine, 5.0 mg/kg, or olanzapine, 2.5 mg/kg or 5.0 mg/kg, was administered to rats. Control rats received neither drug. Rats were housed singly or in groups of 3 for 8 weeks and were tested every 2 weeks. Startle response was elicited by 120 dB pulses with or without prepulses of 3, 6, or 12 dB above background noise.

Results.—Rats reared in isolation showed consistent deficits in prepulse inhibition and occasionally showed increased startle reactivity. In control rats reared socially, quetiapine reversed these deficits without affecting prepulse inhibition. Olanzapine, 2.5 mg/kg, reversed deficits in prepulse inhibition in rats reared in isolation and increased basal prepulse inhibition levels. Both drugs antagonized the increase in startle reactivity seen in rats reared in isolation.

Discussion.—In rats, atypical antipsychotic drugs can reverse deficits in sensorimotor gating caused by isolation rearing. These results confirm previous findings that quetiapine and olanzapine antagonize deficits in prepulse inhibition caused by psychotomimetic agents. Preliminary results of clinical studies suggest that both of these antipsychotic drugs reduce symptoms in individuals with schizophrenia. The isolation-rearing model of prepulse inhibition deficits seems to be sensitive to typical and atypical antipsychotic agents. These findings may help in the development of new treatment for schizophrenia.

▶ An animal model of prepulse inhibition is another useful model of a deficit present in schizophrenia. It can be produced by amphetamine, serotonin, receptor agonist hallucinogen, and phencyclidine, as well as isolation rearing. Isolation rearing may be considered a surrogate for early childhood stress. Regardless of the means of inducing deficits in prepulse inhibition, available evidence suggests that some of the newer antipsychotic agents are able to prevent them. Effects on dopaminergic, glutamatergic, and serotonergic systems, as well as noradrenergic (α-1) antagonism, may mediate the benefits of olanzapine and quetiapine in restoring prepulse inhibition to normal levels.

H.Y. Meltzer, M.D.

Phencyclidine-induced Deficits in Prepulse Inhibition of Startle are Blocked by Prazosin, an Alpha-1 Noradrenergic Antagonist

Bakshi VP, Geyer MA (Univ of California at San Diego, La Jolla)
J Pharmacol Exp Ther 283:666–674, 1997   7–17

Background.—In prepulse inhibition, a form of plasticity of the startle response, a weak stimulus immediately preceding an intense startle stimulus reduces the startle response. Deficits in prepulse inhibition are seen in individuals with schizophrenia and can be demonstrated in rats by phencyclidine (PCP), a psychotogen. In rats, such PCP-induced deficits in prepulse inhibition are resistant to dopamine and serotonin antagonists, but not to the antipsychotics clozapine, olanzapine, and quietiapine, which have antagonistic actions at various receptors, such as alpha-1 and alpha-2 adrenergic, M1 muscarinic, and γ-aminobutyric acid-A (GABA-A) receptors. Phencyclidine indirectly activates multiple neurotransmitter systems, and it is believed that the direct actions of PCP are mediated by noncompetitive antagonism of N-methyl-D-aspartate sites. In this study, the possibility that an antagonist action at a specific receptor subtype causes an interaction between PCP and the clozapine-like antipsychotic drugs was investigated by testing whether a selective antagonist at alpha-1, alpha-2, M1, or GABA-A receptors would block the deficit in prepulse inhibition induced by PCP in rats.

Methods.—Rats were pretreated with the alpha-1 antagonist prazosin at 0, 0.5, 1, or 2.5 mg/kg; the alpha-2 antagonist RX821002 at 0, 0.2, or 0.4 mg/kg; the M1 muscarinic antagonist pirenzepine at 0, 10, or 30 mg/kg; or the GABA-A antagonist pitrazepin at 0, 1, or 3 mg/kg. Animals were then treated with saline or PCP at 1.5 mg/kg. Because of the ability of prazosin to block the effects of PCP, an additional experiment determined the ability of prazosin at 0, 1, or 2.5 mg/kg to prevent deficits in prepulse inhibition induced by the dopamine agonist apomorphine at 0 or 0.5 mg/kg. Animals were tested in startle chambers after drug administration.

Results.—Phencyclidine consistently decreased prepulse inhibition. In 2 separate experiments, prazosin at 1.0 mg/kg and 2.5 mg/kg prevented this deficit but did not increase baseline levels of prepulse inhibition. The effects on prepulse inhibition were distinct from changes in startle reactivity. Prazosin did not antagonize apomorpine-induced disruptions of prepulse inhibition. This indicted that the antagonism of the effect induced by PCP did not simply result from a general improvement in deficient prepulse inhibition. No effect on baseline prepulse inhibition or PCP-induced disruptions in prepulse inhibition was seen from the antagonists for alpha-2, M1, or GABA-A receptors.

Discussion.—These findings suggest that the disruptive effect of PCP on prepulse inhibition may be partially mediated by alpha-1 adrenergic receptors. The antagonism of alpha-1 receptors may be important in mediating the prevention of PCP-induced deficits in prepulse inhibition by antipsychotic agents.

▶ The complex pharmacology of the new antipsychotic drugs has generated no shortage of suggestions as to which elements of their pharmacology contribute to their effectiveness and their side effects. Most attention has focused on their actions on serotonin, dopamine, and acetylcholine systems. However, many of the compounds are powerful adrenergic-receptor blockers. Clozapine, risperidone, olanzapine, and quetiapine (Seroquel) are all powerful antagonists of the α-1 receptor. Risperidone, clozapine, and quetiapine are also powerful α-2 receptor blockers.

This study shows the contribution of α-1 receptor blockade to the PCP-induced prepulse inhibition deficit, whereas the blockade of the apomorhpine-induced deficit is probably caused by dopamine receptor blockade. It is of interest that 5-HT$_{2A}$ receptor blockade may worsen prepulse inhibition deficits, indicating the trade-off between good and bad effects of particular pharmacologic features and the importance of the balance among them for clinical effectiveness.

H.Y. Meltzer, M.D.

Cognition

Functional MR Imaging of the Prefrontal Cortex: Specific Activation in a Working Memory Task
Kammer T, Bellemann ME, Gückel F, et al (Univ of Heidelberg, Germany; Max-Planck-Inst for Biological Cybernetics, Tübingen, Germany; German Cancer Research Ctr, Heidelberg, Germany; et al)
Magn Reson Imaging 15:879–889, 1997   7–18

Background.—In working memory, information is continuously updated and actively maintained to guide subsequent behavior. In the current study, functional MRI was used to identify cortical areas activated by a working memory task involving letter detection.

Methods and Findings.—Twenty-four normal persons underwent scanning with a conventional 1.5 T magnet while performing 1 of 2 tasks. During the activation task, the subjects pressed a button when any presented letter was the same as the second to last in the sequence. In the control condition, the subjects responded to a single predefined letter without memory update requirements. Perceptual input and motor output were identical in the 2 conditions. Movement artifacts were minimized using a 2-way strategy. Eight subjects were excluded from the final analysis. Analysis of the functional MR data from the remaining subjects was based on anatomic regions of interest defined manually in each individual. Engaging working memory was associated with significant activation in the dorsolateral prefrontal cortex (Brodmann's areas 9, 10, 46, and 47) and in both hemispheres.

Conclusions.—This study demonstrates the applicability of this paradigm in a clinical MRI setting. Findings were consistent with previous results of nonlateralized dorsolateral prefrontal activation during continuous context updating and active maintenance.

▶ Working memory deficits are among the most severe and functionally important cognitive deficits in schizophrenia. They may be responsive to treatment with some of the newer antipsychotic drugs (e.g., risperidone). Functional MRI localized working memory for a visual task in the dorsolateral prefrontal cortex in both hemispheres, further evidence that the dorsolateral prefrontal cortex may be abnormal in schizophrenia. The technique developed here will be useful in determining whether patients with schizophrenia have a characteristic impairment in carrying out working memory tasks and whether this can be normalized with antipsychotic drugs.

H.Y. Meltzer, M.D.

Cognitive Deficits in Obsessive-Compulsive Disorder on Tests of Frontal-Striatal Function
Purcell R, Maruff P, Kyrios M, et al (Univ of Melbourne, Australia; Mental Health Research Inst of Victoria, Parkville, Australia)
Biol Psychiatry 43:348–357, 1998   7–19

Background.—Neuropsychological and neuroimaging studies of obsessive-compulsive disorder (OCD) show that the frontal cortex and subcortical structures are involved in the pathophysiology of this disorder. However, few studies have addressed cognitive function in patients with OCD on tasks validated in the assessment of frontal lobe and subcortical dysfunction.

Methods.—Twenty-three patients with OCD but no depression and 23 healthy individuals matched by age, sex, education, and estimated IQ were studied. The accuracy and latency of executive and visual memory function were determined.

Findings.—The performance of patients with OCD was within the normal range in tasks of short-term memory capacity, delay dependent visual memory, pattern recognition, attentional shifting, and planning ability. However, the patients had specific cognitive deficits associated with spatial working memory, spatial recognition, and motor initiation and execution. These deficits were unrelated to aspects of patients' intellectual functioning or comorbid psychological symptoms, which suggests that the impairments were associated with the specific clinical characteristics of OCD.

Conclusions.—Patients with OCD have specific cognitive deficits on executive and visual memory function tasks. The pattern of impairment in these patients was qualitatively similar to that of patients with frontal lobe excisions and subcortical abnormalities on the same battery of tests. This suggests that the underlying pathophysiology of OCD may be best conceptualized as reflecting dysfunction of frontal-striatal systems.

▶ The Cambridge Neuropsychological Test Automated Battery computerized assessment of cognitive function identified a pattern of cognitive impairment suggestive of both frontal lobe and subcortical pathology in patients with OCD. However, there was no relationship to severity of OCD symptoms, suggesting that the symptomatology of the illness and, hence, functional impairment, is not a direct consequence of cognitive impairment. There are no data yet as to whether pharmacotherapy improves the cognitive dysfunction of OCD.

H.Y. Meltzer, M.D.

Frontal-Striatal Cognitive Deficits in Patients With Chronic Schizophrenia
Pantelis C, Barnes TRE, Nelson HE, et al (Univ of Melbourne, Australia; Charing Cross and Westminster Med School, London; Horton Hosp, Surrey, England; et al)
Brain 20:1823–1843, 1997   7–20

Background.—Although hypotheses have been proposed for the observed hypofrontality in schizophrenia, few recent studies have directly compared schizophrenic patients with those with disorders of the neocortex or subcortical structures. The neuropsychologic profiles of patients with chronic schizophrenia were established on a battery of tests sensitive to impairments of set shifting, working memory, and planning.

Methods.—Results of the computerized Cambridge Neuropsychological Test Automated Battery (CANTAB) were compared with 36 hospitalized patients with chronic schizophrenia, patients with neurologic disorders, and healthy persons. The groups were matched for age, sex, and intelligence quotient.

Findings.—Patients with temporal lobe lesions had no impairment in spatial working memory and planning abilities. Schizophrenic patients were impaired in visuospatial memory span when compared with the other groups. Severity of Parkinson's disease (PD) was associated with the degree of impairment in this task. Schizophrenic patients and those with frontal lobe lesions were impaired on a spatial working memory task, with increased between-search errors. Patients with PD did this task poorly in comparison with younger control subjects. Schizophrenic patients could not develop a systematic strategy to complete this task, relying instead on a limited visuospatial memory span. Although all groups were equally able to complete a task requiring higher-level planning ability, the schizophrenic patients and patients with frontal lobe lesions produced fewer perfect solutions and needed more moves to complete the task. Movement times were significantly longer for the schizophrenic patients, suggesting impairment in the sensorimotor skills needed for the task. Although the schizophrenic patients were unimpaired in their planning latencies, they had significantly prolonged execution latencies. Their pattern was similar to that of patients with frontal lobe lesions and contrasted with the prolonged planning time in patients with PD.

Conclusions.—Schizophrenic patients appear to have an overall deficit in executive functioning which is even greater than that in patients with frontal lobe lesions. However, the pattern of findings in these schizophrenic patients resembled that in patients with frontal lobe lesions or basal ganglia dysfunction, which supports the notion of disturbed frontal-striatal circuits in schizophrenia. In addition, schizophrenic patients have a loss of normal relationships between different domains of executive function, which has implications for impaired functional connectivity between different regions of the neocortex.

▶ The data from this study are the product of an elegant, computerized, cognitive assessment battery, CANTAB, which provides a powerful tool for dissecting the types of cognitive deficits present in neuropsychiatric disorders. Comparisons with patients with known lesions—such as frontal lobe lesions and PD—provide a means of identifying the primary site of the dysfunction. The results of this study clearly demonstrate a severe frontal lobe abnormality in schizophrenia, with additional disturbances in the basal ganglia and possible problems in connectivity between these areas. Approaches like the CANTAB are too complex for ordinary clinical practice, but have the potential to be simplified for office use.

H.Y. Meltzer, M.D.

Enduring Cognitive Deficits and Cortical Dopamine Dysfunction in Monkeys After Long-term Administration of Phencyclidine

Jentsch JD, Redmond DE Jr, Elsworth JD, et al (Yale Univ, New Haven, Conn)
Science 277:953–955, 1997   7–21

Introduction.—The effects of the psychotomimetic drug, phencyclidine, on the neurochemistry and function of the prefrontal cortex were examined in monkeys.

Findings.—In vervet monkeys that were treated with phencyclidine twice a day for 2 weeks, performance deficits were noted on a task sensitive to prefrontal cortex function. These deficits were improved by clozapine, an atypical antipsychotic drug. After repeated treatment with phencyclidine, a decrease was observed in basal and evoked dopamine utilization in the dorsolateral prefrontal cortex, a region of the brain associated with cognitive function. The behavioral deficits and decreased utilization of dopamine persisted, even after treatment was discontinued, suggesting that they did not result from direct drug effects alone.

Discussion.—These findings indicate that repeated exposure to phencyclidine in monkeys may help the study of psychiatric disorders, such as schizophrenia, associated with cognitive dysfunction and dopamine hypofunction in the prefrontal cortex.

▶ This study intrigues me because it shows the ability of chronic phencyclidine to produce prolonged deficits during a working memory task, comparable with those present in schizophrenia, and their reversal with short-term clozapine treatment. The study further links the deficit to the ability of phencyclidine to diminish basal and evoked dopamine utilization. This is a valuable model for studying the development of cognitive impairment in schizophrenia, its etiology, and various treatment strategies.

H.Y. Meltzer, M.D.

Differential Effect of a Dopaminergic Agonist on Prefrontal Function in Traumatic Brain Injury Patients

McDowell S, Whyte J, D'Esposito M (Moss Rehabilitation Research Inst, Philadelphia; Temple Univ, Philadelphia; Univ of Pennsylvania, Philadelphia)
Brain 121:1155–1164, 1998   7–22

Background.—Nonhuman primate studies suggest that dopamine is an important neurotransmitter for prefrontal function. The effects of low-dose bromocriptine, a D_2 dopamine receptor agonist, on processes thought to be subserved by the prefrontal cortex, such as working memory and executive function, were studied in persons with traumatic brain injury.

Methods and Findings.—Twenty-four patients were assessed in a double-blind, placebo-controlled, crossover trial. Bromocriptine improved performance on some, but not all, tasks thought to be subserved by prefrontal function. Performance was improved on clinical measures of executive function and dual-task performance, but not in measures of the ability to maintain information in working memory without significant executive demands. There was no improvement in control tasks thought to be independent of the prefrontal cortex.

Conclusions.—Bromocriptine has a selective effect on cognitive processes that involve executive control. The current findings provide a foundation for potential treatments for patents with prefrontal damage causing dysexecutive syndromes.

► The finding that bromocriptine, a D_2 dopamine receptor agonist, was able to selectively improve executive function, but not working memory, is of keen interest and provides further support that the ability of atypical antipsychotic drugs such as clozapine, risperidone, and olanzapine to increase extracellular dopamine levels in the prefrontal cortex may be the basis for their ability to improve cognitive function in patients with schizophrenia. However, bromocriptine improved virtually all frontal lobe tests, including the Wisconsin Card Sorting test, which is not sensitive to these agents in most studies. This may be related to the dopamine receptor-blocking properties of these agents. If so, it suggests that other means of enhancing prefrontal dopamine release without concomitant dopamine receptor blockade, even weak blockade, may be desirable in schizophrenia. It also suggests that strategies of treating schizophrenia which depend upon decreasing dopamine synthesis and release (e.g., autoreceptor stimulation), may have deleterious effects on cognition.

H.Y. Meltzer, M.D.

Dose-dependent Effects of the Dopamine D_1 Receptor Agonists A77636 or SKF81297 on Spatial Working Memory in Aged Monkeys
Cai JX, Arnsten AFT (Kunming Inst of Zoology, China; Yale Univ, New Haven, Conn)
J Pharmacol Exp Ther 283:183–189, 1997   7–23

Background.—Aged monkeys have deficits in spatial working memory similar to the deficits induced by lesions of the prefrontal cortex. Aged monkeys also have significant loss of dopamine from the prefrontal cortex, an important transmitter in proper prefrontal cortex functioning. Results of previous studies in aged monkeys indicate that treatment with D_1 agonists can improve spatial working memory, although the studies used drugs with either partial agonist actions or significant D_2 receptor actions.

Methods.—Aged monkeys were treated with the selective dopamine D_1 receptor full agonists A77636 and SKF81297 to determine effects on working memory functioning of the prefrontal cortex.

Results.—Both A77636 and SKF81297 produced a significant dose-dependent effect on delayed response performance. There was no evidence of side effects. Performance was improved by low doses, but was not affected or was impaired by higher doses. Improvement in and impairment of performance were reversed by pretreatment with SCH23390, a D_1 receptor antagonist.

Discussion.—These findings indicate that very low doses of D_1 receptor agonists may improve cognitive functioning in the elderly. The findings support the results of previous studies showing a narrow range of D_1-receptor stimulation for optimal prefrontal cortex cognitive function.

► Dopamine D_1 receptor function has been much less studied than D_2 and D_4 receptor function D_1 agonists may be useful in Parkinson's disease. Goldman-Rakic and colleagues have provided extensive data about the role of D_1 receptors in working memory in monkeys. It is crucial to obtain some data regarding this issue in humans. The study by McDowell et al. (Abstract 7–22) finds that D_2 receptor stimulation was helpful in a test that partially involves working memory: the Stroop. However, this is also a test of executive function, so further study of bromocriptine with more specific memory tests are needed. D_1 agonists may be tolerable in humans and could be used in the numerous conditions, including normal aging, where working memory is impaired.

H.Y. Meltzer, M.D.

The Influence of Odansetron and m-Chlorophenylpiperazine on Scopolamine-induced Cognitive, Behavioral, and Physiological Responses in Young, Healthy Controls

Brocks A, Little JT, Martin A, et al (Natl Inst of Mental Health, Bethesda, Md; Goettingen Univ, Germany; Emory Univ, Atlanta, Ga)
Biol Psychiatry 43:408–416, 1998   7–24

Background.—Learning and memory appear to be under the separate influence of cholinergic and serotonergic pathways. Whether serotonergic agents can attenuate or exacerbate the memory-impairing effects of anticholinergic blockade in humans was determined.

Methods.—Ten young, healthy volunteers were given either 0.15 mg/kg of IV odansetron, a selective serotonin 5-hydroxytryptamine$_3$ (5-HT$_3$) receptor antagonist, plus 0.08 mg/kg IV of m-chlorophenylpiperazine (m-CPP), a serotonergic agent, combined with 0.4 mg PO scopolamine, an anticholinergic agent, or scopolamine alone. The subjects were assessed on 3 separate days.

Findings.—Scopolamine administration significantly impaired episodic memory and processing speed. These deficits were neither attenuated by ondansetron pretreatment nor exacerbated by m-CPP administration plus scopolamine. However, m-CPP administration resulted in a significant increase in self-rated functional impairment, altered self-reality, and dysphoria ratings. In addition, the effect of scopolamine on pupil size was potentiated.

Conclusions.—The serotonergic effects of ondansetron and m-CPP only minimally modulate scopolamine-induced changes in cognitive performance in young, healthy persons. Further research with older persons is needed to determine whether age influences these findings.

▶ This article is noteworthy for raising the issue of the combined effects of cholinergic blockade on cognition and the possible influence of the serotonergic system on the memory impairment that ensues with muscarinic antagonists. While it would appear that 5-HT_{2c} agonists and 5-HT_3 antagonists are without major influence, the effects of selective serotonin reuptake inhibitors, of buspirone, a 5-HT_{1a} partial agonist, and of the new antipsychotics, which have variable effects on 5-HT_{2a}, 5-HT_{1a}, 5-HT_6, and 5-HT_7 receptors, need to be studied to define the role of 5-HT in cognition.

H.Y. Meltzer, M.D.

Ex Vivo Nerve Growth Factor Gene Transfer to the Basal Forebrain in Presymptomatic Middle-aged Rats Prevents the Development of Cholinergic Neuron Atrophy and Cognitive Impairment During Aging

Martínez-Serrano A, Björklund A (Univ of Lund, Sweden; Autonomous Univ of Madrid)
Proc Natl Acad Sci U S A 95:1858–1863, 1998   7–25

Background.—Studies in rodents have shown that advanced age is accompanied by progressive degenerative changes in the basal forebrain cholinergic system. The degree of change is correlated with the severity of behavioral impairment in learning and memory tasks. Injection or infusion of exogenous nerve growth factor has been shown to reverse these age-dependent atrophic changes in the cholinergic forebrain neurons and to improve spatial learning in rodents.

Methods.—Behaviorally normal middle-aged rats (14 to 16 months old) received bilateral transplants of ex vivo transduced clonal nerve growth factor-secreting immortalized neural progenitor cells in the nucleus basalis and septum.

Results.—During the 9 months after transplant, aged control animals developed impairment in spatial learning in a water maze task. The performance in the water maze task of the study animals with nerve growth factor-secreting grafts was comparable with the performance of 12-month-old control rats. The significant age-induced atrophy of the cholinergic neurons in medial septum and nucleus basalis in the aged control rats was not seen in rats treated with nerve growth factor. ^{3}H-labeled thymidine autoradiography revealed that survival of the transduced cells was good and that the cells had become integrated into the host tissue around the injection sites. Analysis by reverse transcription-polymerase chain reaction analysis showed expression of the nerve growth factor transgene in grafted tissue at 4 and 9 months.

Discussion.—These findings suggest that long-term supply of nerve growth factor from ex vivo transduced immortalized neural progenitor cells in the nucleus basalis and septum can prevent age-related neuronal atrophy and behavioral impairment.

▶ This elegant study shows the power of neurotrophic brain growth factors to prevent some of the degenerative changes of aging. There are numerous families of such growth factors that are being characterized, and this has been accompanied by an extensive effort to mimic their effects pharmacologically. As yet, there has been little success in that regard. Synthetic, stable growth factors that can pass the blood-brain barrier and gain entry to neurons could be of great value in a variety of neurodegenerative disorders.

H.Y. Meltzer, M.D.

Mood Disorders

Expanded Trinucleotide CAG Repeats in Families With Bipolar Affective Disorder

Mendlewicz J, Lindbald K, Souery D, et al (Free Univ of Brussels, Belgium; Karolinska Hosp, Stockholm; Univ of Umeå, Sweden; et al)
Biol Psychiatry 42:1115–1122, 1997   7–26

Background.—Expanded trinucleotide repeats may be associated with anticipation and transmission patterns in families with bipolar affective disorder (BPAD). This hypothesis was tested using the repeat expansion detection method.

Methods.—Eighty-seven 2-generation patient pairs were recruited from 29 families with BPAD. The repeat expansion detection method was used to determine cytosine adenosine guanosine (CAG) repeat expansions between successive generations.

Findings.—Significant changes were noted in age at onset and episode frequency in successive generations. The mean trinucleotide CAG repeat length between parents and offspring increased significantly when the phenotype was more severe, changing from major depression, single episode or unipolar recurrent depression, to BPAD. There was also a parent-of-origin effect, with a significant increase in the CAG median length between G_1 and G_2 with maternal inheritance, especially in female offspring.

Conclusion.—Expansion of CAG repeat length may explain the clinical observation of anticipation in families with BPAD. The data further support the notion of expanded trinucleotide repeat sequences as risk factors in major affective disorders.

▶ This is the third report on this topic and offers by far the strongest evidence that trinucleotide repeat expansions may be 1 of the genetic bases for bipolar disorder. This is the first study to show relevant clinical correlates of this genetic defect (i.e., earlier age at onset and more severe disorder in the second generation studied). This study is also important because it links the genetics of unipolar and bipolar depression. The authors note many reasons for caution about their findings. As usual, genetic studies of this type must be replicated with increasingly stringent methodology before the conclusions can be accepted.

H.Y. Meltzer, M.D.

Serotonin 5-HT$_2$ Receptor Imaging in Major Depression: Focal Changes in Orbito-Insular Cortex
Biver F, Wikler D, Lotstra F, et al (Free Univ of Brussels, Belgium)
Br J Psychiatry 171:444–448, 1997   7–27

Background.—Serotonin receptors may be involved in the pathophysiology of affective disorders. Type 2 serotonin (5-HT$_2$) receptors in the brains of patients with major depression were studied.

Methods and Findings.—Positron emission tomography and selective radioligand [18]altanserin were used to assess 5-HT$_2$ receptor distribution in 8 drug-free patients with unipolar depression and 22 healthy persons. [18]Altanserin uptake was decreased significantly in an area of the right hemisphere in the depressed patients. This area included the posterolateral orbitofrontal cortex and the anterior insular cortex. A trend toward similar changes was noted in the left hemisphere. Uptake was not associated with Hamilton rating scale score.

Conclusion.—The pathophysiology of unipolar depression may involve changes in 5-HT$_2$ receptor in areas of the brain selectively implicated in mood regulation. Further research is needed to determine whether the different agents that enhance serotonin transmission exert their antidepressant effects at this level.

▶ This is the first study of 5-HT$_2$ receptor density in depression using positron emission tomography (PET). Previous postmortem and one single photon emission (SPECT) study have found increased 5-HT$_{2a}$ receptor density in various cortical regions, not a decrease as was found in this study. This study also points to the orbito-insular cortex as a region of interest in depression. The number of patients in this study was small, but this may be a major breakthrough in understanding the decreased serotonergic activity in depression.

H.Y. Meltzer, M.D.

Recovery From Major Depression Is not Associated with Normalization of Serotonergic Function
Flory JD, Mann JJ, Manuck SB, et al (Univ of Pittsburgh, Pa; New York Psychiatric Inst)
Biol Psychiatry 43:320–326, 1998   7–28

Background.—Compared with healthy persons, patients with moderate-to-severe depression typically have blunted plasma prolactin responses to fenfluramine, a serotonergic drug. However, whether this dysregulation represents an acute change during symptomatic depression or a chronic disturbance is unclear.

Methods.—The prolactin responses to D,L-fenfluramine in 29 adults who had had at least 1 major depressive episode, but not in the preceding year, were compared with those of 58 adults with no history of major depression. The groups were matched for age, sex, and socioeconomic status.

Findings.—Peak prolactin responses were significantly lower in persons with a positive history of major depression than in healthy subjects. This difference was not explained by weight, fenfluramine bioavailability, or baseline prolactin levels.

Conclusion.—These findings support the hypothesis that central serotonergic activity is persistently disturbed in adults with depressive episodes. The authors suggest that genetic factors and early social stressors influence serotonergic activity in an enduring manner, which results in vulnerability to depression.

▶ Fenfluramine is now the standard pharmacologic challenge for the serotonergic system. It is not ideal by any means, because it acts indirectly to make more serotonin available and is, thus, dependent upon a host of both presynaptic- and postsynaptic factors. It may also influence prolactin secretion through a dopaminergic mechanism. Despite these caveats, the data showing a persistent abnormality in the response to fenfluramine in recovered depressed patients requires us to reconsider the role of serotonin in depression as a vulnerability factor rather than only the disease process. Further studies with other serotonergic probes are important to clarify which elements of the serotonergic system (e.g., 5-HT_{1a} and 5-HT_{2a} receptors) may be persistently abnormal despite apparent recovery of mood.

H.Y. Meltzer, M.D.

Dexfenfluramine Enhances Striatal Dopamine Release in Conscious Rats via a Serotoninergic Mechanism
Balcioglu A, Wurtman RJ (Massachusetts Inst of Technology, Cambridge)
J Pharmacol Exp Ther 284:991–997, 1998   7–29

Introduction.—The release of brain dopamine (DA) or serotonin (5-HT) into synapses and blocking of the reuptake of these monoamines appears to be the method by which existing weight-reducing drugs produce their effects. In contrast, dexfenfluramine (d-fen) releases 5-HT, but not DA, from synaptosomes. The d-fen also increases 5-HT levels in dialysates from cortex, hypothalamus, and nucleus accumbens. Whereas amphetamine suppresses appetite, d-fen enhances satiety. The d-fen also differs in that it selectively inhibits the overconsumption of carbohydrates. An animal study was conducted to examine the effects of d-fen on the release of DA and 5-HT into striatal dialysates.

Methods.—Amphetamine and d-fen, dissolved in saline, were administered intraperitoneally in male Sprague Dawley rats. Tetrodotoxin and 5-HT were dissolved in artificial CSF (aCSF). Control animals received only the saline vehicle or the aCSF perfusate. Probes implanted into the striatum collected samples every 20 minutes, and the samples were analyzed immediately by high-performance liquid chromatography.

Results.—Mean baseline levels of DA and 5-HT in striatal dialysates collected before drug administration were 74.5 and 3.8 fmol/20 µL, respectively. Administration of a lower anorectic dose of d-fen (0.5 or 1.0 mg/kg) significantly increased dialysate 5-HT concentrations without affecting those of DA. A higher dose (2.5 mg/kg) increased both 5-HT and DA. The DA increase could be blocked by administering the mixed-acting 5-HT antagonist methiothepin (20 µM) and was reproduced by the application of 5-HT (3–10 µM) directly to striatal neurons. Tetrodotoxin (1 µM) decreased the basal release of DA and 5-HT, blocked the effect of d-fen on DA release, and decreased the increase in 5-HT release by approximately 70%. Both amphetamine and phentermine increased dialysate DA concentrations without affecting those of 5-HT; tetrodotoxin did not block the response to amphetamine.

Conclusion.—Data provide the first evidence that lower doses of d-fen (0.5 or 1.0 mg/kg) enhance 5-HT release in the rat striatum. The d-fen can increase DA release at higher (2.5 mg/kg) doses, and 5-HT is likely to mediate this response.

▶ This article provides strong evidence that fenfluramine can increase the release of dopamine in some brain regions at high doses in rats. The issue remains whether it does this at doses that are used in humans for pharmacologic challenge studies and for the now-banned purpose of weight reduction. It further illustrates the important interaction between serotonin and dopamine. In this model, serotonin release increases dopamine release in the striatum, but serotonin can also inhibit striatal dopaminergic function.

H.Y. Meltzer, M.D.

Effects of Tryptophan Depletion vs Catecholamine Depletion in Patients with Seasonal Affective Disorder in Remission with Light Therapy
Neumeister A, Turner EH, Matthews JR, et al (Natl Inst of Mental Health, Bethesda, Md; Vienna Univ; Univ of Erlangen, Germany)
Arch Gen Psychiatry 55:524–530, 1998   7–30

Background.—Hypotheses regarding the mechanism of action underlying light therapy have focused on serotonergic mechanisms. The possible role of catecholaminergic pathways has not been thoroughly studied.

Methods.—Sixteen patients with seasonal affective disorder were enrolled in a double-blind, placebo-controlled, randomized, crossover trial. All patients had previously responded to a standard regimen of daily 10,000-lux light therapy. The effects of tryptophan depletion were compared with catecholamine and sham depletion. Depressive symptoms were measured on the Hamilton Depression Rating Scale, Seasonal Affective Disorder Version.

Findings.—Tryptophan depletion significantly reduced plasma total and free tryptophan levels, and catecholamine depletion significantly reduced plasma 3-methoxy-4-hydroxyphenylethyleneglycol and homovanillic acid concentrations. Compared with sham depletion, both trytophan and catecholamine depletion resulted in a robust increase in depressive symptoms.

Conclusion.—Both tryptophan and catecholamine depletion reverse the beneficial effects of light therapy in patients with seasonal affective disorder. These findings are consistent with previous research showing that serotonin has an important role in the mechanism of action underlying light therapy. In addition, these data provide new evidence that brain catecholaminergic systems may be involved.

▶ The ability of depletion of serotonin or catecholamines to reverse the effect of antidepressant drugs in recovered patients with seasonal affective disorder has shown that patients respond to 1 or the other bioamine depletion, depending on which type of antidepressant has been used. Thus, patients who have responded to a fluoxetine-like antidepressant will usually, but not always, relapse after tryptophan depletion but not after catecholamine depletion. Thus, it is of interest that patients who responded to light therapy were sensitive to both types of depletion, suggesting that both catecholamines and serotonin may be important to its efficacy.

H.Y. Meltzer, M.D.

Effects of Acute Tryptophan Depletion in Lithium-remitted Manic Patients: A Pilot Study

Cappiello A, Sernyak MJ, Malison RT, et al (Yale Univ, New Haven, Conn; Brown Univ, Providence, RI)
Biol Psychiatry 42:1076–1078, 1997   7–31

Background.—Although the efficacy of lithium in the acute treatment of mania has been well established, its mechanism of action is not fully understood. Lithium may enhance serotonin (5-HT) function. The authors of this study hypothesize that intact 5-HT function is needed to maintain the antimanic effects of lithium and that rapid tryptophan (TRP) depletion would temporarily reverse the recovered state of acutely remitted manic patients.

Methods and Findings.—Seven patients who had just completed an open-label course of lithium for bipolar manic episode were subjected to TRP depletion. Ingestion of a low-TRP diet combined with TRP-free amino acid drink significantly decreased plasma free and total TRP levels. Depletion of TRP was correlated with increased manic symptoms for 3 days after the test. All patients returned to baseline conditions within 5 days after the test.

Conclusion.—Maintaining clinical improvement in some acutely remitted bipolar patients may require the short-term availability of the 5-HT precursor TRP. Further research is now needed to determine the role of 5-HT function in the antimanic effects of lithium in bipolar patients.

▶ This is the first study of tryptophan depletion in recently remitted lithium-treated manic patients. At least 2 of the 7 patients studied had a full-blown relapse, as did 1 patient during the placebo challenge. Whether the stress of the study produced the mania or there is a need for adequate serotonergic stimulation for the action lethium requires further study. If deficient serotonin is an element of both depression and mania, then some other factor must be central to producing the direction of mood changes.

H.Y. Meltzer, M.D.

Clinical and Psychometric Correlates of Dopamine D_2 Binding in Depression

Shah PJ, Ogilvie AD, Goodwin GM, et al (Royal Edinburgh Hosp, Scotland)
Psychol Med 27:1247–1256, 1997   7–32

Background.—Although the roles of the serotonergic and noradrenergic neurotransmitter systems in the pathogenesis of depression are widely accepted, evidence also suggests a role for dopaminergic mechanisms. Clinical and psychometric correlates of dopamine D_2-binding in depressed patients were investigated.

Methods.—Fifteen patients with major depressive illness and 15 healthy, age- and sex-matched volunteers underwent a clinical and neuropsychological battery of tests in addition to high-resolution single photon emission tomography (SPECT) with the dopamine $D_{2/3}$ ligand ^{123}I-3-iodomethoxybenzamide (IBZM). Specific binding was estimated by averaging striatum to whole slice or frontal uptake ratios over 8–10 scans obtained from 70 minutes after tracer injection.

Findings.—With whole slice used as a reference, left striatal uptake ratios did not differ significantly between patients and control subjects. Patients had significantly greater right ratios. In addition, IBZM binding in left and right striatum were significantly correlated with measures of reaction time and verbal fluency.

Conclusion.—Increased IBZM binding in striatum probably indicates decreased dopamine function, either because of reduced dopamine release or secondary upregulation of receptors. Whether the abnormalities observed are trait or state related requires further research, as does the possible role of medication as a confounding variable.

▶ Papers that remind us of the role of dopamine in depression are important. As indicated here, neurochemical evidence for decreased dopaminergic activity in depression is fairly robust. The selective serotonin reuptake inhibitors all enhance dopamine release in various forebrain areas. This may be a big part of their antidepressant action. The new antipsychotics have a similar effect, and these drugs are useful as antidepressants. The fact that D_2 blockers like haloperidol do not usually cause depression suggests that other types of dopamine receptors may be involved, the leading candidates being the D_1 and D_3 receptors.

H.Y. Meltzer, M.D.

Increase in the Cerebrospinal Fluid Content of Neurosteroids in Patients With Unipolar Major Depression Who Are Receiving Fluoxetine or Fluvoxamine
Uzunova V, Sheline Y, Davis JM, et al (Univ of Illinois, Chicago; VA Med Ctr, West Haven, Conn; Washington Univ, St Louis)
Proc Natl Acad Sci U S A 95:3239–3244, 1998   7–33

Background.—Recent research suggests that fluoxetine and paroxetine, 2 selective serotonin reuptake inhibitors (SSRIs), increase the brain content of the neurosteroid 3α-hydroxy-5α-pregnane-20-one (3α5α-ALLO) in rats without changing the brain content of other neurosteroids. The 3α5α and 3α5β isomers (ALLO) bind with high affinity to various γ-aminobutyric (GABA) receptor A subtypes and facilitate GABA action at these receptors. The increase in ALLO brain content induced by SSRI treatment may contribute to the anxiety and dysphoria relief associated with the symptomatology of major unipolar depression.

Methods and Findings.—The ALLO content was measured in 4 cisternal-lumbar fractions of CSF before and 8 to 10 weeks after treatment with fluoxetine or fluvoxamine in 15 patients with unipolar major depression.

Compared with control values, ALLO concentrations in depressed patients were reduced by about 60%. Fluoxetine or fluvoxamine treatment in these patients normalized the CSF ALLO content. Symptomatology improvement was significantly correlated with the increase in CSF ALLO after treatment.

Conclusion.—Normalizing CSF ALLO content in depressed patients seems to be adequate for mediating the anxiolytic and antidysphoric actions of fluoxetine or fluvoxamine treatment. Mediation appears to occur through positive allosteric modulation of GABA type A receptors.

▶ The neurosteroids, derived from cholesterol, are formed in the brain and are able to facilitate some of the actions of $GABA_A$ receptor-mediated chloride currents. They also regulate gene expression through the progesterone receptor. Systemic administration in rats reveals anxiolytic and hypnotic properties. They may be of value in disorders of memory, stress, anxiety, sleep, depression, and seizures. The findings that levels of a key neurosteroid ALLO are decreased in the CSF of depressed patients, and that the increase in CSF ALLO levels produced by fluoxetine and fluvoxamine is correlated with improvement in depression ratings is the first direct clinical evidence of the importance of neurosteroids in psychiatric disorders. Comparable studies in anxiety disorders are needed.

H.Y Meltzer, M.D.

Obsessive-Compulsive Disorder and Stress

Hypercortisolism Associated With Social Subordinance or Social Isolation Among Wild Baboons
Sapolsky RM, Alberts SC, Altmann J (Stanford Univ, Calif; Harvard Univ, Cambridge, Mass; Univ of Chicago)
Arch Gen Psychiatry 54:1137–1143, 1997   7–34

Background.—The causes and consequences of basal hypercortisolism and dexamethasone resistance in various neuropsychiatric disorders are still largely unknown. Basal cortisol concentrations and adrenocortical responsiveness to dexamethasone were studied in wild baboons living in a national park in Kenya.

Methods.—Seventy yellow baboons were studied to determine whether social subordinance in a primate is associated with dexamethasone resistance and whether individual differences in adrenocortical measures could be predicted by the extent of social affiliation. The animals were anesthetized and injected with 5 mg dexamethsaone. Cortisol responses were monitored for 6 hours.

Findings.—The socially subordinate baboons were less responsive to dexamethasone than were the dominant baboons. Postdexamethasone cortisol values were more than 3 times greater in the lowest-ranking compared with the highest-ranking animals. In addition, socially isolated males had increased basal cortisol levels and a trend toward relative dexamethasone resistance.

Conclusion.—Social status and degree of social affiliation can affect adrenocortical profiles in nonhuman primates. In this study of baboons, social subordination and isolation were associated with hypercortisolism or feedback resistance.

▶ While patients with chronic fatigue syndrome may suffer from too little output of adrenocorticoids (see Scott et al.), the opposite may be true for subordinate males, at least among the wild baboons. The stress of being in such a position from a survival and sexual perspective produces a substantial outpouring of adrenocorticoids and resistance to suppressing that output. Clearly, it may have some survival benefits but, as Sapolsky and colleagues have pointed out in many articles, there is a potentially neurotoxic price extracted for this adaptive response. At the end, "chronic fatigue" and much worse may result. The moral of the story: keep your cortisol within the normal range by successfully mastering the challenges of your environment.

H.Y. Meltzer, M.D.

Long-term Stress Degenerates, but Imipramine Regenerates, Noradrenergic Axons in the Rat Cerebral Cortex
Kitayama I, Yaga T, Kayahara T, et al (Mie Univ, Tsu, Japan)
Biol Psychiatry 42:687–696, 1997   7–35

Background.—Previous experimental research has indicated that noradrenergic degeneration may play a role in the pathophysiology of depression. The density of noradrenergic axons in the cerebral cortex was measured using the rat model of depression, with or without imipramine.

Methods.—Retrograde labeling of locus coeruleus neurons with horseradish peroxidase and immunohistochemical staining of cortical axons with a dopamine β-hydroxylase antiserum were used. The density of noradrenergic axon profiles of rats exposed to a short-term forced walking stress and of rats recovering from prestress activity after a long-term forced walking stress were assessed. The correlation between the density of noradrenergic axon profiles and the recovery rate of spontanoeus activity was also noted.

Findings.—The density of noradrenergic axons was significantly lower in the depression-model rats. This density tended to be higher in the recovering and short-term stressed rats. The density of noradrenergic axons was associated with the recovery rate of activity.

Conclusion.—Cortical noradrenergic degeneration appears to be involved in the pathogenesis of depression. Prolonged antidepressant treatment may induce regeneration of noradrenergic axons.

▶ In accord with Sapolsky et al.'s (Abstract 7–34) work in primates, severe, chronic stress can be shown to produce long-term changes in rodent brain structures as well as function. The stress used in this study is shown to be related to major depression in that some of its effects are prevented by concomitant treatment with antidepressant drugs. Recent studies of neural size and density in postmortem specimens and of cognition in patients recovered from mood disorders provide data suggestive of long-term damage in the brains of depressed patients. The neuroprotective effects of imipramine are interesting. Whether the many strategies to develop neuroprotective drugs for stroke and degenerative disease may lead to drugs useful in depression is worthy of direct study.

H.Y. Meltzer, M.D.

Blunted Adrenocorticotropin and Cortisol Responses to Corticotropin-releasing Hormone Stimulation in Chronic Fatigue Syndrome
Scott LV, Medbak S, Dinan TG, et al (St Bartholomew's and the Royal London School of Medicine)
Acta Psychiatr Scand 97:450–457, 1998   7–36

Background.—Hypofunctioning of the pituitary-adrenal axis may be the pathophysiologic basis for chronic fatigue syndrome (CFS). Studies have demonstrated blunted adrenocorticotropin (ACTH) responses, but normal cortisol responses to exogenous corticotropin-releasing hormone (CRH), the main axis regulator, in patients with CFS, some of whom had a comorbid psychiatric disorder. Corticotropin-releasing hormone activation of this axis was examined in patients with CFS and no concurrent psychiatric illness.

Methods and Findings.—Fourteen patients with CFS were compared with 14 healthy volunteers. Ovine CRH, 100 µg, was administered, and ACTH and cortisol responses were measured. Basal ACTH and cortisol values were comparable in the 2 groups. In the CFS group, both ACTH and cortisol release were significantly attenuated after CRH administration.

Conclusions.—The blunted ACTH response to exogenous CRH stimulation in patients with CFS may result from an abnormality in CRH levels, leading to a change in pituitary CRH receptor sensitivity, or it may reflect dysregulation of vasopressin or other factors involved in hypothalamo-pituitary-adrenal (HPA) regulation. A reduced output of neurotrophic ACTH, causing a decrease in adrenocortical secretory reserve insufficiently compensated for by adrenoceptor upregulation, may account for the decrease in cortisol production seen in this study.

▶ Diminished output of the HPA axis has been proposed as a cause of CFS.[1] This study is the first replication of that original report of diminished HPA axis responsivity to CRH in this common ailment. The results here replicate a blunted ACTH response but differ in that, in this study, the cortisol response was also diminished. This could be the basis for inadequate trophic effects of glucocorticoids in patients with CFS. Whether glucocorticoids have therapeutic value in this syndrome requires further study.

H.Y. Meltzer, M.D.

Reference

1. Demitrack M, Dale J, Straus S, et al: Evidence for impaired activation of the hypothalamic-pituitary-adrenal axis in chronic fatigue syndrome. *J Clin Endocrinol Metab* 73:1224–1234, 1991.

A Preliminary Study of Tryptophan Depletion on Tics, Obsessive-Compulsive Symptoms, and Mood in Tourette's Syndrome

Rasmusson AM, Anderson GM, Lynch KA, et al (Yale Univ, New Haven Conn; Med College of Georgia, Augusta; Univ of Florida, Gainesville)
Biol Psychiatry 41:117–121, 1997   7-37

Background.—Evidence suggests that altered tryptophan (TRP) metabolism or underactivity of the brain serotonin (5-HT) system has a role in the pathophysiology of Tourette's syndrome (TS). The effects of acute TRP depletion in patients with TS were reported.

Methods.—Six medication-free patients with TS were enrolled in a randomized, double-blind, placebo-controlled study. All had been given a primary diagnosis of TS with obsessive-compulsive disorder or obsessive-compulsive features. On day 1, the patients received a diet containing 160 mg TRP supplemented with 3 500-mg TRP capsules. On day 2, a 16-amino acid drink containing 2.3 g TRP was ingested. During TRP depletion, TRP was limited to 160 mg.

Findings.—Depletion of TRP did not result in worsening of tics, obsessive-compulsive features, or mood symptoms in these patients. No significant differences occurred between the control and TRP-depletion conditions in symptom changes over time. In both conditions, patient-rated tics declined over time.

Conclusion.—Reductions in plasma TRP—which presumably decrease CNS levels of TRP and 5-HT—apparently do not affect TS symptoms. However, because the number of patients studied was small, these results should be interpreted with caution. Further research is warranted.

▶ The failure of tryptophan depletion to worsen the obsessive-compulsive, tic, or mood symptoms in TS contrasts with the previous article by Neumeister et al. (Abstract 7–30) regarding the effects of tryptophan depletion in seasonal affective disorder. It should be noted that none of the patients in this study was currently receiving treatment. Further, the extent of interference with serotonin synthesis may be insufficient. Studies in patients who have partially responded to selective serotonin reuptake inhibitors may be more informative. It would also be useful to test the role of dopamine in TS by a catecholamine depletion regimen. Conceivably, interference with both catecholamine and sertonin neurotransmission are needed to modulate TS.

H.Y. Meltzer, M.D.

Effect of Prefrontal Repetitive Transcranial Magnetic Stimulation in Obsessive-Compulsive Disorder: A Preliminary Study

Greenberg BD, George MS, Martin JD, et al (Natl Inst of Neurological Diseases and Stroke, Bethesda, Md)
Am J Psychiatry 154:867–869, 1997   7–38

Background.—Prefrontal mechanisms appear to play a role in the development of obsessive-compulsive disorder (OCD). Whether prefrontal repetitive transcranial magnetic stimulation affects OCD symptoms was investigated.

Methods.—Twelve patients with OCD underwent repetitive transcranial magnetic stimulation to a right lateral prefrontal site, a left lateral prefrontal site, and a midoccipital site on separate days in random order. Symptoms and mood were assessed for 8 hours after stimulation.

Findings.—Compulsive urges declined significantly for 8 hours after right lateral prefrontal repetitive transcranial magnetic stimulation. Nonsignificant increases in compulsive urges after repetitive transcranial magnetic stimulation of the midoccipital site were noted. After left lateral prefrontal repetitive transcranial magnetic stimulation, there was a briefer, modest, nonsignificant decrease in compulsive urges. Patients' mood improved during and 30 minutes after right lateral prefrontal stimulation.

Conclusions.—Right prefrontal stimulation may disrupt compulsion-related activity. The current preliminary findings suggest that repetitive transcranial magnetic stimulation, which appears to be a safe probe of cortical mechanisms, affects the structures that influence OCD symptoms.

▶ Transcranial magnetic stimulation (TMS) of the right prefrontal cortex, but not other region was able to reduce but not eliminate compulsions, but not obsessions, in this preliminary study. The regional and symptom specificity argues against a placebo effect, but results need to be replicated in a controlled study. The mechanism of TMS is unknown.

H.Y. Meltzer, M.D.

8 Psychopharmacology

Introduction

There has been continued progress in the field this year. The biggest problem for me was choosing the selections to appear in the present volume. This year's selections cover treatment issues in various areas. Of note, the substance abuse literature review was quite rich this year, including some interesting articles on imaging. The majority of the articles here are of clinical importance, and I have included a few relating more to methodological or biological psychiatry which I thought were important in the context of clinical practice. I hope you agree, and I look forward to a new year of progress in the field.

R. Bruce Lydiard, Ph.D., M.D.

Anxiety Disorders

Brofaromine for Social Phobia: A Multicenter, Placebo-controlled, Double-blind Study

Lott M, Greist JH, Jefferson JW, et al (Ciba–Geigy Corp, Summit, NJ; Dean Found for Health, Research and Education, Middleton, Wis)
J Clin Psychopharmacol 17:255–260, 1997   8–1

Background.—Social phobia has been treated with monoamine oxidase inhibitors, benzodiazepines, and β-adrenergic receptor blockers. However, the associated adverse effects of these drugs limit their use. Brofaromine is a selective reversible inhibitor of monoamine oxidase type A and a selective serotonin reuptake inhibitor. These authors studied the effectiveness and safety profile of brofaromine in the treatment of social phobia.

Methods.—The subjects were 102 outpatients (62 men and 40 women, mean age 36.5) with a diagnosis of primary social phobia of $\geq$ 6 months of duration. Patients were randomized to placebo (n = 50) or brofaromine (n = 52), beginning at 50 mg/day and up to a maximum of 150 mg/day depending on response. Laboratory tests, electrocardiograms, physical examinations, and the Liebowitz Social Anxiety Scale were performed at intervals during the 10 weeks of treatment.

Findings.—The mean brofaromine dose was 107.2 ± 27.9 mg/day. Mean Liebowitz Social Anxiety Scale scores decreased significantly in both groups, from 81.8 to 62.6 in the brofaromine group and from 79.8 to 70.7

in the placebo group. The decrease in the brofaromine group was significantly greater than in the placebo group. Significantly more patients in the brofaromine group reported "much" or "very much" improvement than in the placebo group (50% vs 19%). There were 14 dropouts (27%) in the brofaromine group and 17 dropouts (34%) in the placebo group. Adverse events were the dropping out reason for 11 of those receiving active drug and 4 of those receiving placebo; the most common reason was insomnia (reported by 7 of 11 patients taking brofaromine and all 4 patients taking placebo). Among the patients who remained in the study, insomnia, dizziness, dry mouth, anorexia, tinnitus, and tremor were significantly more common in those taking brofaromine. Vital signs or laboratory values did not differ significantly during the trial.

Conclusions.—Brofaromine was an effective treatment for social phobia, with half of the patients reporting they were "much" or "very much" improved. Its side effects were generally tolerable. However, its effectiveness was modest compared with results of other double-blind studies of drug treatments for social phobia.

▶ The report by Noyes et al. (Abstract 8–3) indicates that moclobemide is, at best, an inconsistent and perhaps less potent treatment for social phobia than phenelzine. This report details a small clinical trial employing either brofaromine, a selective monoamine oxidase A inhibitor, or placebo. Interestingly, brofaromine is also a selective serotonin reuptake inhibitor, and thus is somewhat different than its RIMA counterpart moclobemide. Brofaromine was significantly better than placebo on most outcome measures. Of note, the response rate at 50% was modest; this was similar for the findings in the moclobemide studies. This agent has a clinical reputation for being useful because it has a broad spectrum of action and relatively benign side effects and safety profile. There is no reason to become excited yet, since the development of this agent has been suspended. Whether these newer agents are truly as potent as the standard monoamine oxidase inhibitors remains unclear. Hopefully, newer agents will be developed and have sufficient promise to be marketed for anxiety and depression, thus allowing for direct comparisons between these agents and the standard MAOIs to allow us to determine their comparative clinical use.

R.B. Lydiard, Ph.D., M.D.

Moclobemide in Social Phobia: A Controlled Dose-response Trial
Noyes R Jr, Moroz G, Davidson JRT, et al (Univ of Iowa, Iowa City; Hoffmann-La Roche, Nutley, NJ; Duke Univ, Durham, NC; et al)
J Clin Psychopharmacol 17:247–254, 1997   8–2

Background.—Social phobia affects up to 13% of the general population. General social phobia is associated with substantial social and occupational impairment, and even subsyndromal forms are associated with morbidity. Monoamine oxidase inhibitors (MAOIs) are effective in treating this disorder, and phenelzine sulfate is the most commonly used MAOI. However, phenelzine is associated with a significant risk of hypertension. These authors examined moclobemide, a reversible inhibitor of mono-amine oxidase type A with less potential for hypertensive crises, in patients with social phobia.

Methods.—Thirteen centers enrolled a total of 583 patients with primary social phobia according to DSM-III-R criteria. The major exclusion criteria were panic disorder, agoraphobia, obsessive–compulsive disorder, major depressive disorder, suicidal ideation, and substance abuse. All patients had a score $\geq$ 4 on the 7-point Clinical Impression of Severity–Social Phobia scale. During a 1-week placebo trial, 60 patients dropped out. Five hundred six patients (290 men and 216 women, mean age 38.1 $\pm$ 10.4 years) were randomized to placebo (n = 85) or 75 (n = 84), 150 (n = 86), 300 (n = 86), 600 (n = 82), or 900 (n = 83) mg of moclobemide and completed at least 1 assessment. The trial continued for 12 weeks, and safety and efficacy were assessed at regular intervals.

Findings.—Almost one third of the patients (158 of 506) dropped out before the end of the study (no significant differences between groups). Although scores on the Patient Impression of Change Social Phobia scale tended to be higher for patients taking higher doses of moclobemide, differences were statistically significant only at 8 weeks. Similarly, individual pairwise comparisons of Liebowitz Social Anxiety Scale scores differed significantly only at 8 weeks between the placebo and the 150- and 900-mg groups, and at 12 weeks between the placebo and 900-mg group. By 12 weeks, 35% of patients taking 900 mg of moclobemide were "much" or "very much" improved—but so were 33% of patients taking placebo. Adverse effects caused 8.8% of the patients taking moclobemide to drop out and 10.6% of those receiving placebo. Insomnia and dry mouth were more frequent in the patients taking active drug.

Conclusions.—At doses up to 900 mg/day, moclobemide did not differ significantly from placebo in treating patients with social phobia. Although there was no moclobemide-induced hypertension in these patients, the efficacy results do not compare favorably with those of phenelzine, which is associated with a clinical response rate of 55% to 81%. These results vary from other studies that have found moclobemide better than placebo and comparable to phenelzine in patients with social phobia.

▶ Clinicians have been anxiously awaiting the availability of reversible monoamine oxidase inhibitors (MAOIs) in hopes of finding a safe and tolerable alternative to the currently available nonselective MAOIs. This carefully designed and conducted multicentered study was, to say the least, a disappointment. Despite using dosages as high as 900 mg/day, moclobemide did not meaningfully separate from placebo during the course of this study. Placebo response rates were comparable to previous studies, but the response rates were somewhat less than studies that used phenelzine. Of note, the placebo response rate in individuals with avoidant personality disorder was only half that of individuals without avoidant personality disorder. Since avoidant personality disorder and generalized social phobia tend to co-occur frequently, one could speculate that the placebo response rate was higher in patients with nongeneralized social phobia. Even though there were no apparent distinctions when analyzing by severity, most clinicians agree that nongeneralized social phobics are more likely to respond to all treatments, including placebo, than generalized social phobics. This report did not appear to analyse by social phobia subtype. Unfortunately, these results were at odds with 2 previous studies indicating probable efficacy for moclobemide at doses of ≈600 mg/day; this failure to find a drug-placebo difference essentially ended the development of moclobemide in the United States for this indication. Nevertheless, some individual patients might benefit from one of these selective MAOIs, and some enterprising clinicians and patients have been able to arrange to obtain moclobemide from Canada or other countries in which it is available as a treatment for depression and anxiety. Hopefully, nonselective MAOIs will be developed in the future that have the same potency as the available nonselective agents, but a side effects profile comparable to moclobemide.

R.B. Lydiard, Ph.D., M.D.

Clonazepam in the Treatment of Panic Disorder With or Without Agoraphobia: A Dose-response Study of Efficacy, Safety, and Discontinuance

Rosenbaum JF, Moroz G, and Bowden CL, for the Clonazepam Panic Disorder Dose-response Study Group (Harvard Med School; Hoffman–La Roche, Inc., Nutley, NJ; Univ of Texas Health Science Ctr at San Antonio; et al)
J Clin Psychopharmacol 17:390–400, 1997   8–3

Background.—Although clonazepam is effective in treating panic disorder, neither the lowest effective dose nor the dose-response relationships have been determined. These authors undertook to do just that in a multicenter, parallel-group, placebo-controlled, fixed-dose study.

Methods.—Twelve centers enrolled outpatients ≥ 18 years old who had primary panic disorder with or without agoraphobia. Patients with depression, substance abuse, or other anxiety disorders were excluded. Four hundred thirteen patients took ≥1 dose of the study drug; 404 had at least 1 visit; 293 completed the dose-maintenance phase; and 222 completed the 16-week study (74% of the placebo group and 59% to 85% of the clonazepam groups). Patients were randomized to placebo (n = 69) or clonazepam at 0.5 (n = 68), 1.0 (n = 67), 2.0 (n = 66), 3.0 (n = 63), or 4.0 (n = 71) mg/day. Doses were escalated throughout 3 weeks, maintained for 6 weeks, then tapered for 7 weeks. Weekly logs of panic attacks and the Clinician's Global Impression of Severity (CGI-S) scale were used to assess efficacy at regular intervals. Also assessed were the degree of disability, phobic avoidance, and anticipatory anxiety. Clonazepam's effects at each dose were compared with those of placebo; the sample size was not sufficient to detect differences between active drug doses.

Findings.—At the end of the dose-maintenance phase, clonazepam was associated with a decrease in panic attacks; the difference was significant for the 1.0 dose and for all doses combined. Patients taking clonazepam also had improvement in their panic disorder rating (significant for the 1.0 mg dose), phobic avoidance (significant for the 2.0 and 4.0 mg doses), and anticipatory anxiety (significant for the 0.5, 1.0, and 4.0 mg doses). All patients improved according to the CGI-S: "minimal" or better improvement occurred in 68% of the placebo group, 77% of patients taking the 0.5 mg dose, and between 89% to 91% of patients taking higher doses. Significantly more patients taking higher doses had "much" or "very much" improvement. Most patients in all 6 groups reported $\geq$ 1 adverse event, which were generally mild or moderate. Higher doses were associated with more prevalent somnolence (38% for 0.5 mg and 69% for 4.0 mg) and ataxia (1.5% for 0.5 mg and 22% for 4.0 mg). Other adverse effects more prevalent in the clonazepam groups were dizziness, fatigue, and irritability. Also, more patients taking clonazepam (7%-13%) reported depression than patients taking placebo (3%). During the taper phase, although the patient's condition worsened compared with his or her status during the dose-maintenance phase, it did not decrease to baseline levels. Tolerance to clonazepam discontinuation was good.

Conclusions.—The 1- and 2-mg doses of clonazepam were as efficacious as higher doses for treating panic disorder. Adverse events were generally mild or moderate, although patients taking clonazepam reported depression more often. The tapering schedule was well tolerated and safe.

▶ The overall design of this large study, which took nearly 3 years to complete, is very similar to the Cross-national alprazolam studies. What we can learn is that patients with uncomplicated panic disorder respond well to daily doses more than 1 mg, and little additional benefit is derived from higher doses. This was a well-conducted and well-powered study, which is very useful in providing dose-response information for the treating clinician. However, as is a problem with most efficacy studies for which indication is being contemplated by the Food and Drug Administration, the patient group was not representative of the patients we see. Specifically, primary diagnoses of depression and other anxiety disorders were excluded, and patients with Hamilton Depression Rating scores >18 were excluded. Thus, we can only extrapolate treatment information that relates to a relative minority of patients with panic disorder seen in clinical practice. Another feature of this study does not mimic the "real world"—patients were given 9 weeks of treatment, including a 3-week upward titration, and then were tapered off after an additional 6 weeks of treatment throughout 7 additional weeks.

Some rebound in the clonazepam-treated group was no surprise, but we have no way of knowing if a study designed in this way can meaningfully inform the clinician. Specifically, nobody treats a patient for 9 weeks and then tapers medication for 7 weeks. The frustrating aspect of efficacy studies is that some of the flaws (such as having patients with panic disorder but no depression or other important comorbid diagnoses) are driven by regulatory requirements or the corporate sponsor's concern over what may or may not appear on the package insert of the approved agent.

We can take useful clinical information from this study, however. Firstly, a gradual taper is generally associated with a more benign post-discontinuation course; apparently affirmed by this study once again. Also, in this study, depression emerged as a patient complaint (as opposed to a formal diagnosis) in nearly 10% of patients receiving clonazepam vs. 3% receiving placebo. This adverse event was listed 39 times for 36 patients; 12 were discontinued from the study, but only 1 was discontinued for depression. An additional 9 patients, however, required treatment for depression even though they may not have left the study because of it. The authors provide a thoughtful discussion of this issue, and left open the issue of whether depression may have been caused by clonazepam, unmasked by clonazepam, or by a combination of these and possibly other factors. This well-designed, well-conducted study adds some useful clinical information to the literature, with the caveats previously noted. It also underscores our need to be cautious in extrapolating studies conducted in highly refined diagnostic groups, which are not representative of the general patient population with mood or anxiety disorders for which this treatment is intended.

R.B. Lydiard, Ph.D., M.D.

Clinical Improvement With Fluoxetine Therapy and Noradrenergic Function in Patients With Panic Disorder
Coplan JD, Papp LA, Pine D, et al (Columbia Univ, New York; Long Island Jewish Med Ctr, New York; SUNY Health Sciences Ctr, Brooklyn, NY et al)
Arch Gen Psychiatry 54:643–648, 1997   8–4

Background.—Central noradrenergic (NA) dysregulation is believed to be involved in the pathogenesis of panic disorder. This dysregulation can be downmodulated directly (through inhibitory serotonergic projections from brain stem raphe nuclei to NA neurons in the nucleus locus coeruleus) or indirectly (through downregulation of neurotransmitters that stimulate brain-stem NA activity). This study evaluated whether a selective serotonin reuptake inhibitor (SSRI) can mediate antipanic effects by downmodulating the "volatile" NA system in patients with panic disorder.

Methods.—The test group was 17 patients (mean age 40.5 ± 10.2) with panic disorder according to DSM-III-R criteria, and the control group was 16 healthy subjects (mean age 33.9 ± 10.5 years). At the first challenge, clonidine was administered and blood samples were drawn at regular intervals to measure plasma levels of 3-methoxy-4-hydroxyphenylglycol (MHPG). The extent of MHPG oscillatory activity in plasma was used as a measure of NA volatility. Then, the patients were treated with fluoxetine HCl for 12 weeks (mean dose 17.7 ± 16.7 mg/day), and 13 of the 17 patients were rechallenged with clonidine. Thirteen of the 16 controls were rechallenged at 12 weeks, although they had not received fluoxetine between challenges. Subjects were assessed by the Hamilton Depression

Scale, Hamilton Anxiety Scale, Clinical Global Assessment Scale, and a log of the number of panic attacks during the previous week.

Findings.—At the first clonidine challenge, the patients with panic disorder had substantial within-subject fluctuations in plasma MHPG levels (i.e., increased plasma MHPG volatility), while MHPG levels in controls were steady. Two patients did not respond to fluoxetine. Of the 11 patients who did, their MHPG levels dropped to a much greater extent after fluoxetine treatment (6.65-4.46 ng/mL) compared with levels in controls (4.37-3.67 ng/mL). Patients who had the most reduction in MHPG levels between the 2 clonidine challenges had significantly better clinical global improvement scores.

Conclusions.—At the first clonidine challenge, patients with panic disorder had greatly increased within-subject plasma MHPG volatility. This finding supports the hypothesis that NA dysregulation occurs in panic disorder. Furthermore, the improvement in MHPG volatility after 12 weeks of the SSRI fluoxetine was associated with a return toward more normal MHPG fluctuations. However, other studies have shown that some effects of clonidine (i.e., the decreased response of human growth hormone) persist after fluoxetine treatment of patients with panic disorder. Nonetheless, the finding of increased MHPG volatility in patients with panic disorder parallels other work by these authors showing these patients also have great variability of tidal volume. Further work to examine ventilatory, serotonergic, and NA effects may shed more light on the complex relationships between NA dysregulation and SSRIs.

▶ Yet another report has recently appeared that addresses some interesting theoretical questions. First, "selective" serotonin reuptake inhibitors are commonly thought to affect only serotonin. What is clear from this study is that fluoxetine, like the other SSRIs, is not selectively active on serotonin systems with chronic administration, and can have relatively broad effects on monoamine function. In this case, noradrenergic function was assessed in individuals with panic disorder. The finding that "volatility" of noradrenergic function in this paradigm is reduced in those individuals who are responders, but not in those who are not responders. This supports a concept of noradrenergic dysfunction in panic disorder—a biological theory that many have forgotten. Because we now have evidence that fluoxetine is a good treatment for panic disorder, this paper brings noradrenergic function as an aspect of panic disorder pathophysiology back into focus. This is consistent with some of our earlier work in looking at cerebrospinal fluid, in which panic disorder patients' cerebrospinal fluid concentrations of the noradrenergic metabolite correlated poorly with 2 other monoamine metabolites of serotonin and dopamine. It also underscores the need for all of us to think beyond the first level of pharmacological effect of the therapeutic agents that we use. It indicates that we are not dealing with 1-transmitter disorders, even with the most "selective" of agents.

R.B. Lydiard, Ph.D., M.D.

Effects of Cholecystokinin Tetrapeptide on Respiratory Function in Healthy Volunteers

Bradwejn J, LeGrand J-M, Koszycki D, et al (McGill Univ, Montreal; St Mary's Hosp, Montreal; Centre Hospitalier Paul Guiraude, Villejiuf, France; et al)
Am J Psychiatry 155:280–282, 1998   8–5

Introduction.—Previous studies indicate that panic disorder is associated with disturbances in central respiratory function, and respiratory changes are considered as core symptoms of panic attacks. Central cholecystokinin (CCK) receptor agonists are potent panicogenic agents. In humans, systemic CCK tetrapeptide (CCK-4) induces dyspnea at a high frequency. A study in healthy volunteers evaluated respiratory response to CCK-4.

Methods.—Thirty healthy individuals with no history of psychiatric disorders took part in the study. The 14 men and 16 women (mean age, 23 years) were randomized to either a CCK-4 (a bolus injection of 50 µg) or placebo challenge. Behavioral response to the challenge was assessed with the Panic Symptom Scale. A panic attack was defined according to *Diagnostic and Statistical Manual of Mental Disorders,* 3rd edition, revised criteria.

Results.—All of the study participants who received CCK-4, but only 1 of 15 who received placebo, reported dyspnea. Placebo had no effect on any of the respiratory measures, but CCK-4 caused a significant increase in tidal volume. Respiratory rate was not affected by CCK-4. Panic attacks occurred in 60% of the CCK-4 group vs. 7% of the placebo group. The increase from baseline in minute ventilation was almost twice as great in panickers as in nonpanickers.

Conclusion.—The administration of CCK-4 to healthy volunteers produced marked increases in ventilation, a response caused by an increase in tidal volume. Experimental studies suggest that CCK interacts with brain stem mechanisms in altering respiratory function.

▶ This is part of an ongoing series of investigations conducted by Dr. Bradwejn and colleagues. The finding is of particular interest because respiratory function in panic disorder appears to be abnormal in a substantial percentage of subjects. Increases in tidal volume are typically seen before naturally occurring panic attacks as well as those provoked by panicogenic agents. This is another piece in the puzzle in the search for better understanding of the neurobiology of panic disorder.

It is also worth mentioning that several agents have been developed that block the CCK-B receptor, which is the pressured site of action of the tetrapeptide. Unfortunately, these agents never made it to the marketplace, but we have opened the possibility that agents with CCK-B receptor-blocking activity may be useful anxiolytics. There is also some evidence that these agents may help suppress alcohol withdrawal and may have other therapeutic uses as well. Let's stay tuned on this one.

R.B. Lydiard, Ph.D., M.D.

Efficacy of Divalproex Sodium in Patients With Panic Disorder and Mood Instability Who Have Not Responded to Conventional Therapy

Baetz M, Bowen RC (Univ of Saskatchewan, Saskatoon)
Can J Psychiatry 43:73–77, 1998   8–6

Introduction.—Individuals with panic disorder often experience depressive symptoms as well, and their response to treatment is poorer than that of patients with panic disorder alone. An 8-week trial was conducted to determine the efficacy of divalproex sodium in the treatment of patients with panic disorder refractory to conventional therapy and co-morbid mood instability.

Methods.—Patients in the open trial, flexible dose study received divalproex sodium at 250 mg twice daily, increased by 250 mg increments to reach serum levels of 300 to 600 µmol/L. Assessments were conducted at baseline, at 4 weeks, and at 8 weeks by self- and rater-administered questionnaires.

Results.—Ten patients, 6 women and 4 men, completed the study. The mean age of the group was 43.9 years, and the mean duration of panic disorder was 19.3 years. All patients had previously been treated by a psychiatrist and had taken several antidepressants and benzodiazepines in the past. All had panic disorder and symptoms of mood instability; 7 had agoraphobia. Divalproex sodium brought about significant improvement in depressive and anxiety symptoms and mood instability. The average number of panic attacks decreased from 4.3 full attacks and 4 limited attacks weekly to 1.5 full attacks and 1.0 limited attack at the end of the 8-week study, a statistically significant and clinically important change. By week 8, 80% of patients reported being much or very much improved.

Conclusion.—Divalproex sodium proved useful in the treatment of patients with panic disorder and concomitant mood instability. All patients had failed to respond to the standard treatment of antidepressants and cognitive behavioral therapy.

▶ This interesting case series from Canadian researchers is 1 of several suggesting that valproic acid may be useful for panic disorder. Although this, in itself, is not much in the way of news, the growing evidence that there is an interface between bipolar disorder and panic disorder is of clinical significance. This is where an anticonvulsant mood stabilizer may play an important therapeutic role. Many panic patients talk about mood swings (and it is easy to dismiss this as something related to their disorder) when, in fact, they may be describing bipolar disorder type II symptoms. As the authors noted, a double-blind study is indicated to test this possibility further. Interestingly, there was a recent study of cocaine abusers who were treated with carbamazepine; those with "mood spectrum" symptoms in addition to the cocaine abuse did better with carbamazepine treatment overall than did those patients who did not have any evidence of a mood disorder.[1]

R.B. Lydiard, Ph.D., M.D.

Reference

1. Brady, KT: Bipolar disorder and substance abuse. Presented at the Annual Meeting of the American Psychiatric Association, May 30-June 12, 1998, Toronto, Ontario.

Patient Treatment Insistence and Medication Craving in Long-term Low-Dosage Benzodiazepine Prescriptions

Linden M, Bär T, Geiselmann B (Free Univ of Berlin)
Psychol Med 28:721–729, 1998   8–7

Introduction.—Community surveys indicate that benzodiazepine (BZ) prescription practices depart from prescription recommendations. Most patients take these drugs on a long-term basis. Not many studies have evaluated why many patients, long before withdrawal symptoms have developed, oppose stopping benzodiazepines. Patient variables associated with problems in stopping BZ therapy include older age, female gender for short-term outcome, male gender for long-term outcome, and lower education. The percentage of patients on long-term BZ therapy who have never started a withdrawal program is unknown. The characteristics of these patients, compared to the characteristics of patients who cooperate with a withdrawal program, have not been determined. The scope of and factors associated with prewithdrawal insistence were assessed in a series of 122 patients receiving long-term BZ treatment through primary care physicians.

Methods.—Patients receiving long-term therapeutic treatment with BZ were asked to participate in a drug holiday for 3 weeks. Patients were excluded if they showed any signs of addiction, were taking doses higher than 20 mg diazepam-equivalent, were taking more than 1 BZ, or were also taking other hypnotics or tranquilizers. Patients were informed of the benefits and possible withdrawal symptoms and were offered medical and psychological support. It was recommended that patients taper off the BZ, but they could also choose to discontinue the drug abruptly. This action was strongly supported by their general practitioners. Data were gathered about sociodemographic, medication, morbidity, and attitudinal variables. General practitioners reported their perceptions of their patients.

Results.—Average age of this mostly female cohort (78.7%) was 67.2 years. Almost 64% of patients had at least 1 psychiatric disorder (24% anxiety disorder, 25% depressive disorder, 9% organic mental disorder, and 8% somatoform disorder). Nearly 51% reported earlier attempts to discontinue BZ medication. Eighty-four (69%) patients rejected the idea of discontinuing BZ to see if the medication was still needed. In patients who agreed to participate, a tapering program was begun. Eighteen patients (47%) interrupted their withdrawal program and took BZs again as before. Only 12 patients (10%) were able to cease taking BZs. Age, gender, and marital status did not differ significantly between patients who participated and those who refused. A significantly higher proportion of patients with over 9 years of school education agreed to participate.

General practitioners reported that, in their view, patients who refused to participate had a greater variety of complaints, were less cooperative, were harder to satisfy, and usually relied more on medications.

Conclusion.—A major problem with a BZ withdrawal program occurs before the program begins: patients don't want to discontinue their low-dosage BZ prescriptions. Withdrawal problems have been correlated with depressive or dependent personality characteristics. Benzodiazepine low-dosage dependence should be considered a real form of drug dependence.

▶ Primary care physicians are often reluctant to prescribe benzodiazepines to patients because of concern about long-term effects. Research psychiatrists from Berlin enlisted 39 primary care practitioners, who were supportive of the experimental procedure, which was to discontinue medications, either abruptly or gradually, with patients given the choice of abrupt discontinuation or 3- to 4-week taper. Perhaps the most striking thing about this article is the general impression that using benzodiazepines over the longer term is a bad thing. The majority (two thirds) of the patients taking benzodiazepines had at least 1 psychiatric disorder; about a quarter of the sample had an anxiety disorder. The patients who refused to try to discontinue medication had more psychological complaints, were less cooperative, and relied more on medications than those who accepted the agenda. It seems odd that the authors did not consider that the refusers were more anxious, and perhaps more in need of benzodiazepines, than more cooperative patients. Half the refusers had tried to stop their medication previously without success.

One glaring omission is the authors' failure to discuss the possibility that some patients needed ongoing treatment for their anxiety symptoms. Remarkably, there is no assessment of vital signs or new-onset symptoms of withdrawal anywhere in this article, although the researchers themselves recognized that such symptoms occurred in a number of patients. The authors also included 9% of patients with organic mental disorders, according to the results section, but indicated in the methods section that these patients would be excluded from this study. Further, the authors attributed resistance to stopping medication more to attitude than to anything else, calling it "treatment insistence." The patients were taking a modest (approximately 7½ mg of diazepam-equivalent) dose of benzodiazepines. The authors also referred to the patients' refusal to stop benzodiazepines as evidence of psychological dependence and drug-seeking behavior. Relatively little, as noted above, was discussed about either physical dependence or therapeutic need. This is surprising, because the American Psychiatric Association has publicly stated that patients with long-term anxiety disorders may derive benefit from long-term benzodiazepine treatment. There have been no adverse effects which outweighed the benefit in any benzodiazepine study I have seen. In this age of herbal medicines and disdain for benzodiazepines, we should remember that these agents are widely prescribed because they are safe and effective, often making the difference between the ability and inability to function. Chronic anxiety in the patients receiving psychiatric care predominantly from primary care physicians who agree with the authors may suffer unnecessarily.

As psychiatrists, we can help our primary care colleagues through their concern, by noting the chronicity of these disorders, the therapeutic benefit of benzodiazepines for many patients, and by suggesting intermittent consultation with a psychiatric specialist about whether medication use is indicated for patients receiving long-term benzodiazepines.

R.B. Lydiard, Ph.D., M.D.

Mood Disorders

Comparison of Paroxetine and Nortriptyline in Depressed Patients With Ischemic Heart Disease
Roose SP, Laghrissi-Thode F, Kennedy JS, et al (Columbia Univ, New York; Univ of Pittsburgh, Pa; Vanderbilt Univ, Nashville, Tenn; et al)
JAMA 279:287–291, 1998   8–8

Background.—Ischemic heart disease and depression are often co-morbid. In patients who have had a recent myocardial infarction, the occurrence of depression is associated with increased mortality. Thus, a safe, effective treatment for depression is needed for such patients.

Methods and Findings.—Eighty-one outpatients with major depressive disorder and documented ischemic heart disease were randomly assigned to 6 weeks of paroxetine, 20 to 30 mg/day, or nortriptyline targeted to a therapeutic plasma level of 190 to 570 nmol/L. In an intent-to-treat analysis, 61% of 41 patients improved with paroxetine and 55% of 40 improved with nortriptyline. Neither agent significantly affected blood pressure or conduction intervals. Paroxetine showed no sustained effects on heart rate or rhythm or indices of heart rate variability. Nortriptyline was associated with a sustained 11% increase in heart rate, from a mean 75 to 83 beats per minute, and with a decrease in heart rate variability, from 112 to 96. Two percent of paroxetine recipients and 18% of nortripyline recipients experienced adverse cardiac events.

Conclusions.—Both paroxetine and nortriptyline are effective in the treatment of depression in patients with ischemic heart disease. Nortriptyline is associated with a rate of serious adverse cardiac events significantly higher than the rate associated with paroxetine.

▶ This very useful article interplays nicely with the article about hip fracture in elderly patients (Abstract 8–34), who are also likely to have ischemic heart disease as well. We know that treating depression in patients who are recovering from a myocardial infarction reduces the likelihood of cardiac death in the 6 months after the event. These careful investigators included all the relevant variables in their study. The findings confirm most clinicians' impression that paroxetine is a safe treatment in patients with ischemic heart disease. The article about hip fracture in the elderly showed no difference in risk between secondary tricyclics, such as nortriptyline, and the selective serotonin reuptake inhibitors. One should temper findings such as these by suggesting that there may be other reasons for prescribing selective serotonin reuptake inhibitors in some patient groups.

R.B. Lydiard, Ph.D., M.D.

Rapid Conversion From One Monoamine Oxidase Inhibitor to Another
Szuba MP Hornig-Rohan M, Amsterdam JD (Univ of Pennsylvania, Philadelphia)
J Clin Psychiatry 58:307–310, 1997   8–9

Background.—Monoamine oxidase inhibitors (MAOIs) are commonly used to treat depressive disorders, yet not all patients respond to the first MAOI they are administered. When switching from one MAOI to another, current practice is to include a 14-day wash-out period between drugs. These authors used a shorter wash-out period between MAOIs and report their results in patients with depression.

Methods.—Eight patients (3 men and 5 women, from 22 to 67 years old) with depression were evaluated. Two patients had unipolar depression alone; 3 had bipolar depression alone; 1 had unipolar depression and was HIV positive; 1 patient had bipolar depression, cerebrovascular disease, hypertension, and diabetes mellitus; and 1 patient had bipolar depression, posttraumatic stress disorder, and dysmenorrhea. Patients were switched from one MAOI to another with either no wash-out period (4 patients) or a wash-out of only 1 to 8 days (4 patients). The switch was from phenelzine to tranylcypromine in 5 patients and vice versa in 3 patients. During the switch, patients were taking between 1 and 5 other drugs, including benzodiazepines (5 patients), mood stabilizers (5), neuroleptics (3), and a bedtime sedative (1).

Findings.—Half the patients (4 of 8) had no adverse physical symptoms after the MAOI switch. Another patient had transient systolic hypotension upon standing but was otherwise asymptomatic. Three of these 5 patients had been switched from phenelzine to tranylcypromine, and 2 had been switched from tranylcypromine to phenelzine. Wash-out periods were 0 days in 2 patients, 5 days in 2 patients, and 8 days in 1 patient. Three patients had symptoms after the MAOI switch. One patient with bipolar depression alone, who switched from tranylcypromine to phenelzine, immediately had anxiety, nausea, flushing, hyperventilation, a sense of doom, and increased insomnia (i.e., mild serotonin syndrome); she had been taking lithium. The patient with bipolar depression and cerebrovascular disease switched from phenelzine to tranylcypromine immediately; and afterward, he experienced increased anxiety, restlessness, and palpitations. One patient with unipolar depression who switched from phenelzine to tranylcypromine with a 1-day wash-out experienced mild postural lightheadedness. Four of the patients ultimately responded to the new MAOI.

Conclusions.—Other reports of rapid switches between MAOIs include 2 case reports in which the switch resulted in elevated blood pressure (240/130 mm Hg) or was followed by a cerebral hemorrhage. In another report, no adverse effects were seen after an immediate switch from phenelzine to tranylcypromine. In this study, during wash-out periods of 0 to 8 days, switching from phenelzine to tranylcypromine or from tranylcypromine to phenelzine was associated with minimal or no adverse effects. One case of serotonin syndrome was evident, and physicians must be aware of this possibility when MAOIs are combined with serotonin-enhancing drugs.

▶ This clinical report, although limited to observations, addresses the issue of switching from 1 monoamine oxidase inhibitor (MAOI) to another (i.e., phenelzine to tranylcypromine or the reverse). The 8 patients in this study were far from uncomplicated: 5 of the 8 had bipolar depression, and 1 patient with unipolar depression was HIV-positive. Additionally, numerous other medications were given during the switch. In a nutshell, the authors describe little to no difficulty in switching patients with wash-out periods ranging from 0 to 8 days. Only minimal serotonin syndrome and mild postural hypotension were observed; there did not appear to be any direction for the switch that was less favorable. One glaring limitation in this study was the failure to mention the dosage of the MAOIs taken and the dosage switched to. However, we can take away from this clinical report some cautious optimism for those few patients who are faced with a difficult decision about rapidly changing MAOIs. Unfortunately, the paper failed to mention whether the switch was a clinically useful manipulation. If they did not have the information available, it would have been useful to indicate this so the reader was not left wondering whether this switch might be safe, but the clinical payoff was also worthwhile.

R.B. Lydiard, Ph.D., M.D.

Efficacy and Tolerability of Once–daily Venlafaxine Extended Release (XR) in Outpatients With Major Depression
Thase ME, for the Venlafaxine XR 209 Study Group (Univ of Pittsburgh, Pa)
J Clin Psychiatry 58:393–398, 1997   8–10

Background.—Venlafaxine is an antidepressant that inhibits serotonin and norepinephrine uptake, but does not affect other receptors associated with side effects typical of tricyclic antidepressants. Most patients take the drug twice daily (the half-life of its active metabolite is 11 hours). These authors evaluated a new formulation of venlafaxine that allows once-daily dosing in patients with major depression.

Methods.—Twelve different study sites enrolled a total of 197 outpatients ≥ 18 years old with major depression defined by the DSM-IV. Each patient scored at least a 20 on the 21-item Hamilton Rating Scale for Depression (HAM-D), and none had a decrease in score of >20% between screening and the start of the study. Subjects were also assessed by the Montgomery-Asberg Depression Rating Scale (MADRS) and the Clinical Global Impressions (CGI) severity scale. Patients were randomized to receive either a microsphere-encapsulated formulation of 75 mg of venlafaxine (n = 95) or placebo (n = 102). Drug responses were monitored, and an extra 75-mg capsule was allowed after 14 days and after 28 days if needed to achieve a response (i.e., the maximum drug dose was 225 mg/day). Dosing continued up to 8 weeks.

Findings.—The mean dose of venlafaxine between weeks 3 and 8 ranged from 172 to 177 mg. For the venlafaxine group, CGI severity scores were significantly improved by the second week of treatment, HAM-D scores were significantly better by the third week of treatment, and the MADRS score was significantly improved by the fourth week compared with the placebo group. Furthermore, these improvements were maintained throughout the study. There were 26 dropouts in the venlafaxine group (27%) and 41 dropouts in the placebo group (40%). Significantly more patients withdrew because of unsatisfactory response from the placebo group than from the active drug group (22% vs. 5%). Six patients taking placebo (6%) and 10 patients taking venlafaxine (11%) withdrew because of adverse events (mainly nausea and insomnia). Side effects were also common in the patients who remained in the study, and consisted mainly of nausea (36% of venlafaxine group and 18% of placebo group), insomnia (35% and 15%, respectively), and somnolence (27% and 11%, respectively). With active drug, nausea was greatest during the first week of treatment, but by the third week the incidence was similar to that with placebo. There was a small but significant increase in supine blood pressure in the venlafaxine group (from 75.3 ± 7.5 mm Hg at baseline to 78.4 ± 9.2 mm Hg at week 8); 4 patients had an increase of ≥ 10 mm Hg to a value > 90 mm Hg at some time during the study.

Conclusions.—Once-daily dosing with an extended release formulation of venlafaxine effectively treated depression without major side effects. Once-daily dosing is more convenient than the twice-daily regimen currently used, which would be expected to improve patient compliance. Patients taking venlafaxine experienced an increase in supine blood pressure, and thus blood pressure should be monitored.

▶ Venlafaxine is 1 of those agents which did not catch on quickly, in part because it has been generally assumed that it requires twice-daily administration. This study, while not particularly exciting otherwise, does indicate that the extended-release form of the drug is superior to placebo in a double-blind, well-powered study. We have yet to see enough direct comparative studies to see relative side effects profiles, and short-term studies of this nature do not really tell the whole story. Nausea has probably been the most prominent side effect associated with venlafaxine treatment, and this study was really not much different. However, with a more gradual dosing strategy (in the real world, one is not required to push the dose as fast as in a trial like this 1) may be more tolerable. Interestingly, dropouts for side effects were limited: 11% total, 4% for nausea. Sexual side effects, which have been discussed as being perhaps better with this agent, were no greater than with its competitors, but long-term studies will really tell the story on this issue, and it remains an open question. At any rate, the agent will now be easier to use if we have a once-daily administration schedule. More long-term data will be useful in truly assessing this agent.

R.B. Lydiard, Ph.D., M.D.

A Double-Blind, Placebo-controlled Trial of Nefazodone in the Treatment of Patients Hospitalized for Major Depression

Feighner J, Targum SD, Bennett ME, et al (Feighner Research Inst, San Diego, Calif; Crozer-Chester Med Ctr, Upland, Pa; Bristol-Myers Squibb Company, Wallingford, Conn)
J Clin Psychiatry 59:246–253, 1998   8–11

Background.—Few placebo-controlled clinical trials indicating the efficacy of the newer antidepressants in markedly or severely depressed hospitalized patients have appeared in the literature. The efficacy of nefazodone was compared with that of placebo in patients with major depression.

Methods and Findings.—One hundred twenty patients with major depression hospitalized at 2 centers were given nefazodone or placebo in a 6-week trial. Nefazodone was better than placebo in reducing total score

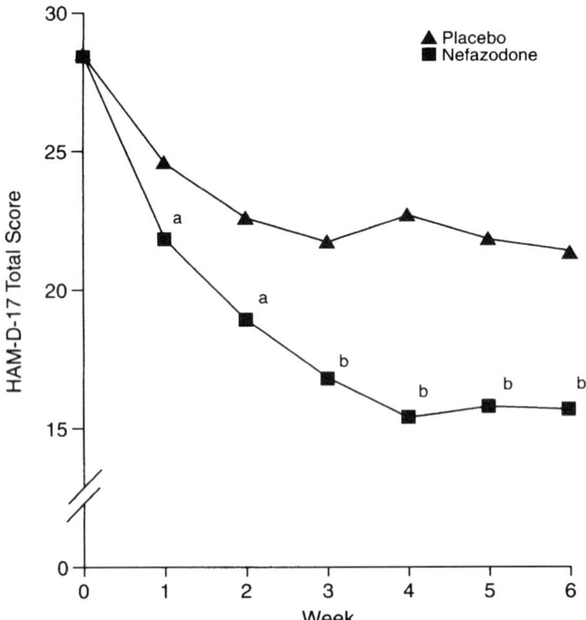

FIGURE 1.—Mean change in HAM-D-17 total score by weekly visit. * $P < 0.05$; † $P < 0.01$; both probabilities based on ANOVA of mean change from baseline scores. *Abbreviations: HAM-D-17,* Hamilton Rating Scale for Depression; *LOCF,* last observation carried forward, intent-to-treat data set. (Courtesy of Feighner J, Yargum SD, Bennett ME, et al: A double-blind, placebo-controlled trial of nefazodone in the treatment of patients hospitalized for major depression. *J Clin Psychiatry* 59:246-253, 1998. Copyright 1998, Physicians Postgraduate Press. Reprinted by permission.)

on the 17-item Hamilton Rating Scale for Depression (HAM-D). Response rates were 50% in the nefazodone group and 29% in the placebo group. Nefazodone was also superior in improving scores on the Montgomery-Asberg Depression Rating Scale; the HAM-D retardation, anxiety, and sleep disturbance factors; and HAM-D depressed mood. Dysthymic patients with major depression also significantly improved with active treatment. Significant differences in response rates were seen as early as week 2 through the end of the study. Mean nefazodone dose was 491 mg/day at the end of week 2 and 503 mg/day at the end of treatment (Fig 1).

Conclusions.—Nefazodone is significantly better than placebo in the treatment of marked to severe major depression in hospitalized patients. The clinical benefits of nefazodone appear as early as the first week of treatment.

▶ The "take-home" message from this study is that severe depression is responsive to nefazodone in patients requiring hospitalization. Certainly this study is not typical in that most patients are not held in a hospital for 1 to 4 weeks for observation. However, patients in this sample were very depressed and in need of hospitalization as indicated by the criteria (suicidal, treatment-resistant, noncompliant, or severe functional disability requiring hospitalization). It is notable that 80% of these patients had melancholic depression, and Hamilton Rating scores around 28 supports this (see figure). The dose of nefazodone by week 2 was about 500 mg and was 500 to 600 mg daily at study's end. Is nefazodone effective for severe depression? Apparently. Practitioners need to use this medication at a higher dosage than they normally use. The study is informative because many practitioners with whom I have talked have suggested that nefazodone may be "weaker" than other antidepressants. This does not appear to be the case so long as an appropriate intensity of treatment is maintained.

R.B. Lydiard, Ph.D., M.D.

Methodological Problems in the Estimation of the Onset of the Antidepressant Effect
Müller H, Möller H-J (Univ of Bonn, Germany; Ludwig-Maximilian-Univ, Munich)
J Affect Disord 48:15–23, 1998   8–12

Introduction.—The time to onset of activity is an important consideration in selecting an antidepressant. Agents with a late onset of activity could reduce patient compliance and lead to premature disruption of therapy. There is little solid evidence, however, that some agents or classes of agents produce a faster onset of activity.

Methods and Findings.—Using MEDLINE, investigators reviewed the literature published since 1975 to determine whether a specific pattern could be observed in the onset of antidepressant effect. Several factors contribute to shortcomings in the evaluation of the onset of activity. The time interval between successive observations is usually at least 1 week, providing only a rough estimate of time to onset of the antidepressant effect. Different strengths of a medication can affect estimates of its speed, as can the chosen efficacy criteria used in a study. More modern approaches to the question of onset of activity—including time series analysis, the survival analytical approach, and clinical global impressions—also have limitations.

Discussion.—Statements on the time of onset of the antidepressant effect are often a byproduct of efficacy studies and contain methodologic weaknesses. The mean and the distribution of the onset of activity are needed, not the onset of the mean. Observer rating scales have a problem of interrater reliability, and studies likely to be more reliable have specially trained raters.

▶ This article points out the significant variations in the evaluation of new agents in regard to the important clinical feature of speed of onset of antidepressant effect. This has been an area of controversy for many years. The authors point out the various statistical manipulations—sometimes innocent, other times perhaps less so—that underlie claims that a newer agent may be more quickly effective than an older one. Basically, the evidence that there is any agent that acts more quickly than any other is not convincing, but from year of the introduction of desipramine to the present, these claims have been thrown about. We, as clinicians, must be shrewd and even suspicious when anyone tells us that they have an agent which treats depression more quickly than older agents do. So far, the newer agents provide comfort, but not speed.

R.B. Lydiard, Ph.D., M.D.

Effects of Trazodone and Fluoxetine in the Treatment of Major Depression: Therapeutic Pharmacokinetic and Pharmacodynamic Interactions Through Formation of Meta–Chlorophenylpiperazine
Maes M, Westenberg H, Vandoolaeghe E, et al (Clinical Research Ctr for Mental Health, Antwerp, Belgium; Vanderbilt Univ, Nashville, Tenn; Univ of Utrecht, The Netherlands; et al)
J Clin Psychopharmacol 17:358–364, 1997   8–13

Background.—Trazodone is a heterocyclic antidepressant that is a relatively weak serotonin (5-HT) reuptake inhibitor. Previous research suggests that its antidepressant effects are at least partly attributable to its metabolite, meta-chlorophenylpiperazine (mCPP). Previous reports also indicate that fluoxetine, a selective 5-HT reuptake inhibitor, increases plasma levels of trazodone. This study was undertaken to determine if fluoxetine or pindolol (a 5-HT antagonist) would affect plasma levels of trazodone and mCPP in patients with depression who were taking trazodone.

Methods.—The subjects were 27 inpatients with major depression. After a drug-free period of 10 days, all subjects began taking oral trazodone, 100 mg/day. One week later, plasma trazodone and mCPP levels were measured, and subjects were assessed by the Hamilton Rating Scale for Depression (HAM-D). Then, while continuing trazodone dosing, subjects were randomized to placebo, 20 mg/day of fluoxetine, or 7.5 mg/day of pindolol. Blood assays and the HAM-D were repeated 2 and 4 weeks later.

Findings.—Placebo and pindolol had no affect on plasma levels of trazodone and mCPP. However, fluoxetine significantly increased trazodone and mCPP levels after 2 and 4 weeks of dosing. As plasma levels of both compounds increased, the HAM-D score improved significantly. Thirteen of the 27 patients responded to trazodone treatment; trazodone and mCPP plasma levels were significantly greater in responders than in nonresponders. Plasma levels of trazodone changed in a parallel manner with those of its metabolite, and the metabolite concentrations were a mean of 7.2% ± 3.7% of those of the parent compound.

Conclusions.—Adding fluoxetine to trazodone significantly increased plasma levels of trazodone and its active metabolite mCPP. Furthermore, increases in plasma concentrations of these compounds were associated with improvements in depression. In fact, the fluoxetine-induced changes in mCPP levels had a closer association with clinical improvement than changes in trazodone levels. These findings confirm that mCPP has an antidepressant effect, possibly by augmenting trazodone's capacity to inhibit 5-HT reuptake. Both mCPP and fluoxetine desensitize 5-HT_{2C} receptor function, and this may contribute to their antidepressant effects when combined.

▶ Maes and coworkers conducted an interesting study of inpatients, which was of interest to me because of the common clinical practice of combining trazodone and selective serotonin reuptake inhibitors (SSRIs) for SSRI–related insomnia. The authors measured clinical outcome and pharmacokinetic parameters for 4 weeks of combined administration of trazodone with either fluoxetine, placebo, or pindolol. The groups were really too small to conclude anything meaningful about augmentation strategies, although it appeared that the combination of fluoxetine and trazodone in this study may have been better than either of the other 2 treatments (which included such small sample sizes that no statistical analysis would have been meaningful). The study demonstrated that fluoxetine administration in combination with trazodone can cause significant increases in the metabolite mCPP, which is 1 of the main metabolites of trazodone. One might expect this anxiogenic trazodone metabolite, in combination with fluoxetine, to cause significant jitteriness in subjects. Although the report mentioned this, the authors clearly demonstrate that this combination can drive mCPP up to levels that can cause acute anxiety and provoke neuroendocrine responses when given to anxious patients. The authors speculated this increased mCPP level, as well as an increased trazodone level, may have contributed to the enhanced effect of the combination.

Because of the limited number of observations during the combination treatment, it is not clear whether trazodone and mCPP levels were still rising after 4 weeks, which appeared to be the case in 5 of 11 patients, or whether they had plateaued. These findings suggest that mCPP may possibly underlie activation seen in patients who had been intolerant of or unresponsive to fluoxetine and were subsequently treated with nefazodone, which is also metabolized (although to a lesser extent) to mCPP. The authors also discuss the interesting pharmacodynamic theory, based on the preclinical literature, that the SSRIs, trazodone, and mCPP all may affect desensitizing 5-HT_{2c} receptors—an effect believed to contribute to the therapeutic effects of antidepressants. Thus, while not a particularly useful study of augmentation strategies, this article presents evidence that a combination of fluoxetine (and probably other SSRIs) with trazodone (or maybe nefazodone) can cause significant increases in the metabolite mCPP. This pharmacokinetic interaction may mediate some of the early adverse effects seen in this combination, as well as a pharmacodynamic interaction that could theoretically enhance the antidepressant effects of a combination.

It is worth mentioning that the authors based this study on their previous observations that combining trazodone with fluoxetine or trazodone with pindolol was more effective than using trazodone alone in the treatment of major depression. Interestingly, the authors used only 100 mg/day of trazodone, which is less than the usual effective antidepressant dose of this agent. One reason for the findings of better improvement in depression during the course of 4 weeks of combined treatment was that patients receiving fluoxetine were also receiving an effective dose of an antidepressant, which also appeared to increase the plasma levels of trazodone itself, as well as a potentially active metabolite.

R.B. Lydiard, Ph.D., M.D.

Dose Escalation vs. Continued Doses of Paroxetine and Maprotiline: A Prospective Study in Depressed Out-patients With Inadequate Treatment Response
Benkert O, Szegedi A, Wetzel H, et al (Univ of Mainz, Germany; Smith Kline Beecham Pharma GmbH, Munich)
Acta Psychiatr Scand 95:288–296, 1997   8–14

Introduction.—The therapeutic response to some antidepressant agents improves as the dosage is increased within certain limits, whereas dosage escalation offers no advantage with other antidepressants. A study of 544 outpatients with various degrees of depression compared the possible benefits of dosage escalation of paroxetine and maprotiline.

Methods.—The multicenter study was conducted in a randomized, double-blind manner. Eligible patients were aged 18 to 71 and had major or minor depression and a total score of 13 or greater on the 17-item Hamilton Depression Rating Scale. Paroxetine was started at 20 mg daily, given in a single oral dose in the morning; the other patients received maprotiline (100 mg) divided into 3 doses per day. Patients who failed to have sufficient clinical improvement after 3 weeks had the dosage increased or continued with the previous dosage for an additional 3 weeks.

Results.—Response rates were 40% mg at week 3 in the paroxetine 20 mg and maprotiline 100 mg group. At 6 weeks, approximately 75% to 80% of all groups (those increased and those maintained at the initial dose) had responded. Thirty-six nonresponders to paroxetine were randomized to continue the previous dosage and 50 to receive an increase to 40 mg daily; 48 nonresponders continued to receive 100 mg of maprotiline and 40 were given the increased dosage (150 mg). Dose escalation did not significantly increase therapeutic response with either antidepressant. Response was defined as a reduction of 50% or greater in the Hamilton Depression Rating Scale. Results were unchanged after patients were stratified according to baseline severity of depression. The incidence of adverse events was not increased by the larger dosage.

Conclusion.—This prospective study using explicit criteria for dosage escalation found no significant benefit when the dosages of paroxetine and maprotiline were increased for nonresponders (from 20 mg to 40 mg and from 100 mg to 150 mg daily, respectively). For most patients with acute depression, a dosage of 20 mg of paroxetine a day is optimal.

▶ This article provides an example of a good idea that was limited by an inadequate experimental design. The authors are clearly aware of the limitations of this study of dosage escalation vs. continuation of the same dosage of either paroxetine or maprotiline in nonresponsive patients with major or minor depression. This is a particularly important problem which clinicians often face, and this study had a chance to provide some useful information. Unfortunately, the authors included a broad spectrum of patients and used only a 3-week observation period for assessing initial response, followed by a second 3-week period for assessing the effects of the second manipulation (dosage escalation vs. no change). Although it could be argued that the robust endpoint response rates in this group of patients should address my concern about the short initial treatment period, there was not adequate observation time for the patients who are randomized to an increased dosage vs. no dosage change. There may have been more resistant patients, and these patients may have required a longer period to become responders.

Of course, the lack of a placebo control, which the authors note, is another limitation of this study. The diagnostic categorization of these patients was not clear. They were assessed through "modified research diagnostic criteria," and for many patients all procedures were apparently carried out by experienced research assistants. This leaves open the question of both diagnostic and assessment capabilities, and since these individuals were not more thoroughly characterized in the article, the reader is left wondering whether this was another problematic aspect in the methodology. I selected this article because if 1 were to read quickly through it, one could easily walk away with the impression that in clinical practice it is not worthwhile to increase the dosage of an antidepressant if patients haven't responded after 3 weeks; this does not correlate with my clinical experience. This was clearly a study which involved a great deal of effort, and one which could have been made much better with closer attention to methodology.

R.B. Lydiard, Ph.D., M.D.

Pharmacological Choices After One Antidepressant Fails: A Survey of UK Psychiatrists
Shergill SS, Katona CLE (Maudsley Hosp, London; UCL Med School, London)
J Affect Disord 43:19–25, 1997   8–15

Introduction.—Approximately one third of patients with depression fail to respond to first-line antidepressants, and up to 21% have not recovered after 2 years of adequate dosage and compliance. A popular option in such cases is lithium augmentation, but it is not known whether most psychiatrists are aware of treatment choices for refractory depression. This question was examined in a survey of practicing psychiatrists in the United Kingdom.

Methods.—The survey, sent to 300 randomly selected physicians on the membership roll of the Royal College of Psychiatrists, presented a detailed vignette of a "typical" case of depression with initial treatment failure. The patient was a white woman, aged 40, who had been depressed for about 4 months. She sought treatment after intrusive suicidal thoughts led her to consider crashing her car. Her history included sexual abuse by her stepfather, migraine headaches, and a sister who had been treated for an episode of major depression. Treatment consisted of amitriptyline, 150 mg daily; and intensive individual, group, marital, and occupational therapy. No improvement was seen after 6 weeks.

Results.—Surveys were returned by 175 psychiatrists (63%). Respondents were predominantly men (61%) working as consultants (51%) in general psychiatric practice (62%). They had spent a mean of 13 years in the field and saw a mean of 9 patients per year with refractory depression. The most popular treatment choices in such cases were increasing dosages of tricyclic medication and change of medication to selective serotonin reuptake inhibitors; augmentation with tri-iodothyronine or with tryptophan or monoamine oxidase inhibitors was rarely chosen. Psychiatrists with elderly patients were more likely to choose lithium augmentation; electroconvulsive therapy was the preferred choice of those seeing more patients with resistant depression.

Conclusion.—The best established treatments for resistant depression were underused by psychiatrists in the United Kingdom, many of whom (39%) expressed a lack of confidence in treating this problem. Resistant depression should be included as a topic in continuing professional development courses.

▶ In this survey of Fellows of the Royal College of Psychiatrists in the United Kingdom (all of whom would be considered well-trained, often-senior people) regarding their choice of treatment after initial antidepressant failure, almost half the respondents would have increased the dosage, and another third would have switched from the tricyclic antidepressant used as the initial treatment in the case vignette to a selective serotonin reuptake inhibitor. However, the findings that only 1% of respondents would potentiate with tri-iodothyronine and that only 12% would have chosen to augment with lithium were surprising. Although most of these psychiatrists had executed most of the treatment choices, a third of the respondents were not confident treating resistant depression. The need for information in this clinical area is clear. There are very few data by which to guide these treatment decisions, and unfortunately the literature is not always useful to the practicing clinician. The authors suggest that additional training and postgraduate education are important in enhancing the skills of psychiatrists—even the best-educated ones—in the management of this population. Because psychiatrists in the United States as well as the United Kingdom will be increasingly asked to see these resistant patients, this article underscores our need for solid scientific information, ongoing education, and more standardized outcome measures to help us communicate with one another.

R.B. Lydiard, Ph.D., M.D.

Should Anxiety and Insomnia Influence Antidepressant Selection: A Randomized Comparison of Fluoxetine and Imipramine
Simon GE, Heiligenstein JH, Grothaus L, et al (Group Health Cooperative, Seattle; Lilly Research Lab, Indianapolis, Ind; Univ of Washington, Seattle; et al)
J Clin Psychiatry 59:49–55, 1998   8–16

Introduction.—The more sedating antidepressants are frequently recommended for patients with significant anxiety or insomnia. Few experimental data are available to support these recommendations. A large primary-care–based randomized trial was undertaken to assess how initial symptom patterns predict early response to fluoxetine or imipramine.

Methods.—Three hundred thirty-six patients from a health maintenance organization were randomized to treatment with fluoxetine or imipramine. The primary care physician managed all subsequent care. Before randomization and again 1 month after treatment initiation, patients completed the 17-item Hamilton Rating Scale for Depression and the Hopkins Symptom Checklist anxiety and depression subscale.

Results.—There were no significant between-group differences in rates of improvement of insomnia, agitation, or anxiety at 1-month evaluation. Neither baseline level of insomnia nor baseline level of anxiety was predictive of differences between groups in overall Hamilton or Hopkins depression subscale. Patients in the fluoxetine group were significantly less likely than patients in the imipramine group to change or discontinue medication during the first month; baseline levels of insomnia or anxiety had no effect on this finding.

Conclusion.—Baseline levels of insomnia or anxiety should not influence the choice of fluoxetine or imipramine as initial treatment in patients with moderate depression.

▶ Much is made, by pharmaceutical representatives as well as expert psychopharmacologists, of the activating effects of the selective serotonin reuptake inhibitors (SSRIs), in this case fluoxetine. Noting that Lilly funded this research, I should comment that it appears that the science is solid and the study was conducted by a group of highly respected clinical investigators (which lowers my paranoia titer). The finding of an equally good outcome for depression in the 2 groups was not surprising. Interestingly, high anxiety or high insomnia at baseline was not differentially affected by either imipramine or fluoxetine. This is important because we are often concerned that agitation, insomnia, and anxiety are indications for more sedating agents. This article nicely shows that effective treatment of depression is really the key. On the clinical level, one can provide sedation initially with a fairly reasonable assumption that, in the longer term, both the anxiety and insomnia will improve. With the additional safety features associated with the SSRIs in the depressed population, it appears that these drugs remain the treatment of choice for depression, and that tricyclics should be reserved for those patients who are unresponsive to or intolerant of SSRIs.

R.B. Lydiard, Ph.D., M.D.

Fluoxetine in Breast-Milk and Developmental Outcome of Breast-fed Infants
Yoshida K, Smith B, Craggs M, et al (Univ of London)
Br J Psychiatry 172:175–179, 1998   8–17

Introduction.—Some women who experience postnatal depression are treated with antidepressants. The effect of fluoxetine on the development of infants exposed to the drug during breast feeding was examined in a study of 4 mothers and infants.

Methods.—One women was given a diagnosis of obsessive-compulsive disorder, and 3 had major depressive disorder. All infants were born at full term and were healthy at delivery. In 3 cases, the infants were born by normal vaginal delivery; 1 was delivered by Cesarean section. Breast-feeding was started after delivery and continued after the mothers began taking fluoxetine (20-40 mg/day). The mean age of the infants at the start of medicated breast-feeding was 7 weeks; the mean duration of medicated breast-feeding was 21 weeks. Plasma, breast milk, and urine samples were assayed for transfer of fluoxetine and its principal metabolite, norfluoxetine. Infants were assessed during the first year of life using the Bayley Scales of Infant Development.

Results.—All samples of maternal plasma and breast milk contained fluoxetine and norfluoxetine. The range of fluoxetine in plasma was 138 to

272 ng/mL in the 3 women prescribed 20 mg/day; the concentration was 427 ng/mL in the woman taking 40 mg/day. Breast milk contained 39 to 177 ng/mL. Amounts of the drug in infants' plasma were below the limit of quantitation (5-20 ng/mL). Assessment with the Bayley Scales yielded no signs of abnormal development in the infants, and all were neurologically normal.

Conclusion.—Breast-fed infants whose mothers were treated with fluoxetine ingested 3% to 10% of the maternal dose of 20 to 40 mg/day, but the drug and its principal metabolite were below their limit of detection in infants' urine and plasma. In the few cases reported thus far, no acute toxic effects have been attributed to fluoxetine in this setting.

▶ Although this is a very small case series, the authors provide useful information on the clinical impact of prescribing fluoxetine (and by extrapolation, other selective serotonin reuptake inhibitors) on the concentrations of drug in breast milk and also on the neurologic development in the infant. Importantly, they found no significant effects during approximately 1 year of infant development. This has been the impression of clinicians, but the study adds some reassurance to those of us who sign prescription forms with trembling hands because of worry about possible adverse drug effects on an infant. Further studies will be important in clearing the way for optimal treatment, both during gestation and postnatally, if it appears that this is a safe therapy.

R.B. Lydiard, Ph.D., M.D.

Serum Sertraline and *N*-Desmethylsertraline Levels in Breast-feeding Mother-Infant Pairs

Wisner KL, Perel JM, Blumer J (Case Western Reserve Univ, Cleveland, Ohio)
Am J Psychiatry 155:690–692, 1998   8–18

Background.—The use of selective serotonin reuptake inihibitors (SSRIs) during pregnancy has not been well studied. Serum sertraline levels of breast-feeding women and their infants were analyzed.

Methods and Findings.—Nine mother-infant pairs were studied. Serum levels of sertraline and N-desmethylsertraline were measured. Seven infants had very low sertraline levels (less than 2 ng/mL), and 1 had a low level (3 ng/mL). In addition, low N-desmethylsertraline levels (6 ng/mL or less) were observed in 7 infants. One infant had a high level of N-desmethylsertraline. Another infant had unusually high serum sertraline and N-desmethylsertraline levels—half the mother's concentrations. However, all the babies were thriving (Table 1).

Conclusions.—Most of the infants in this series had very low serum levels of sertraline and N-desmethylsertraline, consistent with previous reports. However, 1 infant had unusually high levels of both. Although

TABLE 1.—Serum Concentrations of Sertraline and N-Desmethylsertraline in 9 Pairs of Nursing Mothers and Infants

Case	Infant's Age (Weeks)*	Infant's Sex	Infant's Birth Weight (Lb, Oz)	Maternal Dose of Sertraline (Mg/Day)	Number of Days Dose Was Given	Hours After Last Dose*	Maternal Serum Level (Ng/Ml) Sertraline	Maternal Serum Level (Ng/Ml) N-Desmethyl-sertraline	Infant Serum Level (Ng/Ml)† Sertraline	Infant Serum Level (Ng/Ml)† N-Desmethyl-sertraline
1	22	F	6, 10	50	7	7	13	28	<2	<2
2	13	M	7, 03	100	14	5	60	94	<2	4
3	5	M	7, 11	100	21	4	62	96	<2	5
4	5	F	6, 02	200	14	5	120	285	<2	24
5	15	M	7, 10	125	48	8	66	90	<2	<2
6	22	F	8, 06	150	16	4	134	184	<2	3
7	4	F	6, 07	75	21	2	12	31	0	3
8	4	M	7, 13	200	11	5	112	140	3	6
9	4	M	6, 10	100	21	2	117	114	64	68

*At serum sampling.
†<2 denotes that the serum concentration was below the limit of quantifiability; 0 denotes that it was not detectable.
(Courtesy of Wisner KL, Perel JM, Blumer J: Serum sertraline and N-desmethylsertraline levels in breast-feeding mother-infant pairs. *Am J Psychiatry* 155:609-692, 1998. Copyright 1998, the American Psychiatric Association. Reprinted by permission.)

sertraline use during breast-feeding is apparently acceptable, a safe exposure level to any agent is difficult to establish. Whether chronic exposure to even very low doses of antidepressants may affect infant neurodevelopment, is a possibility which has not been studied systematically.

▶ Wisner and colleagues studied concentrations of sertraline in *N*-desmethylsertraline in clinically remitted mothers who were receiving sertraline for depression. As noted, there were very low levels of sertraline in 8 of 9 infants; discussion of the infant with higher levels has been reviewed above and was considered spurious. Clinical studies of this nature are useful to practitioners who treat women in the childbearing years who are at the greatest risk of depression. Specifically, they indicate that breast-feeding is probably safe in infants whose mothers are receiving sertraline as an antidepressant. Although we cannot extrapolate to the general population the healthiness of these infants, the study supports the concept of treating patients through gestation and through breast-feeding with the SSRIs in general. For this class of medications, the data strongly indicate that they are safe with respect to organogenesis. What we do not yet know is what the intellectual development (ie., behavioral teratology) effect of these agents might be. Considering this unknown risk along with the risks of *not* treating mothers for depression adds both ethical strength and medicolegal protection to those of us who are forced to make difficult choices along with our patients. Thus, with appropriate consultation and truly informed consent, we can help advise our patients more emphatically that continued treatment may allow them to enter the daunting role of motherhood free of the significant impairments associated with depression.

R.B. Lydiard, Ph.D., M.D.

Serum Levels of Valproate and Carbamazepine in Breast-feeding Mother-Infant Pairs

Wisner KL, Perel JM (Case Western Univ, Cleveland, Ohio; Univ of Pittsburgh, Pa)
J Clin Psychopharmacol 18:167–169, 1998   8–19

Background.—The possible adverse effects of anticonvulsant use during breast-feeding have not been established. Three women with bipolar disorder who insisted on breast-feeding their infants were assessed in the current study.

Methods and Findings.—One woman was taking carbamazepine (CBZ) and 2 were taking valproate (VLP). Serum levels in the mothers and infants were determined after maternal steady-state was achieved. In the infant of the mother taking CBZ, the serum level of the drug was 15% of the total maternal CBZ. Free CBZ in this infant was 20% of the mother's values. The 2 infants of the mothers taking VLP had low serum levels of that agent—1.5% and 6% of maternal values, respectively.

Conclusions.—The serum levels of both CBZ and VLP in these infants were lower than previously reported values. However, careful monitoring is still recommended, as information is limited.

▶ Because of the small amount of studies to date on SSRIs, we know next to nothing about the concentrations of anticonvulsant in breast milk of breast-feeding mothers taking these agents. Wisner and Perel present a review of the literature from epileptics and then present 3 cases describing their patients who were breast-feeding while taking anticonvulsant, and they report the concentrations in the serum of those infants. Again, the balance between what is optimal for the mother and child vs. medicolegal risks bears mention. The American Academy of Pediatrics indicates that lithium is contraindicated, which is no surprise. I was, however, surprised that the article does not indicate that carbamazepine or valproate is incompatible with breast-feeding. To add some support to this, Wisner reports relatively low serum levels in her patient children. The appropriate caveats regarding individual cases are made. Again, as with the sertraline study by Wisner et al previously mentioned (Abstract 3–35), information such as this is useful in both assuring mothers as well as nervous clinicians about the relative safety of mood stabilizers in patients who might otherwise be unable to care for their infants in the critical postpartum period and beyond. Articles like this also demonstrate to many of us practitioners that reporting clinically relevant information derived from our practice may be helpful to others as well.

R.B. Lydiard, Ph.D., M.D.

Pregnancy Outcome Following Maternal Use of the New Selective Serotonin Reuptake Inhibitors: A Prospective Controlled Multicenter Study
Kulin NA, Pastuszak A, Sage SR, et al (Univ of Toronto; Teratogen Information Service, Tampa, Fla; Pennsylvania Hosp, Philadelphia; et al)
JAMA 279:609–610, 1998   8–20

Background.—Selective serotonin reuptake inhibitors (SSDIs) were introduced about 10 years ago and are now used for depression by millions of individuals around the world. Fetal safety is a major concern, because more than 50% of all pregnancies are unplanned, and an estimated 8% to 20% of all women have depression. Studies of pregnancy outcome after maternal exposure to fluoxetine have reported no evidence of major malformations or behavioral teratology, although women exposed to fluoxetine throughout their pregnancy did have more perinatal complications and minor malformations. New SSRIs have been introduced recently and there are no data on their reproductive safety in human beings.

Methods.—Nine Teratology Information Service centers in the United States and Canada participated in a study of fetal safety and risk of fluvoxamine, paroxetine, and sertraline. The rate of major congenital malformations was determined in women who were counseled during pregnancy and evaluated after exposure to fluvoxamine, paroxetine, or sertraline. The rate of major congenital malformations was also determined in a group of control participants who were counseled after exposure to nonteratogenic agents.

Results.—There were 267 women who took fluvoxamine, paroxetine, or sertraline for depression in the first trimester of pregnancy; 267 control participants. Exposure to the SSRIs was not associated with a higher risk of major malformations or with a higher rate of miscarriage, stillbirth, or prematurity. The mean birth weight and gestational age were similar in the study and control groups.

Discussion.—These findings indicate that fluvoxamine, paroxetine, and sertraline, when used at recommended doses, do not increase the risk of major congenital malformations in pregnant women. On all measured pregnancy outcomes, these results were well within the range of results reported for the general population.

▶ This article should be welcomed by clinicians who wrestle with the use of antidepressants in pregnant patients. These clinicians often have to balance the risk of fetal harm against the risk of not treating depressive illness, and to consider what effects no treatment might have on fetal development, because problems with nutrition and other aspects of poor self-care are associated with depression. These investigators found no adverse effect from newer SSRIs. We may not be able to breathe easy based solely on studies like this, but these data certainly add to the rationale for use of these agents in depressed pregnant mothers, and also provide good medical/legal defense for those of us who bite the bullet and do the right thing. The apparent lack of industry support for this particular study is also comforting. The authors report that anatomically correct children were born to mothers taking these agents. It would be useful to push this envelope a little further by assessing postnatal development (cognitive and perceptual/motor skills) for at least 3 to 5 years, in children who were exposed in utero. I applaud the authors for their careful work, which is likely to benefit both clinicians and patients by assuring us that treatment of depression in pregnant women does not appear to be dangerous to the fetus.

R.B. Lydiard, Ph.D., M.D.

Safety of Abrupt Discontinuation of Fluoxetine: A Randomized, Placebo-controlled Study
Zajecka J, Fawcett J, Amsterdam J, et al (Rush-Presbyterian-St Luke's Med Ctr, Chicago; Univ of Pennsylvania, Philadelphia; Columbia Univ, New York; et al)
J Clin Psychopharmacol 18:193–197, 1998   8–21

Introduction.—Several recent reports have indicated that abrupt discontinuation of the newer antidepressants, including the selective serotonin reuptake inhibitors, may cause adverse effects. Abrupt discontinuation of paroxetine, but not of sertraline or fluoxetine, has been described. Since fluoxetine has a half-life longer than paroxetine's or sertraline's, its discontinuation may produce fewer clinical complications, a difference resulting from the more gradual readjustment it allows. Adverse events during the 6 weeks after abrupt discontinuation of 12 weeks of fluoxetine (20 mg/day) treatment are reported.

Methods.—Three hundred ninety-five research participants who met Diagnostic and Statistical Manual-III-R criteria for major depression and had a 17-item Hamilton Rating Scale for Depression score of 16 or higher were randomized to continuation of treatment with fluoxetine or placebo (299 and 96 patients, respectively). Patients were evaluated at weeks 1, 2, 4, and 6 after randomization.

Results.—Mean Hamilton Rating Scale for Depression score (of 274 women and 121 men) was 20.9. At every evaluation point, the groups were similar in their reports of new or worsened adverse events. Rates of patient discontinuation because of adverse effects were similar in the 2 groups. A small percentage of patients who discontinued fluoxetine experienced mild, self-limited lightheadedness or dizziness of little clinical significance. No cluster of symptoms suggesting a discontinuation syndrome was observed.

Conclusion.—Abrupt discontinuation of fluoxetine is not correlated with a clinically significant discontinuation syndrome. Among the selective serotonin reuptake inhibitors, fluoxetine may be a good choice for patients likely to forget doses.

► This article describes findings that fall under the category of things My Mother Could Have Told Me. However, science is almost invariably better than opinion. Most clinicians share the impression that fluoxetine is not likely to be associated with adverse effects after abrupt discontinuation. This patient sample was mildly depressed (Hamilton score averaged around 20). The large sample size, however, suggests that the findings are probably reliable and supports the clinical impression that fluoxetine is easier to discontinue than shorter-acting selective serotonin reuptake inhibitors. This is a study that probably needn't be repeated, but this large, carefully conducted clinical trial does add a much-needed confirmation to the clinical impression regarding differences among the selective serotonin reuptake inhibitors.

R.B. Lydiard, Ph.D., M.D.

Meta-analysis of Trials Comparing Antidepressants With Active Placebos

Moncrieff J, Wessely S, Hardy R (Inst of Psychiatry, London; Kings College School of Medicine, London; Univ College London)

Br J Psychiatry 172:227–231, 1998   8–22

Introduction.—The use of active placebos can help to prevent subversion of double-blind design, because unblinding effects can introduce bias

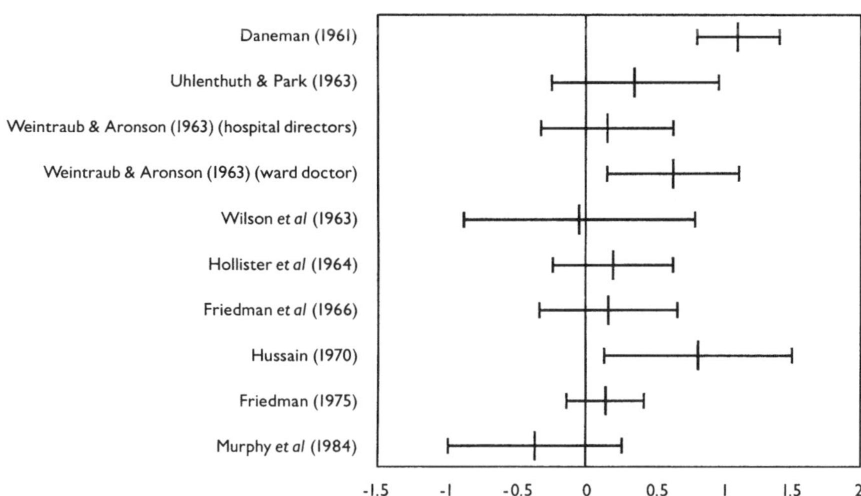

FIGURE 1.—Effect size. (Courtesy of Moncrieff J, Wessely S, Hardy R: Meta-analysis of trials comparing antidepressants with active placebos. *Br J Psychiatry* 172:227-231, 1998.)

into clinical trials. It has already been demonstrated that antidepressants can be distinguished from placebos. Active placebos can be used to mimic side effects of medications. Reported is a meta-analysis of controlled trials using active placebos to help determine efficacy of antidepressants.

Methods.—Databases of Medline, Embase, and PsychLit, key terms *active placebo* and *atropine*, hand searches of major psychiatric journals, and reference lists of previous published reports were used to find trials comparing antidepressants with active placebos. Heterogeneity was analyzed and sensitivity analyses were done. A subgroup analysis of inpatient and outpatient trials was performed.

Results.—Only 2 of 9 trials satisfying inclusion criteria demonstrated a consistent difference in favor of the active drug (Fig 1). Combining all trials provided pooled effect size estimates of between 0.41 and 0.46, with high heterogeneity caused by 1 strongly positive trial. Sensitivity analyses excluding this and 1 other trial diminished the pooled effect to between 0.21 and 0.27.

Conclusion.—Meta-analysis is very sensitive to determinations about exclusions. The pooled estimates of effect changed according to which combination of trials was used. The most and least conservative estimates were 0.21 and 0.47, respectively. These findings indicate that unblinding effects and expectations of treatment could influence results of antidepressant trials. The specific effects of antidepressants could be smaller, with the placebo effect being responsible for more of the clinical improvement, than is generally believed. Comparisons should be made between new antidepressants and inert and active placebos to determine the antidepressants' effects.

▶ I think this article is interesting because these authors address the issue of discriminating between placebo and active drug in studies assessing the efficacy of antidepressants. The article describes a meta-analysis of studies which included "active placebos," placebos that exerted effects consistent with the agents being studied, which in this case were tricyclics. Although this may not seem relevant to current psychiatry, since most of us use selective serotonin reuptake inhibitors as standard treatments, the authors still make some important points that are highly relevant to clinical psychopharmacology. The authors conclude that there is relatively little difference between active agents and "active placebos" in the handful of studies which they were able to find.

These studies, all of which were determined to be of reasonable clinical design, had durations ranging from as short as 3 weeks (in 2 studies) to as long as 12 weeks (in 2 studies). In all studies except 1, there was a small, usually nonsignificant difference between the drug and active placebo. In a meta-analysis that included only active placebo, which might mimic the side effects of the agent being tested, raters in both groups who are aware of these effects experience an inflation of their expectation. Thus, a confounding factor of observing side effects in both placebo recipients and patients receiving active drugs tends to minimize the difference between these effects and points to expectation on the parts of the participants in the clinical trial. This thoughtful study gets to the heart of the problems with doing clinical trials accurately. One solution is to have independent raters who do not discuss side effects or medications with clinical volunteers in these antidepressant trials. Even with these near-perfect circumstances, there is some "bleed-over" of side effects that are detected simply by asking questions related to symptoms of depression included on clinical rating scales. The authors also mention a possibility that atropine itself has antidepressant effects, which may have obscured differences between active drug and placebo. In our experience, raters who have assessed patients receiving imipramine and placebo can fairly accurately pinpoint those patients (85% accuracy, unpublished observations) taking imipramine, whereas there was an extremely low rate of discrimination between a selective serotonin reuptake inhibitor and placebo in that same study (unpublished observations). Furthermore, many clinical trials using imipramine, many of which have remained unpublished, have failed to discriminate between placebo and active drugs. Thus, the enthusiasm for investing in studies which include "active placebos," especially studies of newer agents, is limited at best.

In my opinion, the placebo effect experienced in clinical trials extends well beyond subjective effects of the placebo, which might be minimized by having an active substance that mimics the side effects of the agent to be tested. So many other factors, including clinical setting, patient expectations, and rater expectations, also enter into the picture and appear to be even more important sources of heterogeneity. Readers of clinical trials should pay attention to the methods used to evaluate outcome. These vary widely among studies, some of which use mean decreases and a depression rating score, while others use percentages of participants classified as responders on the Clinical Global Impression Scale. We are far from using standardized approaches to this, and if there is to be a next step, I would be most in favor of standardization of outcome measures across the industry, using clinically determined anchor points for determining responders. For example, a new patient who should be rated as a responder would be 1 in whom the rating clinician would not change the treatment based on the degree of clinical response. Although this clearly leaves some partial responders in the nonresponder category, it serves to enhance our ability to discriminate active agent from placebo. Given the tremendous expense (between $300–$500 million) that it takes to get a new drug to market, other statistical exercises may also be in order. These include meta-analysis of several multi-center studies to add discriminative power to the analysis, and also the ability to throw out a percentage of participants with high placebo response rates, using a set of predetermined rules agreed upon by all parties (including the federal regulatory agencies). Our knowledge of those factors that contribute to the placebo response is rudimentary. These authors make a valiant attempt to understand 1 critical factor, and we need all the help we can get.

R.B. Lydiard, Ph.D., M.D.

ECT Treatment and Cerebral Perfusion in Catatonia

Galynker II, Weiss J, Ongseng F, et al (Beth Israel Hosp, New York)
J Nucl Med 38:251–254, 1997   8–23

Background.—Why and how catatonia occurs is unknown, but it is associated with dysfunction of frontal lobe motor regulation centers. This case report revealed a correlation between substantial improvements in brain perfusion with an improvement in catatonia after electroconvulsive therapy (ECT).

> *Case Report.*—The patient was a 40-year-old woman who had a 25-year history of schizoaffective disorder. She was brought to the emergency department because she became stiff, nearly mute, and had stopped eating and drinking. She had been admitted 2 years previously for catatonic depression, and ECT had been successful. Physical exam revealed severe psychomotor retardation, negativism, and waxy flexibility, with sporadic stupor, a flat affect, and a somewhat depressed mood. Her Hamilton Rating Scale for Depression (HRSD) score was 14 and the Scale for the Assessment of Negative Symptoms (SANS) score was 24. ECT was instituted for 5 treatments. After the fifth treatment, symptoms of catatonia and depression improved, with an HRSD score of 13 and a SANS score of 16. The rigidity, waxy flexibility, and negativism were completely resolved. Single photon emission computed tomography (SPECT) was performed before the first ECT treatment and 2 days after the fifth one. These scans were compared to those of 8 healthy controls without psychiatric or neurologic disorders.

Compared with scans from healthy controls, the patient's first SPECT scan had significantly decreased perfusion in numerous areas: the frontal cortex (left inferior frontal, 21%; right inferior frontal, 15%), the posterior temporal cortex (15% bilaterally), the parietal cortex (left 25%, right 18%), and the posterior frontal lobes corresponding to motor cortex (left 29%, right 20%). The patient's SPECT scan after the fifth ECT treatment showed normal perfusion in the frontal, posterior temporal, parietal, and motor cortices. The right motor cortex and the right parietal cortex had improved substantially, but still had decreased perfusion compared with scans from healthy subjects (13% and 11%, respectively).

Conclusions.—Several psychiatric disorders, including schizophrenia and major depressive disorder, have documented reductions in brain perfusion. In this study, SPECT was able to correlate substantial improvements in perfusion with complete resolution of catatonia and partial resolution of depression. Most of the changes in the scans seemed to be from the resolution of catatonic symptoms rather than depression. These results suggest that catatonia is a state phenomenon, rather than a syndrome of schizophrenia.

▶ This single case report, which used SPECT scanning to monitor the ECT effects in a patient with schizoaffective disorder and catatonia, provides a possible glimpse into the future of biological psychiatry. The description of the affected pattern of brain metabolism suggests some overlap—but not complete overlap—with areas described as abnormal in depressed patients. They noted that the patient's parietal and motor cortex metabolic pattern changed more dramatically in this patient, and they hypothesize that this was a reflection of improvement in catatonia rather than changes in depression. They further note that other studies of catatonia in patients with diagnosis of schizophrenia showed similar patterns to the patient described in this report. While this report will not change my clinical practice, or probably yours, in the very near future, it underscores the advent of an era in which technology that is relatively inexpensive and accessible may be increasingly used, especially as specific patterns of abnormalities and brain metabolism (such as suggested here for catatonia) become more evident. This also helps bring the practice of psychiatric medicine closer to the mainstream of traditional medicine because we have procedures to allow us to assess brain function in addition to symptoms. It also has reduced stigma because it demonstrates biological abnormalities. It helps promote further the concept that psychiatric disorders, like other medical disorders, have a biological basis that reflects change with treatment. This should be good ammunition to use for reluctant third-party payors who often ignore varying degrees of illness severity in the mentally ill.

R.B. Lydiard, Ph.D., M.D.

Psychosis

Hypothesis Testing: Is Clozapine's Superior Efficacy Dependent on Moderate D_2 Receptor Occupancy?

Carpenter WT Jr, Zito JM, Vitrai J, et al (Univ of Maryland, Baltimore; Nathan Kline Inst, Orangeburg, New York)
Biol Psychiatry 43:79–83, 1998   8–24

Background.—The mechanism underlying clozapine's superior antipsychotic efficacy in treatment-resistant schizophrenia has not been defined. Moderate occupancy of D_2 postsynaptic receptors, rather than full occupancy, may be essential, possibly because of a more effective D_1/D_2 or serotonin-2a/D_2 ratio. This hypothesis was tested.

Methods.—Data were obtained from the New York Effectiveness of Clozapine Study. Six-week clozapine treatment results were compared in patients discontinuing oral neuroleptic medication with patients discontinuing long-acting depot neuroleptic. In the latter group, "full" D_2 occupancy was ensured during the 6 weeks of clozapine therapy. If *moderate* occupancy were needed for enhanced efficacy, then the group discontinuing treatment would be expected to show more improvement.

Findings.—Both groups showed the expected improvement after 6 weeks of clozapine therapy. The change in Brief Psychiatric Rating Scale scores did not differ significantly between groups.

Conclusions.—These data do not support the moderate occupancy hypothesis of clozapine efficacy. If these findings are valid, drug development aimed at attaining superior antipsychotic efficacy will be based on other hypotheses of therapeutic action.

▶ William Carpenter, a thoughtful pioneer in schizophrenia research, uses this study to inject (pun intended) some scientific exploration into the literature by reanalysis of this clozapine. All of us as clinicians are inundated by detail men in our offices, at our professional meetings, and in our journals regarding specific advantages of 1 type of agent over another in all of the pharmacologic classes we use. This is particularly so in the antipsychotics with newer agents appearing frequently, making claims based on their receptor activities that they may be better for 1 reason or another. Carpenter and colleagues tested the hypothesis that moderate D_2 receptor occupancy underlies clozapine's superior efficacy. In this nicely done and simple-minded study, they showed that clozapine had its typical effect in the context of what should be high D_2-receptor occupancy. The take-home message from this is that development of new drugs for treating psychotic patients should probably look elsewhere for mechanisms of superiority. I thought this article was worth mentioning because of my impression that information given busy clinicians by eager detailing personnel—however well meaning they may be—may not always be useful. Clozapine has been a very useful and cost-effective treatment for patients who are nonresponsive to other kinds of medications, and there are data to support this. We also must be comfortable with the concept that we really don't know what most of the medications that we use actually do with respect to their therapeutic efficacy, even though it might make us feel better at the time. So, just as mothers give babies acetaminophen, we should give agents that have been shown to be effective and relatively safe and hope that science will prevail in guiding us to developing better therapeutic agents in the future.

R.B. Lydiard, Ph.D., M.D.

A Double-blind, Controlled Comparison of the Novel Antipsychotic Olanzapine Versus Haloperidol or Placebo on Anxious and Depressive Symptoms Accompanying Schizophrenia
Tollefson GD, Sanger TM, Beasley CM, et al (Lilly Research Labs, Indianapolis, Ind)
Biol Psychiatry 43:803–810, 1998   8–25

Introduction.—Co-morbid depression is common in schizophrenia and may actually represent a separate dimension of the illness. A co-morbid mood disturbance in schizophrenia needs a careful differential diagnosis to exclude iatrogenic and other secondary causes. It is commonly believed that conventional neuroleptic drugs can induce or worsen a depressive state in some patients. Olanzapine (OLZ) is a novel thienobenzodiazepine with a broad-based receptor profile and mesolimbic dopaminergic selectivity. The profile of OLZ may offer a superior therapeutic effect. The relative baseline to end point treatment effects were assessed in a 6-week, randomized, multicentered trial comparing OLZ, haloperidol, and placebo.

Methods.—Three hundred thirty-five patients with acute exacerbation of chronic schizophrenia were randomized to 3 fixed dosage ranges of OLZ (5, 10, or 15 mg), haloperidol (10–20 mg), or placebo. An a priori defined anxiety-depression cluster from the Brief Psychiatric Rating Scale was analyzed to determine treatment efficacy.

Results.—Patients assigned to placebo experienced only marginal improvement in anxiety/depression from baseline to end point. Patients treated with haloperidol had some improvement, compared to their counterparts treated with placebo. Patients randomized to treatment with OLZ experienced increasing improvement, according to the Brief Psychiatric Rating Scale anxiety/depression factor, as dosage increased. The 10 and 15 mg dosages of OLZ provided significant improvement in mood status.

Conclusion.—The differential benefit observed with OLZ in the treatment of co-morbid anxious and depressive symptoms in patients with schizophrenia occurs because of contributions from a more selective mesolimbic dopaminerigic profile, and because of D_1 or D_4 activity, release of dopamine/norepinephrine in the prefrontal cortex, and/or serotonin $5\text{-HT}_{2A,C}$ antagonism.

▶ This article, a meta-analysis of efficacy studies comparing olanzapine and haloperidol, provides an interesting clinical discussion point. We often fail to appreciate that schizophrenics are susceptible to other psychiatric disorders such as anxiety or mood disorders. Often these disorders are difficult to detect because of the problems in eliciting a crisp history (for example, discriminating paranoia from rumination or worry can sometimes be a problem). The main finding—that haloperidol was less effective than the 10- and 15-mg dosages of olanzapine in alleviating anxiety symptoms—suggests that the newer medications (in this case olanzapine) with a broader receptor interaction profile may also be therapeutic across a broader range of symptoms. The selective serotonin reuptake inhibitors are broadly effective for mood and anxiety disorders, and represent a real advance over tricyclic antidepressants. More controlled studies examining this important clinical question are warranted. Failure to treat prominent symptoms such as mood or anxiety symptoms can contribute to patients' noncompliance with medications and increase the associated morbidity and relapse rate in patients with chronic psychotic disorders.

R.B Lydiard, Ph.D., M.D.

Clozapine Treatment in Australia: A Review of Haematological Monitoring
Copolov DL, Bell WR, Benson WJ, et al (Mental Health Research Inst of Victoria, Melbourne, Australia; Westmead Hosp, New South Wales, Australia; Univ of Sydney, New South Wales, Australia)
Med J Aust 168:495–497, 1998   8–26

Introduction.—Clozapine is an atypical antipsychotic used to treat patients with schizophrenia in whom conventional antipsychotic drugs, like haloperidol or the phenothiazines, are ineffective. It is also used in patients with intolerable adverse effects to these medications. Treatment with clozapine may be complicated by life-threatening agranulocytosis, so regular hematological evaluations are necessary. The incidence of clozapine-induced agranulocytosis was prospectively assessed, using the formal Clozaril Patient Monitoring System (CPMS), in a large series of Australian patients.

Methods.—The CPMS central database was used to review hematological monitoring for the first 3 years (June 1993 to July 1996) of its operation. All patients treated with clozapine, as well as medical practitioners, pharmacists, and treating centers (4061, 1949, 1017, and 171, respectively) were registered with the CPMS. The incidence of agranulocytosis, neutropenia, and leukopenia combined was 2.6% (104 of 4061 patients). Incidence of agranulocytosis was 0.9% (37 patients). No deaths have been reported in Australia as a result of complications of clozapine-induced agranulocytosis. As has been reported from other countries, most incidences of agranulocytosis occurred within the first 18 weeks of treatment with clozapine. These findings support the current Australian policy of replacing weekly monitoring with monthly monitoring after 18 weeks.

Conclusion.—The stringency of monitoring clozapine treatment and the degree of early warning afforded by the CPMS have paid off: there have been no Australian deaths from complications of clozapine-induced agranulocytosis. Patient protection is assured by the physician and pharmacists and by the CPMS by using monthly hematological testing.

▶ This article describes findings, replicated in the United States and elsewhere, about serious adverse effects associated with clozapine treatment. In this sample of over 4,000 patients, there were no deaths. Two and a half percent had low white blood count and only 0.9% had agranulocytosis. The authors emphasize the need for close monitoring of white blood counts in patients treated with clozapine. Weekly monitoring presents a difficult problem in cost of treatment. Although most of these patients experienced agranulocytosis within the 18 weeks of treatment, 22% of the sample developed this problem *after* 5 months of treatment. The authors used *monthly* blood monitoring after 18 weeks as opposed to *weekly* blood monitoring. The lower frequency reduced costs by 75%. This is grist for the mill of containing health care costs while also maintaining adequate therapeutic benefit in patients receiving clozapine.

R.B Lydiard, Ph.D., M.D.

Pharmacokinetic Interactions of Clozapine With Selective Serotonin Reuptake Inhibitors: Differential Effects of Fluvoxamine and Paroxetine in a Prospective Study
Wetzel H, Anghelescu I, Szegedi A, et al (Univ of Mainz, Germany)
J Clin Psychopharmacol 18:2–9, 1998   8–27

Background.—The use of combined antipsychotic and antidepressant agents is increasing in the treatment of schizophrenic patients unresponsive to monotherapy with typical neuroleptics or clozapine. The pharmacokinetic interactions of clozapine and its metabolites N-desmethylclozapine and clozapine N-oxide with the selective serotonin reuptake inhibitors (SSRIs) fluvoxamine and paroxetine were analyzed.

Methods.—Thirty patients received clozapine at a target dose of 2.5 to 3 mg/kg body weight. The dose was increased gradually, and serum levels of the drug and 2 metabolites were assessed twice at 7-day intervals after steady-state conditions were reached. Fluvoxamine, 50 mg/day, was added in 16 patients, and paroxetine, 20 mg/day, was added in 14. Serum levels of clozapine and its metabolites were measured after the SSRI was coadministered for 1, 7, and 14 days.

Findings.—Average trough concentrations of steady-state serum levels of clozapine, N-desmethylclozapine, and clozapine N-oxide were substantially increased under fluvoaxime by about 3 times baseline levels. By

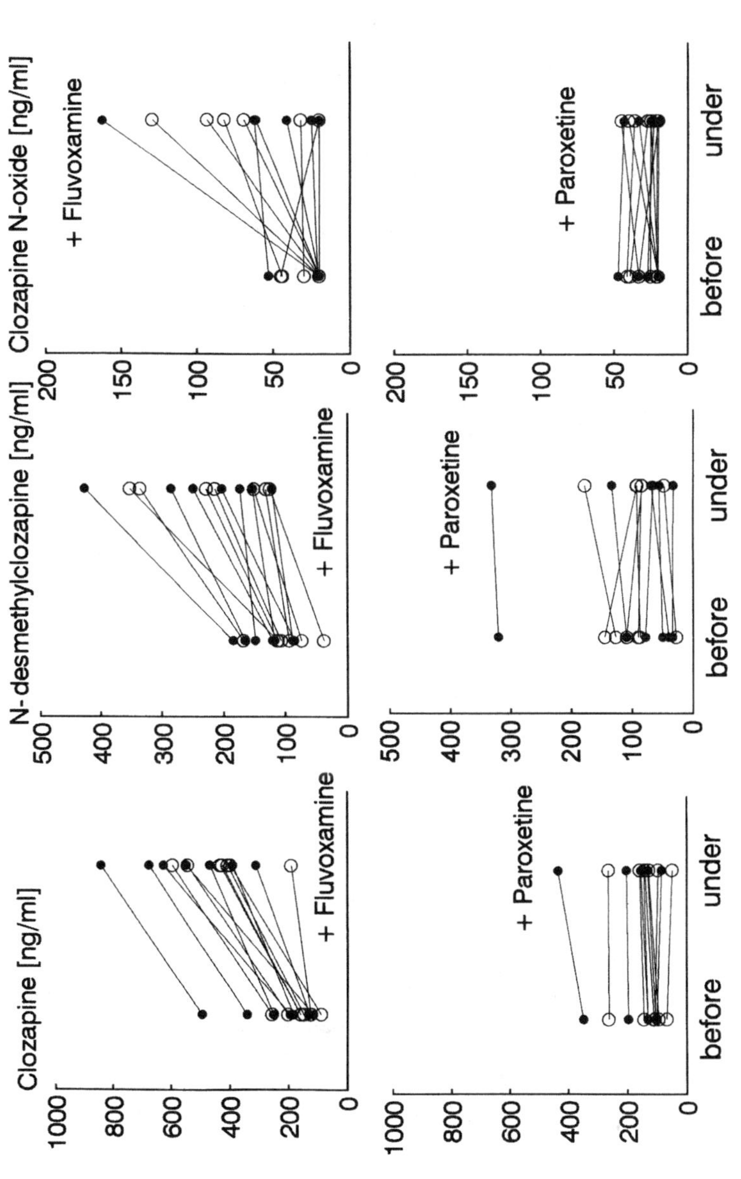

FIGURE 1.—Blood levels of clozapine, N-desmethylclozapine, and clozapine N-oxide before (day 0) and 1 week after start of coadministration of either fluvoxamine or paroxetine in schizophrenic patients. Values given are serum concentrations of individual patients. *Black circles*, nonsmokers; *white circles*, smokers. (Courtesy of Wetzel H, Anghelescu I, Szegedi A, et al: Pharmacokinetic interactions of clozapine with selective serotonin reuptake inhibitors: Differential effects of fluvoxamine and paroxetine in a prospective study. *J Clin Psychopharmacol* 18:2-9, 1998.)

contrast, paroxetine induced minimal, nonsignificant changes. Mean elimination half-life estimation of clozapine 2 weeks after initiation of fluvoxamine comedication showed an increase from 17 to about 50 hours. No change occurred with paroxetine coadministration. The ratio of N-desmethylclozapine to clozapine did not change significantly with the administration of either SSRI. Compared with nonsmokers, mean clozapine serum levels were significantly lower (by 32%) in smokers with monotherapy (Fig 1).

Conclusions.—Fluvoxamine induced relevant increases in serum concentrations of clozapine and its metabolites in these patients. This effect is probably attributable to the inhibition of enzymes catalyzing the degradation of clozapine and N-desmethylclozapine. Paroxetine, at the usual clinically effective dosage of 20 mg/day, did not produce significant pharmacokinetic interactions.

▶ This German research group reports on a well-controlled study of coadministration of the SSRIs fluvoxamine and paroxetine in patients with schizophrenia who are receiving clozapine. The profound effects upon clozapine concentrations caused by coadministration of fluvoxamine could well be clinically significant. This is an important study because it characterizes the effects of the SSRIs both in smokers and nonsmokers, and the effect is apparently the same in smokers (although they do run lower clozapine levels in general). My eyes tend to glaze over when I get information about cytochrome drug interactions, but this one unglazed them because of the clinical implications of this interaction. Although apparently fluoxetine, sertraline, and fluvoxamine all have the effect of increasing clozapine levels, it is clear that fluvoxamine fairly reliably exhibits this phenomenon. There are 2 take-home messages from this. The first, noted by the authors is that caution should be used when fluvoxamine is used in patients with schizophrenia who are also given SSRIs; if one does not wish for a pharmacokinetic interaction, paroxetine is the best choice. Conversely, if patients who are receiving clozapine appear to have very low levels and an increase in clozapine levels would be desirable, it may be that an agent like fluvoxamine may actually be used to increase clozapine levels (although caution should be used in observing clozapine levels if this were to be the clinical choice). Depression and anxiety disorders are common in schizophrenic patients. Clinicians are gradually beginning to appreciate this, and are using agents to treat comorbid psychiatric disorders in the schizophrenic population. Useful reports like this can help enhance our clinical practice. Fluvoxamine also apparently inhibits the metabolism of caffeine, which is commonly consumed in large quantities by schizophrenic patients. An eye on caffeine consumption is probably useful if fluvoxamine is the choice of the practicing clinician for use in a schizophrenic patient.

R.B. Lydiard, Ph.D., M.D.

Treatment of Tardive Dyskinesia

Egan MF, Apud J, Wyatt RJ, et al (Natl Inst of Mental Health Neuroscience Ctr, Washington, DC)
Schizophr Bull 23:583–609, 1997   8–28

Introduction.—The introduction of clozapine and other atypical antipsychotic agents has raised hopes that tardive dyskinesia (TD) may be eradicated someday. For now, this disorder remains a significant clinical problem for patients and physicians. Management approaches to TD are described.

Managing TD.—Most TD is mild. Therapeutic efforts focus on minimizing neuroleptic exposure or changing treatment to atypical agents in patients with mild to moderate TD. Tardive dyskinesia typically does not

---

TABLE 4.—Possible Treatment Approach to Tardive Dyskinesia

A. For mild to moderate TD that does not require suppression
1. Reevaluate need for antipsychotics; use other classes of medications when possible.
2. If an antipsychotic is required, switch to a putative atypical antipsychotic (olanzapine, risperidone, seroquel, sertindole).
3. If typical antipsychotics must be used, taper to lowest possible levels and follow for improvement in TD.
4. Add vitamin E to neuroleptic if TD persists. If no improvement in 3 months, discontinue vitamin E.
5. If symptoms progress, consider clozapine.

B. For suppression of moderate to severe TD
1. Switch to a putative atypical agent; begin with olanzapine. Increase dose until TD is suppressed or maximum dose is reached. Gradually taper to lowest effective dose that suppresses psychosis and TD. Consider other putative atypical agents (resperidone, seroquel, sertindole) if no response is seen to the first.
2. Switch to clozapine.

If steps 1 and 2 fail, try adding the following medications, one at a time, to whatever antipsychotic (typical and atypical) is being used. For careful evaluation of response, antipsychotic dose should remain stable. If no response is seen after an adequate trial, one suppressive agent should be discontinued before trying the next.
3. Add vitamin E to antipsychotic.
4. Add calcium channel blocker (e.g., nifedipine) to antipsychotic.
5. Add noradrenergic antagonist (e.g., clonidine) to antipsychotic.
6. Add benzodiazepine (e.g., clonazepam) to antipsychotic.*, †
7. Add dopamine depleter (e.g., reserpine) to antipsychotic.*
8. Increase dose of typical antipsychotic until TD is suppressed, then very gradually taper dose.‡
9. Try other possible suppressive agents‡; cholinergic agonists (e.g., tacrine), dopamine agonists (e.g., amantadine), buspirone, GABA agonist (e.g., gabapentin), an SRI, cyproheptadine, opioid antagonists, estrogen, steroids, ECT.

C. For suppression of tardive dystonia
1. Add anticholinergics (increase gradually to "high" doses).
2. Add vitamin E.
3. Add clonazepam.
4. Go to steps 1, 2, 4, 7, and 8 in part B.
5. Consider botulinum injections.

*May be tried first, particularly if rapid relief is needed.
†When adding to clozapine, be cautious because of case reports of respiratory depression.
‡These therapies should be considered experimental. Although the other therapies have some support for their efficacy in well-controlled studies, these have less support, in general. Clear benefit and risk data may not be available.
Abbreviations: GABA, gamma-amino-butyric acid, *SRI*, serotonin reuptake inhibitor; *ECT*, electroconvulsive therapy; *TD*, tardive dyskinesia.
(Courtesy of Egan MF, Apud J, Wyatt RJ: Treatment of tardive dyskinesia. *Schizophr Bull* 23:583-609, 1997.)

---

progress, which indicates that the risk of remaining on typical neuroleptics is slight. Moderate to severe TD is more challenging, and patients typically require medication to suppress symptoms (Table 4). Most suppressive agents have limited success. No treatment strategy is clearly superior or even successful in most patients. Raising the doses of typical neuroleptics may be useful for short-term suppression, yet the long-term efficacy and risk of this approach have not been clearly elucidated. Data on atypical neuroleptics are sparse. Clozapine has a short-term suppressive effect that is weak, but patients may experience improvement with long-term treatment.

Other Approaches.—Other medications that have relatively few side effects and may have suppressive properties include calcium blockers, adrenergic antagonists, and vitamin E. Gamma-amino-butyric acid agonists agents and dopamine can be helpful but are accompanied by troubling side effects. Anticholinergic agents and botulism toxin have also been effective in treating TD.

Conclusion.—Despite the new generation of neuroleptics, TD remains a challenging clinical problem. A better understanding of the mechanisms of actions of atypical neuroleptics and of the physiology of the basal ganglia should enhance treatment approaches.

▶ This article was completed by a research team who is well known in the area of antipsychotic medication treatment. This thorough review covers the waterfront of the various options available to us and presents a thoughtful flow diagram (untested) that is useful for clinicians. The authors end with the hope that the newer agents that appear to have a lower risk for development of tardive dyskinesia may provide a brighter future for patients who require treatment with antipsychotics. The article itself is certainly well worth reading, with a take-home message (see table) which will probably be useful to many busy clinicians.

R.B. Lydiard, Ph.D., M.D.

Substance Abuse

Cocaine as a Risk Factor for Neuroleptic-induced Acute Dystonia
van Harten PN, van Trier JCAM, Horwitz EH, et al (Psychiatric Hosp Welterhof, Heerlan, The Netherlands; Overvecht Hosp, Utrecht, The Netherlands; Psychiatric Hosp Curaçao, The Netherlands Antilles; et al)
J Clin Psychiatry 59:128–130, 1998   8–29

Introduction.—The known risk factors for neuroleptic-induced acute dystonia (NIAD) are male gender, younger age, neuroleptic potency, dose, and history of NIAD. Two reports have suggested that cocaine use may also be a risk factor. Cocaine use as a risk factor for NIAD was prospectively assessed in a high-risk cohort.

Methods.—Twenty-nine patients at high risk for NIAD were admitted between June 1, 1993, and June 1, 1995. Patients were male, aged 17 to 45, and received high-potency neuroleptics within 24 hours of hospital admission. None of the patients had used neuroleptics before admission. Patients with neurodegenerative disorders or exposure to anticholinergics, benzodiazepines, promethazine, carbamazepine, phenytoin, or levodopa were excluded. Cocaine use was defined as "the use of cocaine or base within 24 hours before admission" and NIAD was defined as "the sudden onset, within 7 days after the start of neuroleptic treatment, of sustained muscle contractions." Cocaine use was determined by urine samples collected within 24 hours of admission. Follow-up time was 7 days.

Results.—Of 29 patients who met inclusion criteria during the 2-year trial, 9 were cocaine users and 20 were cocaine nonusers. Five, 3, and 1 of the 9 cocaine users were diagnosed with schizophrenia, mania, and cocaine-induced psychosis, respectively. Significantly more cocaine-using psychiatric patients than nonusers developed NIAD. Type of neuroleptic used by the NIAD and non-NIAD group did not differ.

Conclusion.—Cocaine use is a primary risk factor for NIAD and needs to be included in the list of well-known risk factors. Anticholinergics should be administered for at least 7 days to avert NIAD in psychiatric patients who are cocaine-users.

▶ This article describes a small but interesting study intended to evaluate whether recent cocaine users who were admitted to a psychiatric hospital were at greater risk for cocaine-induced dystonia than comparable patients who had not recently used cocaine. Although the numbers were small, the study is relatively clearly described and appropriately criticized by the authors. Regardless of additional psychiatric status, recent cocaine abuse appeared to confirm considerable risk for acute dystonia in individuals recently exposed to cocaine. It was also interesting that schizophrenics appeared in both the cocaine-user and non-user groups. The frequency with which schizophrenics abuse cocaine has been an area of interest lately and the abuse appears to occur in a substantial subgroup of schizophrenic patients. From a clinical perspective, the use of neuroleptics for acute cocaine intoxication or post-cocaine agitation is relatively common, as is the use of high-potency benzodiazepines. This article should alert clinicians who treat these patients that there may be additional risk for neuroleptic-induced dystonic reactions in patients who have recently used cocaine. The authors suggest, and I concur, that some protection from neuroleptic-induced dystonic reactions should be included in the treatment plan for newly hospitalized patients who have recently used cocaine. One good choice might be amantadine, which has relatively few anticholinergic properties and appears to be protective against acute neuroleptic-induced dystonia. The use of anticholinergic agents in these patients may induce some delirium and might be reserved for patients who are nonresponsive to amantadine, or used in combination to avoid high-dose anticholinergic treatment. This is an interesting companion to Abstract 8-30, which shows exaggerated response to benzodiazepines in individuals who had recently been cocaine abusers (reviewed elsewhere in this series). The scientific underpinnings of this clinical observation may result from hyperactivity of dopamine receptors induced by cocaine abuse in this clinical subpopulation. Further information about this apparently common clinical situation would be welcome.

R.B. Lydiard, Ph.D., M.D.

Enhanced Sensitivity to Benzodiazepines in Active Cocaine-abusing Subjects: A PET Study
Volkow ND, Wang G-J, Fowler JS, et al (Brookhaven Natl Lab, Upton, NY; State Univ of New York, Stony Brook)
Am J Psychiatry 155:200–206, 1998   8–30

Introduction.—The findings that dopamine brain activity is enhanced by cocaine and dopamine signals are transferred through γ-aminobutyric acid (GABA) led researchers to hypothesize GABA-ergic disruption in individuals who abuse cocaine. Thirteen current cocaine abusers and 14 healthy volunteers had GABA brain function assessed by positron emission tomography after administration of lorazepam, a benzodiazepine that facilitates GABA neurotransmission.

Methods.—The cocaine-abusing subjects had a mean age of 38 years; all met *Diagnostic and Statistical Manual of Mental Disorders*, 4th edition criteria for active cocaine dependence and were free of current medical illnesses. Neither the healthy volunteers nor the cocaine abusers were taking medication at the time of the study. All participants underwent physical, psychiatric, and neurologic examinations and routine laboratory tests. Two PET scans were obtained with fluorodeoxyglucose, 1 after administration of placebo and the other after administration of lorazepam (30 μg/kg).

Results.—The control group exhibited significantly higher plasma concentrations of lorazepam than the cocaine-abusing group, yet the latter group reported significantly more lorazepam-induced sleepiness. This sleepiness was correlated with lorazepam-induced changes in thalamic metabolism. Decreases in global and regional brain glucose metabolism were significantly larger in the cocaine group than in the comparison group. Regional metabolic measures were significantly higher in the cocaine group in the striatum, thalamus, and parietal cortex during placebo administration. Whole brain metabolism was significantly higher in the cocaine-abusing group than in the comparison group at baseline, but regional metabolic measures were equivalent in the 2 groups after lorazepam administration.

Conclusion.—Cocaine-abusing individuals were found to have an enhanced sensitivity to lorazepam, suggesting disruption of GABA pathways. The intense sleepiness experienced by some abusers after lorazepam administration may contribute to the increased toxicity and mortality seen when alcohol and cocaine are combined.

► Dr. Volkow and her colleagues report on an elegant study demonstrating the consequences of substance abuse on brain metabolism in chronic cocaine abusers. The study also replicates some previously reported effects on brain metabolism (increased metabolism during withdrawal from chronic cocaine), and reports on regional differences in areas affected by lorazepam between normal control subjects and cocaine abusers.

Studies such as this carry the field several steps further in terms of being able to document the profound effects on brain metabolism elicited by chronic substance abuse. The authors carry this even further, in making the clinical point that the increased sedation encountered in the cocaine-abusing subjects—despite lower plasma levels of lorazepam—may carry a risk in administering benzodiazepines after a period of chronic cocaine abuse.

Giving benzodiazepines early in detoxification from cocaine is a common clinical practice, and substance abusers often self-administer benzodiazepines to "come down" after a cocaine binge. This report suggests that caution is indicated in treating individuals or cocaine abusers with what might normally be considered reasonable doses of a benzodiazepine. Hopefully, further information of this kind will emerge to make us smarter regarding the optimal treatments for substance abusers.

R.B. Lydiard, Ph.D., M.D.

Geriatrics

Imipramine Treatment of Opiate–dependent Patients With Depressive Disorders: A Placebo–controlled Trial
Nunes EV, Quitkin FM, Donovan SJ, et al (Columbia Univ, New York; Bridge Plaza Treatment and Rehabilitation Services, New York; Long Island Jewish/ Hillside Hosp, Glen Oaks, NY; et al)
Arch Gen Psychiatry 55:153–160, 1998   8–31

Background.—Depression is frequent in patients who abuse drugs; could it be that they are taking drugs to "feel better"? In 3 previous studies, researchers found a tendency for antidepressants to be more effective in cocaine abusers who were depressed. The current study expanded these findings by evaluating the use of antidepressants in depressed substance abusers who were receiving methadone.

Methods.—Patients attending 2 community-based, university-affiliated methadone maintenance clinics were eligible. Patients could be included if they met the DSM-III-R criteria for a depressive order and had at least 1 of the following features: depression that occurred before the start of regular substance abuse, secondary depression that developed or persisted during a previous 6-month period of abstinence, or secondary depression that persisted for at least 1 month during the current methadone treatment. Ultimately, 169 patients were enrolled. During 1 week of placebo, 26 dropped out and the depression improved in 6, so they were not included in the trial. The remaining 137 patients were randomized to imipramine ($n = 74$) or placebo ($n = 63$); 84 patients completed at least 6 weeks of dosing (42 from each group). At baseline and each week, patients were assessed by the Hamilton Depression Rating Scale and the

Clinical Global Impression scale, and for how often and how much they used or craved the abused substance.

Findings.—Patients taking imipramine had an average highest dose of 268 ± 50 mg/day. Significantly more patients taking imipramine met the global response criterion and the depression symptom scores were significantly lower than patients taking placebo. Overall, 57% (24 of 42) of patients taking imipramine responded to treatment compared to only 7% (3 of 42) of patients taking placebo. No predictors of global response could be identified, although nonresponders tended to use more benzodiazepines and alcohol. Patients with a moderate or high level of substance abuse at baseline tended to improve more than those with a low baseline abuse level. Improvement in depression was significantly associated with less substance abuse at 6 weeks. However, of the 27 global responders, the depression improved before the substance abuse in 33%, and substance abuse improved before depression in 59%. About two thirds of patients in each group continued the substance abuse.

Conclusions.—Imipramine had a strong antidepressant effect in these depressed substance abusers who were undergoing methadone maintenance treatment. These results indicate that targeting treatments to groups of drug abusers who have the same psychiatric comorbidity can be effective. Future studies might include the effects of psychosocial interventions on the effectiveness of antidepressants in this population. However, the lack of causality between improvement in depression and reduction of substance abuse indicates that a patient's mood is only 1 of many factors that lead to substance abuse.

▶ This ambitious study brought the field a little bit further down the road to understanding psychiatric comorbidity. The authors selected a subgroup of patients with depression and opioid dependence who were enrolled in a methadone program. The study suggests that matching patients for treatment is a good idea at least some of the time. Another important feature of this study is that there was no naive search for "a cure" (such as abstinence from substance abuse forever) but rather a reduction in ongoing substance abuse. The study suggests that the substance abuse field has taken a different view of what successful treatment might mean—and that "good outcome" cannot apply to only those individuals who remain abstinent. The dosage of imipramine used indicated a good strength of treatment. Unfortunately, the suicidal idea among some patients probably required excluding individuals who may otherwise have been able to complete treatment and do better clinically. Interestingly, Nunes et al left open the question of whether the self–medication hypothesis applies. This study suggests that even among the subgroup of depressed methadone patients, some may be self-medicating while others may be simply taking the opioid initially for the same reason that most people do—it feels good. It's a complicated world, and Nunes et al point out very well that variability, even within the subgroups of patient groups, is probably likely. I applaud their efforts to understand and rationally approach treatment for this important subgroup of patients.

R.B. Lydiard, Ph.D., M.D.

Potential Role for Estrogen Replacement in the Treatment of Alzheimer's Dementia
Schneider LS, Farlow MR, Pogoda JM (Univ of Southern California, Los Angeles; Indiana Univ, Indianapolis)
Am J Med 103:46S-50S, 1997   8–32

Background.—Patients with Alzheimer's disease have substantial deficits in cholinergic function. Tacrine hydrochloride is an acetylcholinesterase inhibitor that modestly improves the cognitive symptoms of the disease. Estrogen is believed to improve cholinergic function through neurotrophic and neuroprotective effects. Thus, these authors examined whether estrogen replacement therapy (ERT) had any additional effect on the clinical and cognitive responses of women with Alzheimer's disease who were treated with tacrine.

Methods.—The authors analyzed data from a previous 30-week, multicenter, randomized, double-blind, placebo-controlled trial of tacrine in patients with Alzheimer's disease. That study was based on women who were more than or equal to 50 years old, otherwise healthy, and had a caretaker to ensure drug compliance and perform assessments. Forty-six patients had been receiving ERT before the tacrine trial, and 277 were not using ERT. Patients were randomized to placebo or to 1 of 3 doses of tacrine (80-160 mg/day). Thus, on an intent-to-treat basis, 83 patients were taking placebo without ERT, 9 were taking placebo + ERT, 194 were taking tacrine without ERT, and 37 were taking tacrine + ERT. Of patients who completed the 30-week protocol, these groups had 53, 7, 50, and 8 patients, respectively. Every 6 weeks, patients were assessed by the Alzheimer's Disease Assessment Scale-Cognitive Scale (ADASc), the Clinician's Interview Based Impression of Change (CIBI) scale, the Caregiver's Impression of Change (CIC), and the Mini-Mental Status Examination (MMSE).

Findings.—Intent-to-treat analysis indicated a statistically significant difference for the ADASc: Patients taking tacrine + ERT had a significantly better response at 30 weeks than those taking placebo without ERT or tacrine without ERT. Patients taking tacrine + ERT also tended to respond better on the CIBI, CIC, and MMSE. Analysis of the patients who actually completed the trial confirmed these trends, with significant dose-related trends found for the ADASc, the CIBI, and the CIC ($P = 0.07$ for the MMSE) in patients taking tacrine + ERT.

Conclusions.—Based on cognitive measures, clinical assessments, caregiver evaluations, and mental status ratings, women with Alzheimer's disease who were taking ERT had the most improvement during tacrine dosing. Why estrogen enhanced the effects of tacrine is not known, but possible factors include: downregulation or decreases in β-adrenergic receptors and serotonin receptors, neurotransmitter effects, antiinflammatory effects, and decreases in circulating apolipoproteins. These results warrant future randomized trials to explore further the effects of ERT in women with Alzheimer's disease.

▶ This report is derived from a subset of a large multicenter study of the treatment of Alzheimer's. The authors analyzed a group of elderly women with Alzheimer's disease who had received estrogen replacement during the course of this study comparing tacrine and placebo. The results showed that a combination of estrogen replacement therapy with either condition resulted in greater improvement—suggesting this agent may benefit cognitive functioning. While the authors do provide some speculative comments about what the mechanism of action might be, they do not mention depression as a contributing factor. While the literature is far from clear on this issue, it is conceivable that estrogen replacement may benefit depression in these female Alzheimer's patients, which was already effectively at baseline, and thus would not have been detected during the course of this clinical study. In any case, the clinical take-home message is that estrogen therapy is probably under-used, especially in women with cognitive decline. It may be a useful adjunctive treatment for this growing population of individuals.

R.B. Lydiard, Ph.D., M.D.

Valproic Acid Treatment of Agitation in Dementia

Herrmann N (Univ of Toronto; Sunnybrook Health Science Centre, Toronto)
Can J Psychiatry 43:69–72, 1998   8–33

Introduction.—Neuroleptics have been of only modest benefit in patients with behavioral disturbances associated with dementia. Recent reports of small series of patients have indicated that valproic acid may be useful in managing behavioral disturbances associated with dementia, possibly because it enhances gamma-ergic aminobutyric acid neurotransmission. To further document the effectiveness and safety of this medication, valproic acid was administered to a group of 16 very impaired elderly patients with dementia and serious agitation who had not responded to previous psychotropic interventions.

Methods.—Patient age range was 68 to 95. Valproic acid was administered as divalproex sodium, beginning in divided doses starting at 125 mg twice daily. Treatment effectiveness was assessed using the Behave AD, the Cohen-Mansfield Agitation Inventory, and the Clinical Global Impression Scale. Dose ranges were 750 to 2,500 mg, divided, per day, with levels of 184 to 742 µmol/L.

Results.—Scores on the Cohen-Mansfield Agitation Inventory decreased from 68.8 to 61.0 and scores on the Behave AD dropped from 15.8 to 12.3, both significant differences. For the Clinical Global Impression Scale, 1, 3, 4, and 8 patients, respectively, were rated as very much improved, much improved, minimally improved, and unchanged. One patient had to discontinue treatment because of side effects.

Conclusion.—The absence of a control group makes interpretation difficult. Valproic acid was well-tolerated and moderately effective in the treatment of behavioral disturbances in elderly patients with behavioral disturbances associated with dementia.

▶ This article describes 16 elderly patients who had been underresponsive to other pharmacological interventions and who were treated openly with divalproex sodium. Twenty-five percent of patients benefited significantly, another 25% benefited minimally, and 8 patients derived no benefit. The measures for classifying improvement are clearly described. Probably the most important aspect of this study was that there were no serious adverse effects noted in this group of patients, which is an improvement over agents such as haloperidol, low-potency antipsychotic medications or benzodiazepines, all of which have their own set of potential risks in these elderly patients. Using agents such as valproate in this group of agitated patients may be useful either alone or in combination with other commonly used agents such as low dose neuroleptics. There may be relatively little risk in using combinations of divalproex sodium and other agents such as lorazepam or phenothiazines. In this small series, 1 of each type of dementia included appeared to benefit from the treatment. This article adds to the small literature on using divalproex sodium to treat agitation in demented patients. Such a hypothesis-generating study should be followed by a larger, double-blind, placebo-controlled trial.

R.B. Lydiard, Ph.D., M.D.

Benzodiazepines May Have Protective Effects Against Alzheimer Disease
Fastbom J, Forsell Y, Winblad B (Karolinska Inst, Stockholm)
Alzheimer Dis Assoc Disord 12:14–17, 1998   8–34

Background.—Drugs with neuroprotective effects are effective in cerebral ischemia. The neuronal degeneration in patients with Alzheimer disease (AD) is thought to involve similar mechanisms. To date, the neuroprotective effects of gamma-aminobutyric acid (GABA)-mimetic agents have not been studied in patients with dementia. The association between benzodiazepine use and the occurrence of AD and vascular dementia was reported.

Methods.—Longitudinal data from a case-control study were analyzed. The case subjects were 314 elderly persons scoring 23 or less on the Mini-Mental State Examination during screening, and the control subjects were 354 persons scoring 24 or higher. All were aged 75 or older. Subjects with a history of continuous benzodiazepine use were compared with nonusers. The diagnosis of dementia was based on DSM-III-R criteria.

Findings.—At a follow-up of 3 years, benzodiazepine users had a significantly lower incidence of AD than nonusers. The relationship continued to be significant after adjusting for age, sex, education level, use of nonsteroidal anti-inflammatory drugs, and estrogens.

Conclusions.—Benzodiazepines may have a protective effect against the development of AD. A randomized, placebo-controlled clinical trial to confirm these findings is now needed.

▶ This is a very interesting study conducted by researchers in Sweden who observed a cohort of elderly individuals during a 3-year period. Controlling for the appropriate treatment factors in this patient group, including estrogens, use of nonsteroidal anti-inflammatory drugs, age, and gender, they noted a lower incidence of dementia in the group receiving benzodiazepines. This raises the interesting possibility that BZs, through their effects on GABA function, may inhibit glutamate transmission, which has been implicated in the genesis of Alzheimer's dementia through neuronal destruction. The instruments used seemed to be state-of-the-art, and clinical assessments were apparently carefully performed. These individuals, however, did not measure or report on the use of other psychotropic medications which one could predict were also probably used by this elderly population. The finding merits further investigation and goes against the grain of current clinical wisdom regarding the long-term use of benzodiazepines in elderly patients. The finding that there were less cognitive changes in individuals who were users vs. nonusers is intriguing and bears further investigation. This certainly is not a "green light" for prescribing benzodiazepines for every patient aged more than 65 years. It does suggest that there may be important factors that remain unstudied and that could benefit from further scrutiny. I think that studies like this that are counterintuitive are particularly intriguing. Sometimes the truth really is stranger than fiction.

R.B. Lydiard, Ph.D., M.D.

Use of Selective Serotonin-Reuptake Inhibitors or Tricyclic Antidepressants and Risk of Hip Fractures in Elderly People
Liu B, Anderson G, Mittmann N, et al (Sunnybrook Health Science Centre, Toronto; Inst for Clinical and Evaluative Sciences in Ontario, Canada; Univ of Toronto)
Lancet 351:1303–1307, 1998   8–35

Introduction.—Psychotropic drugs increase the risk of falls and hip fractures in elderly people. Mechanisms of increased risk include sedation, orthostatic hypotension, arrhythmias, and confusion. Fewer than 30% of persons with hip fractures return to their normal level of functioning; over 50% need a permanent walking aid. It is possible that depression itself increases risk of fractures. Although bone density is not associated with duration of antidepressant therapy, premenopausal women with a history of depression have bone-mineral density significantly lower than that of

TABLE 3.—Estimated Unadjusted and Adjusted Odds Ratios for Hip Fracture, by Timing of Exposure

Exposure	N	Odds Ratio (99% CI)	
		Unadjusted	Adjusted*
SSRI			
Current	891	3·3 (2·9–3·8)	2·4 (2·0–2·7)
Indeterminate	326	2·3 (1·8–2·9)	1·8 (1·4–2·3)
Former	471	1·6 (1·3–2·0)	1·2 (0·9–1·5)
Secondary-amine TCA			
Current	400	3·0 (2·4–3·7)	2·2 (1·8–2·8)
Indeterminate	104	1·7 (1·1–2·6)	1·2 (0·8–2·0)
Former	169	2·2 (1·6–3·1)	1·4 (1·0–2·0)
Tertiary-amine TCA			
Current	1,715	1·8 (1·6–2·0)	1·5 (1·3–1·7)
Indeterminate	733	1·2 (1·0–1·5)	1·1 (0·9–1·3)
Former	1,029	1·2 (1·0–1·4)	1·0 (0·8–1·2)

*For co-morbidity and previous drug exposure
Abbreviations: SSRI, selective serotonin-reuptake inhibitor; *TCA*, tricyclic antidepressant.
(Courtesy of Liu B, Anderson G, Mittman N: Use of selective serotonin-reuptake inhibitors or tricyclic antidepressants and risk of hip fractures in elderly people. *Lancet* 351:1303-1307, copyright 1998 by The Lancet Ltd.)

nondepressed controls. The selective serotonin-reuptake inhibitors (SSRIs) have been reported to cause fewer cardiovascular and anticholineric side effects than tricyclic antidepressants (TCAs). It is not known if this translates into a lower risk of hip fractures. The risk of hip fracture associated with SSRIs and the risk associated with TCAs were assessed in a case-control investigation.

Methods.—Administrative health care data from the province of Ontario, Canada, were abstracted. A total of 8,239 patients aged 66 or older,

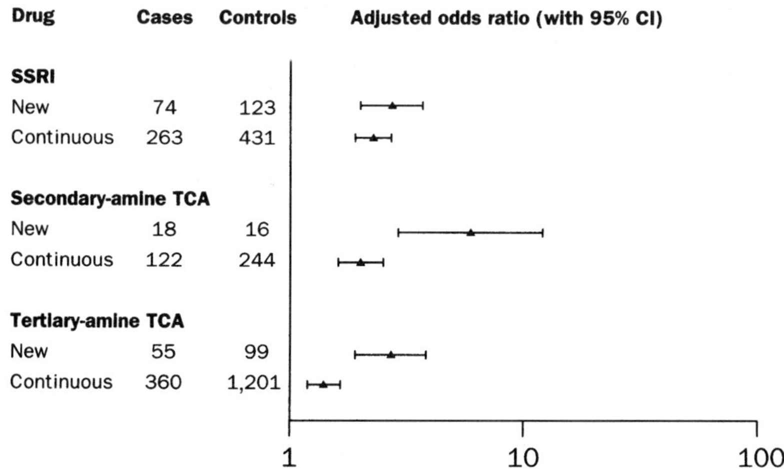

FIGURE 1.—Adjusted odds ratio and 95% confidence interval for current users. *Abbreviations: SSRI*, selective serotonin-reuptake inhibitor; *TCA*, tricyclic antidepressants. (Courtesy of Liu B, Anderson G, Mittmann N: Use of selective serotonin-reuptake inhibitors or tricyclic antidepressants and risk of hip fractures in elderly people. *Lancet* 351:1303-1307, copyright 1998 by The Lancet Ltd.)

who were hospitalized between April 1994 and March 1995 for hip fracture, were age- and sex-matched to 5 controls. Logistic regression was used to determine the odds ratio for hip fracture. Adjustments were made for potential confounding effects produced by concomitant drug use and co-morbidity.

Results.—Using the reference category of participants with no exposure to antidepressants, the adjusted odds ratio for hip fracture was 2.4, 2.2, and 1.5, respectively, for exposure to SSRIs, secondary-amine TCAs, and tertiary-amine TCAs. Current use was correlated with a higher risk of hip fracture than former use, for all types of antidepressants (Table 3). For all 3 drug classes, the odds ratio for hip fracture was higher for new current users than for continuous current users (Fig 1). The proportions of current use in the low-dose range were 22%, 50%, and 58%, respectively, for SSRIs, secondary-amine TCAs, and tertiary-amine TCAs.

Conclusion.—Significant increases in the risk of hip fracture were observed in patients taking any of the 3 classes of antidepressants. In risk of hip fracture, SSRIs do not offer an advantage over TCAs.

▶ My teachers used to tell me that the main cardiovascular risk of the tricyclics was hip fracture. This article presents a large study of the risk of hip fracture in elderly patients taking antidepressants. The authors carefully thought through the variables which could contribute to potential differences, variables such as earlier experience with SSRIs or tricyclics, menopausal status (which might affect bone density), depression, and co-administration of other medications. The surprising finding was that there was no real difference between groups after controlling for all these variables. It should be noted that half of the SSRI-treated patients had been exposed to tricyclics in the past. It may be that this group was sensitive to medication in general and that the SSRI was prescribed in patients with a higher risk. One frustrating aspect of this article is that the authors did not report actual mg per day of these agents, but rather calculated the dosage categories through a method adopted by the World Health Organization.

As a clinician, I am a little befuddled about how to evaluate such reports. I did not see any discussion or measurement of pretreatment orthostatic blood pressure changes, which may be a reasonable factor to consider here as well. Nearly 10% of the group using the tertiary-amine tricyclics, which were allegedly safer than the other 2 classes, were "new users." For both tricyclic groups, new users were at more risk than continual users, again suggesting a selection factor here. Also, 50% to 60% of the patients taking tricyclics were described as being "low dose." This article focuses on safety, and one has to wonder whether the patients receiving low doses were less likely to recover from depression and perhaps less likely to be ambulatory. Although there was no statistical correspondence between dosage and hip fracture, there was a higher risk in the high-dose tricyclic groups, but not in the high-dose SSRI group. Tricyclics were prescribed across a broader diagnostic range in this elderly group. These patients were more likely than younger patients to receive tertiary tricyclics for sedation or relief of pain. Both the lower dosage and differences in concomitant psychiatric disorders could contribute to the absence of drug class differences as well.

The authors conclude that their study showed no difference in risk of hip fracture between tricyclics and SSRIs, and that exposure to any of the 3 classes of drugs examined increases the risk of hip fracture. I can't argue with their statistical treatment, but there seem to be enough factors here to muddy the waters in this counterintuitive finding. Were this study supported by industry or a managed health care organization, I would be much more suspicious; however, this appears to be a carefully conducted scientific study. Of note, new TCA users were likely to have more falls than those who showed tolerability to the TCAs. Also, more patients in the two TCA groups were taking low dosages. The take-home message is that we all need to be careful in treating elderly people with antidepressant medications. I remain unconvinced, as a clinician, that an elderly patient receiving a tertiary tricyclic is at less risk for hip fracture caused by medication than a patient receiving an SSRI. Further attention to important clinical points like this is warranted.

R.B. Lydiard, Ph.D., M.D.

Other

Clinical Efficacy of Methylphenidate in Conduct Disorder With and Without Attention Deficit Hyperactivity Disorder
Klein RG, Abikoff H, Klass E, et al (Long Island Jewish Med Ctr, New Hyde Park, NY)
Arch Gen Psychiatry 54:1073–1080, 1997   8–36

Introduction.—Attention deficit hyperactivity disorder (ADHD), a frequent diagnosis in the United States, corresponds largely to conduct disorder (CD) in the United Kingdom. These contrasting approaches have therapeutic implications, for stimulants are not considered appropriate for children with CD. Researchers examined the hypothesis that methylphenidate hydrochloride, effective in ADHD, would not significantly improve symptoms in CD.

Methods.—Eighty-four children with a diagnosis of CD were randomized in a double-blind manner to receive methylphenidate hydrochloride (up to 60 mg/day) or placebo for 5 weeks. The children ranged in age from 6 to 15 years; two thirds also met criteria for ADHD. Three classroom observations were conducted during the study period and clinical response was recorded weekly.

Results.—Children taking methylphenidate were rated as significantly better by their parents and teachers on all CD measures including antisocial behavior. The drug had positive significant impact on teacher ratings of ADHD symptoms. Overall, improvement rates for children taking methylphenidate vs. placebo were, respectively: teachers, 59% vs. 9%; mothers, 78% vs. 27%; and psychiatrists, 68% vs. 11%. Drug-induced improvement of CD symptoms was significant after partialling out for initial ADHD ratings.

Conclusion.—Hyperactivity and conduct disorders appear to have a close association, and children with both ADHD and CD are at high risk for sustained antisocial behavior, compared with those with CD only. In this group of children, CD symptoms, including antisocial behavior, responded quite well to short-term methylphenidate treatment, and the effects of the drug were not dependent on severity of ADHD symptoms.

▶ This is an important study of an area that is clearly under-studied and poorly understood. The authors observed simultaneous improvement in ADHD and CD ratings in children receiving methylphenidate compared with those receiving placebo. Interestingly, the effects on conduct and attentional function appear to be independent of one another. Although this study was not able to solve the riddle of whether CD and ADHD are really part of the same diagnostic class, it raises the possibility that early intervention for ADHD may have beneficial effects on the subsequent development of anti-social behavior, which has been shown to commonly emerge in children who have attention problems early. The study is an important step forward in our ability to improve the quality of life for children, teachers, and parents. It raises a glimmer of hope that the clinical course of the disorder may be modified, to some extent, by early intervention and consistent treatment thereafter.

R.B. Lydiard, Ph.D., M.D.

Benzodiazepine-receptor Ligands in Humans: Acute Performance-impairing, Subject-rated and Observer-rated Effects
Rush CR, Armstrong DL, Ali JA, et al (Univ of Mississippi, Jackson)
J Clin Psychopharmacol 18:154–166, 1998   8–37

Background.—Benzodiazepines are comonly prescribed for sleep disorders. The acute performance-impairing, subject-rated, and observer-rated effects of different doses of quazepam, triazolam, zolpidem tartrate, and placebo were compared.

Methods.—Nine healthy persons were included in the study. The drugs were administered orally in a double-blind, crossover design.

Findings.—Triazolam and zolpidem produced a dose- and time-related impairment of learning, performance, and recall. In addition, they produced sedative-like subject- and observer-rated drug effects. The behavioral pharmacologic profiles of these drugs were indistinguishable: at peak effect, the absolute magnitude of drug effect was similar across measures. Quazepam did not significantly impair performance nor result in significant sedation.

Conclusions.—Across a 3-fold range of doses, zolpidem and triazolam produced similar dosage-related impairments in learning, recall, and performance and increases a subject- and observer-rated drug effects. Thus, despite the purportedly unique benzodiazepine-receptor binding profile of zolpidem, this drug has performance-impairing, subject-rated, and observer-rated effects that are virtually indistinguishable from those of classic benzodiazepine agonists such as triazolam.

▶ The search for the perfect hypnotic continues. Many clinicians, including myself, are confused about the varying reports of the degree to which agents can produce potentially adverse effects such as impairment of learning, performance, and memory. Remember that the concerns of triazolam-induced amnesia and behavioral disinhibition were so great that in Great Britain the drug was significantly restricted for use as a hypnotic. This within-subject study included both observation by clinicians and subjective responses by patients. Clinically comparable dose ranges of zolpidem, triazolam, and quazepam were used in a placebo-controlled fashion. The take-home message here is that zolpidem apparently had effects similar to triazolam in healthy volunteers. Thus, the purported difference in BZ-receptor interaction for zolpidem, which may in fact be the case, does not translate into less of the adverse effects that we are concerned about when we prescribe a hypnotic. The measures used to ascertain these effects are well standardized and accepted measures, which lend credibility to the findings.

The authors carefully discuss the discrepancies between their study and others who included individuals with a history of substance abuse as well as those without such history. Although normal volunteer studies may be somewhat difficult to translate into clinical practice, this represents one of the better studies that I have seen, and its results suggest that we cannot assume that zolpidem carries a major advantage over triazolam, at least in younger individuals. It should be remembered that early on triazolam was originally prescribed in doses that were substantially higher than those currently used in clinical practice, and this may have been why there was such concern expressed with the adverse effects that emerged. Why haven't we seen these types of effects with zolpidem? I am not sure, but it may be that lower doses are used initially and also that the exposure in the general population is still significantly less than that of triazolam. This phenomenon of number of patient exposures relates directly to the number of reports of adverse effects. Until we have a better idea of the denominator and numerator of the ratio of patients taking the drugs to the numbers of adverse effects, it appears that we should consider zolpidem as potentially capable of producing these unwanted effects, and clinical caution is indicated. Conversely, as the dosages of triazolam have been more judiciously used, the frequency of reports of serious adverse events has apparently decreased also. As I said previously, the search for the ideal hypnotic continues.

R.B. Lydiard, Ph.D., M.D.

Subject Index

Author Index